NEURO-VISUAL PROCESSING REHABILITATION: AN INTERDISCIPLINARY APPROACH

William V. Padula, OD, FNAP, FAAO, FNORA

Raquel Munitz, MS, COVT

W. Michael Magrun, MS, OTR/L

Optometric Extension Program Foundation

Published by Optometric Extension Program Foundation, Inc.
1921 East Carnegie Ave., 3-L
Santa Ana, CA 92705-5811

Managing Editor: Sally Marshall Corngold

Library of Congress Cataloging-in-Publication Data

Padula, William V.
Neuro-visual processing rehabilitation : an interdisciplinary approach / William V. Padula, Raquel Munitz, W. Michael Magrun.
p. ; cm.
Neurovisual processing rehabilitation
Includes bibliographical references and index.
ISBN 978-0-929780-31-3 (alk. paper)
I. Munitz, Raquel. II. Magrun, W. Michael. III. Optometric Extension Program Foundation. IV. Title. V. Title: Neurovisual processing rehabilitation.
[DNLM: 1. Vision Disorders--rehabilitation. 2. Child. 3. Disabled Children--rehabilitation. 4. Psychomotor Performance--physiology. 5. Vision, Ocular--physiology. 6. Visual Perception--physiology. WW 600]

617.7'12--dc23

2011042238

****

Optometry is the health care profession specifically licensed by state law to prescribe lenses, optical devices and procedures to improve human vision. Optometry has advanced vision therapy as a unique treatment modality for the development and remediation of the visual process. Effective vision therapy requires extensive understanding of:

- the effects of lenses (including prisms, filters and occluders)
- the variety of responses to the changes produced by lenses
- the various physiological aspects of the visual process
- the pervasive nature of the visual process in human behavior

As a consequence, effective vision therapy requires the supervision, direction and active involvement of the optometrist.

****

DEDICATION

We dedicate this book to the memory of our dear friend and colleague, Dr. Christine Nelson, whose understanding of neuro-postural development remains a core theme of this book.

With loving thoughts and appreciation, this book is also dedicated to our families for their support and encouragement during the many hours required to complete this work.

WVP

CONTENTS

LIST OF FIGURES

LIST OF TABLES

FOREWORD

In this book Dr. William Padula and his co-authors offer an opportunity for the reader to rethink the very concept of vision and its interrelationship with other brain and sensory systems. The authors, a team of dedicated and caring professionals, draw upon published research, case reports, opinions, decades of combined clinical experiences and out-of-the box thinking. In turn, they ask no more than that the reader keep an open mind.

The field of Neuro-optometric Rehabilitation developed in response to the observations of a group of committed practitioners who experienced limited success when working with brain injured clients using standard techniques. However, this subspecialty is new and, as with any new endeavor, it is still developing models for best clinical practices.

Often persons with traumatic brain injury may look the same physically, and show no signs of their injuries. This leads family and friends to be quite confused about the functional inabilities their loved ones demonstrate. For example, many patients have difficulty counting change or they may be unable to find a desired item on a shelf containing several different objects – activities that could easily be accomplished prior to their injuries. Thus these patients may be consigned to the care of psychiatrists or psychologists. While they often need the guidance and support these caregivers offer, such intervention does not address the profound dysfunction that often occurs in visual processing.

Sadly, the therapeutic options for brain injured patients are currently limited. However, clinicians are increasingly aware of this and are rising to the challenge. Centers of excellence for neurologic disease, brain injury and rehabilitation are emerging within both the military/veterans' healthcare systems and the private sector. New diagnostic methodologies are being tested, and novel interventional techniques are being explored by those in this specialized field. This book is a sampling of the future. In fact, the collaboration required to present this book is probably one of its most important lessons, i.e., that modern science will succeed best when clinicians, researchers, patients and their loved ones interact with a common goal.

Eric Singman, MD, PhD
Director, General Eye Services Clinic
Wilmer Eye Institute at Johns Hopkins University

FOREWORD

I look back on the late 1980's with much pride. It was a time of great excitement and passion which all began one day at work when I received a phone call from Dr. William Padula. He inquired as to my participation in the area of traumatic brain injury and whether I would be interested in sharing my thoughts with other doctors who similarly were treating these patients. Interested? He could not have asked a more timely question. The meeting turned out to be one of the early steps in the formation of the Neuro-Optometric Rehabilitation Association and the beginning of a long and valued friendship.

Bill began to speak of new and innovative ideas that would lead to treatment concepts which extended well beyond the traditional "eyeball" concerns of modern medicine. He started to lead our thinking to look at the traumatically damaged brain as one that often misinterprets visual input in the form of alterations in body posture and, accordingly, alterations in body movement and localization processes. The early meetings with the "giants" in developmental and functional optometry – William Ludlam, OD; John Streff, OD; John Thomas, OD; Gus Forkiotis, OD; and Daniel Gottlieb, OD, – resulted in a fertile soil upon which the seeds of successful treatment of these patients began to germinate. Bill clearly saw that experts in body posture and movement skills were so valuable to the total picture that he invited Christine Nelson, OTR, PhD, and Raquel Munitz, MS, to guide us. They helped us understand the processes associated with body core and midline which extended into the visual-motor and visual-perceptual interpretations of internal and external space. Bill began to speak of the "Visual Midline Shift Syndrome" and "Post Trauma Vision Syndrome" and demonstrated that yoked prisms could be used effectively in the treatment of such dysfunctions. He prudently encouraged us not to just think of ocular alignment dysfunction, but to appreciate the critical nature of sensorimotor processes and visual/postural organization in relationship to the rehabilitation process. Bill's thinking extended far beyond the cookbook models of vision care that are, too often, considered to be modern treatment regimens.

It is truly an honor to have been asked to write this Foreword to Dr. Padula's book, *Neuro-Visual Processing Rehabilitation: An Interdisciplinary Approach.* As the staff consultant and co-founder of Vision Clinics of the Kessler Institute for Rehabilitation (West Orange, Saddle Brook, and Chester, NJ) I could not be a more supportive advocate of the concept of interdisciplinary care for the vision care practitioner who is interested in working with patients who have incurred a neurological event such as a traumatic brain injury, cerebral vascular accident, Lyme disease, Parkinson's disease, as well as other neurological and developmental dysfunctions. The old expression, "No man is an island" is a most appropriate metaphor for the need to work together with the many people who comprise the rehabilitation team that successfully treats these patients. To my many colleagues who believe in sitting back in their offices waiting for these patients to come to them: forget it. Read these pages. *Neuro-Visual Processing Rehabilitation: An Interdisciplinary Approach* is a look at the future, both the future for optometry and for the field of rehabilitation. Ask the right questions, confer with team members, and then get out there and show them what can be done. Learn from others and, most of all, show these patients the respect and provide the care that they deserve. Thank you, Bill, for your leadership and dedication to helping those most in need.

Vincent R. Vicci Jr., OD, DPNAP
Westfield, NJ

PREFACE

Much has been written about the brain and its connectivity. Despite this plethora of information, we still have only a "key-hole" view and understanding about the dynamics of brain processing. We seem to try to relate it to our current level of mastery of technology by comparing the brain to the manner in which computers process information. The computer is based on logic and can be provided with modest dynamics for decision making. Yet even the most sophisticated computers are limited in contrast to the human brain and its ability to process information and make decisions.

Vision is a brain process. Sometimes it appears that we forget that the eyes are only sophisticated cameras. It is amazing that we use the process of vision every day of our lives, but are not able to grasp the profound influence vision has on our thought patterns, cognitive processes, memory, spatial orientation, balance, movement and many other daily functions. We can't even escape this visual influence when we daydream or sleep. For those who are born with vision, images still occupy our attention. Even the adventitiously blinded person continues to have visual images in the dream state.

Vision is dominant in the development of the child. When there is congenital blindness, the child's development will predictably be delayed. While vision soon dominates attention, concentration, and much of cognitive executive functioning, the portion of the visual process that organizes this in the brain isn't even neurologically developed at the time of birth. There are at least two visual processing centers in the brain: one that we can "think" with and the other that happens before we can think. The bimodal visual system has a spatial component that initially processes information to lead and organize relationships of vision, posture, and balance for the purpose of being upright against gravity, and a focal component that eventually develops the domination of attention and concentration.

Yet despite its importance we can't think or attend *through* the spatial process. Thus we become victims of our own visual attention and cognitive orientation toward the image. We become oblivious to the portion of the visual process that enables us to move, maintain posture and balance, and essentially permits us to use the higher part of our vision for cognition, attention and concentration without having to think about how to remain upright, take our next step, or shift from one visual regard to another.

How do we know that there is such a preconscious spatial visual process when we can't think with it? First of all, there is research to document that primates, including humans, process visual information in two different ways. Secondly, neuro-anatomists have shown that there are neurological pathways not only to the occipital cortex but also pathways to a second visual processing site located in the mid-brain in an area known as the superior colliculus. In addition, some of the latest research is recognizing a third level of visual processing located in the thalamus.

More practically, try first balancing on one foot while looking at something across the room and then try it while looking through a pinhole, or while wearing pinhole glasses. Or, try writing someone's name in cursive handwriting and then try it through the same pinhole glasses so that all you can see is the tip of the pen. You will learn that the spatial visual process, provided primarily through the peripheral vision of each eye, is important for posture and balance and works in conjunction with vestibular and sensorimotor systems. Further, writing requires the ability to spatially organize the movement of the pen without conscious visual effort, which also requires support of the spatial visual process and coordination with the sensorimotor systems.

Why is this so important? If we don't "think" in the spatial visual process then the conscious visual process must be the most important part of our vision. This is a partially true statement. Our central visual process is important so long as we have the preconscious visual process established and creating the spatial organization and structure in which the conscious visual process can function. Without this, the detail visual process attempts the organization of our visual world through the conscious mode of cognition, attention and concentration. When this happens we become visually inefficient, ineffective, bound by details, and often feel as if we are living in an altered state. Cognitively our thoughts become jumbled often affecting speech and language capabilities, and skills such as reading become over focalized on letters, causing limited reading speed and affecting comprehension. Without the preconscious spatial visual process we have difficulty aligning our eyes, tracking an object, and shifting our eyes from point to point. We become focally bound on detail.

This is the visual world of many people who have neurological problems such as brain injury, cerebrovascular accidents, multiple sclerosis, cerebral palsy, Parkinson's disease, Lyme disease, autism and other conditions that may affect visual processing in the brain. The harder the person tries to use the focal or detail portion of the visual process the less adaptable vision becomes and the more the symptoms increase.

Binocular vision problems are common following a dysfunction of the visual process associated with a neurological event. Optometrists and ophthalmologists often diagnose conditions of strabismus, convergence insufficiency, and deficiencies of pursuit tracking and saccadic eye movements. With the diagnosis there often are accompanying recommendations to develop therapy programs to improve fixation, pursuit tracking, convergence and saccadic fixations. These programs are usually oriented towards improving the particular skill of using the eyes to create a fixation, pursuit, saccadic movement or convergence ability. Often it seems that the rehabilitation attempt emphasizes the very part of the visual process that is bound, that is, if the person is over-focalizing or demonstrating a problem with visual skills of changing eye position through pursuit movement, saccades, or convergence, then the therapy program is actually designed to *increase the effort to fixate.* This occurs because of a lack of understanding that the problem may actually lie in the patient's inability to release the fixation or organize the spatial field to allow those eye movement skills to take place.

It is interesting to study the development of the visual process in infancy and childhood. A.M. Skeffington, OD, and Arnold Gesell, MD, recognized the profound and intimate relationship of vision to the motor system. Although they made statements such as "vision is motor" (A.M. Skeffington[1]) and "vision is related to thought although it emanates from an action system," (Gesell et al.[2]) the brilliance of these statements is that they were made well before researchers such as Trevarthen, Hein, Liebowitz and Post were able to document the bimodal visual process. Yet their research has not been incorporated into the concept of vision examinations or even into most of the methods of therapy and rehabilitation that have been developed.

The two visual processes are deeply entwined in the motor development of the child. Particularly interesting is the relationship between posture, flexion, extension and the unique development of each child's organization of postural tone. This is responsible for both the organization and balance between the two visual processes.

It is fascinating to observe the relationship of the bimodal visual development to the milestones of motor development. For example, at one month the child extends his visual awareness of the environment. However, this only occurs when he is able to push up from the prone position and extend the upper body, head, and neck as the eyes are directed up to gaze at the more distant environment. The pincer grasp at six months must be accompanied by flexion of the head and neck with eyes directed at the target.

However, the flexion needed for the pincer grasp will most often not occur on developmental schedule unless it is preceded by extension of the wrist and dissociation of wrist movement from arm movement. This is supported by the ambient (spatial) process. Following this, development of focalization will occur in conjunction with flexion of the wrist, head, and neck, leading to the pincer grasp.

The extension and flexion process is not only anterior-posterior but also lateral and diagonal. All movements create balance and new modes of function between the bimodal processes of vision. "Vision is motor" and "it emanates from an action system" through this bimodality. The implications of this statement lead us to new dimensions in understanding the visual dysfunctions that occur following a neurological event as well as those that may occur during a child's development.

My co-authors and I have written this book as a means to create a new perspective on vision and the problems associated with visual dysfunction, including those following a neurological event. The visual process will be discussed with emphasis on its relationship to the motor and other sensory systems. In addition, we have attempted to raise questions about whether we are truly effecting positive change by placing emphasis on what is essentially a commonly employed "focalization therapy." Is there instead a way we can influence change in visual function and performance through balancing the relationship of the bimodal process of vision? And what is the role of yoked prisms in establishing this balance?

The authors invite the reader to attempt to release from preconceptions about vision. Use this as an opportunity to look at visual behavior in a new way and perhaps change your understanding of "vision and the brain."

William V. Padula

ABOUT THE AUTHORS

(In order of appearance in the text)

William V. Padula, OD, FNAP, FAAO, FNORA

William V. Padula, OD, is a graduate of the Pennsylvania College of Optometry at Salus University of Health Sciences. He is a Fellow of the American Academy of Optometry, the Neuro-Optometric Rehabilitation Association International (NORA), and the National Academy of Practice.

Dr. Padula completed a fellowship at the Gesell Institute where he was also Director of Vision Research. He was the founding Chairman of the Low Vision Section for the American Optometric Association, and the founding President of NORA. Dr. Padula was appointed the National Consultant in Low Vision Services for the American Foundation for the Blind. He has also served as Consultant to the Committee on Vision for the National Academy of Sciences in Washington, DC. Recently he has served as a consultant to the Walter Reed Hospital in Washington, DC. He is the Past Chairperson of the National Academy of Practice in Optometry, and is the Treasurer of the National Academy of Practice (NAP).

Dr. Padula founded the first low vision clinic at the Zhongshan Eye Research Hospital in Guangzhou, People's Republic of China, which was named in his honor. He lectures and consults internationally in China, India, Italy, Mexico, etc., with programs regarding children's vision related to learning and development, and adult vision problems related to stroke, TBI and other physical challenges.

Dr. Padula has authored several books and numerous papers. He has developed three award winning educational video format DVDs about vision and Neuro-Optometric Rehabilitation for persons with neurological challenges. He also holds five U.S. patents for instruments related to vision.

Dr. Padula is on staff at the Hospital for Special Care and Gaylord Hospital in Connecticut, and has a private practice in Guilford, CT. He was honored to be chosen Connecticut Optometrist of the Year in 2009 by his colleagues in the Connecticut Association of Optometrists.

Raquel Munitz, MS, COVT

Ms. Munitz earned her MS in Psychology from the National University of Mexico. In 1964 she received her certificate in infant treatment from Mary Quinton and in 1977 she received her certification in Neuro-developmental Treatment.

Ms. Munitz began her professional work as a counselor for the blind. Her interest in vision emerged while she worked with neurologically impaired and learning disabled children. Much of her career has been spent searching for new ways to approach the multi-faceted problems these children present.

W. Michael Magrun, MS, OTR/L

W. Michael Magrun received his MS in Occupational Therapy from the State University of New York at Buffalo in 1974. He is a former instructor of pediatric occupational therapy at the SUNY at New York and the University of Central Arkansas. He holds certifications in neuro-developmental treatment for children and infants. His practice has centered around the understanding, evaluation and treatment of movement and postural disorganization and disability as it relates to developmental disorders and learning disabilities. Mr. Magrun has published in the *American Journal of Occupational Therapy*, *Somatics Journal*, *Occupational Therapy in Health Care* and the *Arkansas Occupational Therapy Association News-Journal*, and has authored books and clinical videos. Mr. Magrun currently is Vice President of Clinician's View, a clinically based continuing education development company.

Christine A. Nelson, PhD, OTR (1937 - 2008)

Christine A. Nelson earned her MS in Child Development from Neurodevelopmental (Bobath) Treatment in 1963. Dr. Nelson was certified as an NDT Coordinator-Instructor by Dr. and Mrs. Karel Bobath in 1973 after completing requirements for her PhD in Human Development at the University of Maryland. She received the NDT Association Award for Excellence in 2004.

Dr. Nelson began her career in occupational therapy, working with physically disabled and blind children, moving from institutional to community to private settings. Her direct treatment of multi-handicapped children, her experience in developmental assessment and her preparation of therapists to work with children with neuromotor disorders prepared her to share her practical insights into problems of posture and movement as they relate to visual impairment. Dr. Nelson authored a chapter on cerebral palsy in *Neurological Rehabilitation* published by Mosby, participated in the making of two films and wrote several other chapters and articles. She was Clinical Coordinator of the Centro de Aprendizaje de Cuernavaca, Mexico.

David F. Delacato, MEd

David F. Delacato has spent the last 25 years working in the field of rehabilitation. He is the Director of Delacato International which provides services to families of individuals suffering from autism, cerebral palsy, and dyslexia.

Mr. Delacato consults internationally with programs for acquired and congenital brain injuries. He has lectured throughout the United States, Europe, and Asia.

Antonio Parisi, MD

Dr. Parisi received his medical degree in 1995 from the University of Naples Federico II. He is a neurologist whose specialty is epilepsy. In 1992 Dr. Parisi began to collaborate with Dr. Carl Delacato and his teams in both Italy and Switzerland, and now also in England. In 2001, he founded and became president of the *Carl and Janice Delacato Study and Research Center for Neuroscience.* Dr. Parisi has published extensively in the field of epilepsy, and has published a book, *Children Who Do Not Look You in the Eye: The Secrets of Autistic Behavior (1999)*, in which he sustains the hypothesis of sensory perceptual dysfunction in the genesis of autism.

Jennifer McCullagh, AuD, PhD

Jennifer McCullagh is an assistant professor of Communication Disorders at Southern Connecticut State University in New Haven, CT. She earned her AuD and PhD degrees from the University of Connecticut, Storrs, in 2009. Dr. McCullagh's areas of interest are neuro-audiology, auditory electrophysiology, and auditory processing disorders.

Stephanie C. Nagle, AuD, PhD

Stephanie C. Nagle received her AuD in clinical audiology and her PhD in Speech, Language, and Hearing Science from the University of Connecticut in 2010. She is currently an assistant professor of Audiology at Towson University in Maryland. Her areas of research and interest include auditory electrophysiology, assessment and treatment auditory processing disorders, and pediatrics. Dr. Nagle has previously published work in the *Journal of the American Academy of Audiology* and the *Hearing Journal.*

Diantha Morse, MA

Diantha Morse earned her MA degree in Speech Pathology and Audiology from the University of Connecticut and completed post graduate work in Audiology at the University of Michigan. She served as a clinical audiologist at Hartford Hospital and the Connecticut Children's Medical Center in Hartford, CT, and was an assistant professor of Audiology with the University of Connecticut's Department of Communication Sciences in Storrs, CT. Although now retired, she continues to be active with Connecticut's Early Hearing Detection and Intervention Task Force, of which she was a founding member.

Frank E. Musiek, PhD

Frank E. Musiek is Professor and Director of Auditory Research, Dept. of Communications Sciences and Professor of Otolaryngology, School of Medicine, University of Connecticut. He is the 2007 American Academy of Audiology recipient of the "James Jerger Career Award for Research in Audiology," the 2010 recipient of "The Honors of The American Speech, Language and Hearing Association," and the recipient of the "Book of the Year Award" for the *Handbook of Central Processing Disorders, Vol. I and II* (with Gail Chermak, co-editor), 2007. He has published over 175 articles and book chapters and 8 books in the areas of auditory evoked potentials, central auditory disorders and auditory neuroanatomy.

Marc Zola, PhD

Dr. Zola received his doctorate in Human Development from the University of Chicago. He subsequently completed post doctoral fellowships in Clinical Research, Statistics, and Methods at Northwestern University; and in Clinical Neuropsychology at the Institute of Living in Hartford, CT.

Dr. Zola has held positions as the Director of Neuropsychology and Rehabilitation Psychology at the Rehabilitation Hospital of Connecticut, and as the Program Director for the Neuropsychiatric Unit at Connecticut Valley Hospital. He served as the Neuropsychologist for a large inner city school district for almost a decade. He has consulted both locally and nationally on clinical issues regarding pediatric and adult neuropsychology, Quantitative EEG, and Neurofeedback. Dr. Zola has written numerous publications and lectures nationally on such topics as autism, Asperger's syndrome, AD/HD, learning disabilities, dyslexia, Lyme disease, and traumatic brain injury. He is currently in private practice in Avon, CT.

Judith A. Padula, BS

Judith A. Padula graduated from Dominican College in Blauvelt, NY, and was a Certified Teacher of the Visually Impaired in Connecticut for over 10 years, working with visually-impaired and multi-handicapped children. She has co-authored publications about low vision rehabilitation for visually-impaired children and its effect on academic performance. She has coordinated visual stimulation and vision therapy programs for low vision children in school systems and optometric private practices.

ACKNOWLEDGMENTS

There are many people who have assisted us in various ways during the production of this book. First, I would like to extend our appreciation and thanks to our patients. We have spent many years working with patients with disabilities of all types, some of whose problems are discussed in various chapters. We continue to learn and grow by listening to and working with them.

We wish to thank Robert Williams, Executive Director of both the Neuro-Optometric Rehabilitation Association (NORA) and the Optometric Extension Program Foundation (OEP), for his encouragement to write this book.

We would also like to extend a special word of thanks to the office staff at the Padula Institute of Vision for their efforts in helping to complete this work.

Last, but clearly not least, we would like to thank Diantha Morse for having edited this book. Diantha's exceptional editing skills, love of learning, and interest in vision and hearing, enabled her to make many valuable contributions. Her dedication to this project has been outstanding. Without her diplomatic and gentle adherence to the concept of this book, it would never have been completed.

Chapter 1

THE BIMODAL RELATIONSHIP BETWEEN FOCAL AND AMBIENT VISION

William V. Padula

> ***"Vision is a dynamic interactive process of motor and sensory function, mediated by the eyes for the purpose of simultaneous organization of posture, movement and spatial orientation, for manipulation of the environment and, to its highest degree, of perception and thought."   WVP***

The visual world occupies a major portion of our attention and cognition, however, vision is often taken for granted. We don't think about how we use our vision to walk, sign our name, or read. Yet how we see leads to and influences our experiences. From the very earliest moments of life children learn to use their vision to create experiences necessary for perceptual development. These experiences then support the development of a unique visual style which will be used to analyze new information and explore relationships throughout life.

What is vision? A common misconception about vision is that our eyes function like cameras in that they admit light rays which are relayed to the brain for interpretation so that we can understand our surroundings, make decisions, etc. But is this actually the way vision works?

As we will explore in this book, that concept involving a passive relationship of vision and sight to the higher brain processes is a simplistic one. It does not acknowledge or take into account the complexity of the motor and sensory processes involved or the relationship of vision to development.

Vision is not the same as sight. We often confuse these two words. Sight is the ability to see and resolve detail. Traditionally, it is examined by optometrists and ophthalmologists by testing one's ability to see and report the smallest detail on a chart at a specific distance. This is called acuity. It does not relate directly to function and performance. Having 20/20 acuity at distance does not mean that a person won't trip over an obstacle or a crack in the sidewalk that he did not see, or that he won't have an accident while driving because he didn't notice an oncoming car as he pulled into traffic. One might argue that these examples are related to the scope of visual field. However, this person may have had an eye exam that showed both 20/20 acuity and a normal scope of visual field. Yet even with so called "perfect" sight he may be unable to find his own keys that are resting on the table in front of him. Thus sight relates to static measurements of acuity which quantify certain aspects of our vision, but it does not directly relate to how we use our vision.

In order to understand the visual process and its relationship to function and performance, we must begin by looking at how the visual process develops and the extent to which vision influences our movements, thoughts, perceptions, posture, balance, etc. Vision is a behavior that is often predictable, but it is too complex a process to be totally predictable. However, by understanding the process of vision as well as its development, we will have a better understanding not only of how vision affects our function and performance, but how it can interfere with our development.

It has been recognized by Gesell, Ilg, and Bullis[1] during extensive studies of child development that vision is a primary process and a mover of development. Vision also plays a critical role in learning. There are over one million nerve fibers that exit each eye. These represent approximately 70% of all the sensory nerves in the entire body.[1] Therefore, a major amount of information is received by the cortex from the two eyes.

During the development of the embryo/fetus the organogenesis of the eyes occurs in the course of which three different embryonic layers participate in the development and support of neural structures that eventually become the eyes.[2] The neuroectoderm gives rise to the retina, epithelium of the ciliary body/iris, and optic nerves. The surface ectoderm contributes to the lens and anterior surface of the cornea, the main elements of the eyes affecting the optics of dioptric power. The mesoderm is responsible for the stromal and vascular elements of the eyes. Of importance is the early appearance (4th week) of bilateral evaginations from the diencephalon which form the optic vesicles.[3] The proximal part of each vesicle constricts and forms the optic stalk connecting the vesicle to the diencephalon, while the distal part expands into a hollow bulb. Through growth and invagination, the distal part will develop into the optic cup forming two layers. The inner layer becomes the neural retina containing the rods, cones, ganglion cells and other neural elements, while the outer layer develops into the retinal pigment epithelium (RPE). By the sixth week axons from the developing retinal ganglion cells will grow into the optic stalk and form the optic nerve (CNII), the optic chiasm and the optic tract, eventually delivering messages from the eyes to the visual cortex. Of interest is the fact that not only does the neuroectoderm develop and contribute to the eye but it also develops into the cortex. Therefore, it must be recognized that the eye, neurologically, is in part an end result of developing brain tissue. Further, the eye is the only sensory organ in which neuroectoderm is involved in development.

Nerve fibers emanate from the central part of the eye called the macula. These fibers align centrally in the optic nerve and the optic tract, and localize themselves in the central area of the visual cortex. Peripheral fibers from the eyes orient themselves in the optic nerve and optic tract around the central fibers. These peripheral fibers eventually align themselves in the peripheral areas of the visual cortex.

Most people think of vision as a sensory function that delivers information to the brain much like a computer or a camera, as was previously stated. However, our understanding of the organization of the higher levels of the visual system and its relationship to cognitive processing and visual imagery has been limited, and thus has restricted our comprehension of how our vision actually works. Instead we are highly involved in the cognitive functions pertaining to the detail to which we attend. We thus limit our awareness of how the systems of movement and posture relate to visual processing and, in turn, how vision affects the motor system.

Our individual sensory processors (eyes, ears, nose, mouth, and fingers) lead us to interpret our own organization as a group of isolated systems. This isolation has brought about the establishment of highly specialized professions such as optometry, ophthalmology, audiology, etc. While such an approach is effective in providing treatment for a specific sensory organ, it is not effective in dealing with problems relating to combinations of sensory and motor functions. Problems that involve sensorimotor coordination have sometimes been considered as difficulties with sensory integration. The term itself causes us to perceive a mismatch of passive sensory information that is delivered to our brain for decision making. It causes us to think that our sensory systems and brain operate by means of a stimulus-response (S-R) model of functioning, that the stimulus must be transferred to the brain in order for a response to occur. This simplistic concept was disproved by psychologists over fifty years ago. Instead, research[4,5] has shown that we learn by organizing the response prior to receiving the stimulus. This may be confusing at first, particularly if one does not have an understanding of how the process of sensory organization occurs. However, since through its neural substrate vision provides a major sensory distribution to the brain, we especially must consider the dynamic role that vision plays in the relationship of establishing a response-stimulus-response (R-S-R) model in order to understand how learning and behavior occur.

All sensory systems are integrated neurologically, as stated by John Streff, OD (Gesell Institute 1976). The nerve fibers from these systems, although initially separate, join together and integrate sensorimotor information in the brain so that this information may be shared and matched. For example, some individuals have stated that if they take off their glasses they have difficulty hearing. This may indicate that for these individuals the visual process needs to match information with the auditory process. However, it is not only the sensory systems that share and match information; the motor process (efferent system) is critical in providing a background for the sensory systems. A good example of this is balance. It can be observed that when standing on one foot balance is diminished for most individuals when their eyes are closed.

The interpretation is that vision shares and matches information with other sensory systems such as the vestibular system and the kinesthetic process and that all provide important components for balance and movement. It can also be demonstrated that for many children, as well as for individuals who have had a neurological event, tracking or following an object with their eyes can be very difficult. However, if the child or the person who had the neurological event points to the target that they are attempting to track, improvement can be observed. This demonstrates that the motor process is reinforcement for sensory function.

When attempting to understand behavior, we must try to think of it as a representation of the way in which a person both interprets and organizes information through all of the sensorimotor processes. This point will become clear as the discussion of the performance of individuals with motor or sensory impairments is analyzed. With this as a background, we will now attempt to understand vision as it relates to behavior, and to then develop a model by which vision can be understood when considering rehabilitation of the neurologically challenged child or adult.

Researchers such as Liebowitz and Post and Trevarthen[6,7] have demonstrated that there are two separate visual processes. Their research has been given greater acclaim in the field of psychology than in the field of vision care. The reason may be that it is easier to understand this research than it is to make their model of vision practical to the clinician practicing optometry or ophthalmology, or to provide a background of information for others involved in rehabilitation such as occupational and physical therapists, and speech/language pathologists. In a general manner, let us consider what the visual process is according to these researchers and attempt to create a behavioral and clinical model.

As was noted, the visual system is composed of not one, but at least two systems: a central or focal visual process and a peripheral or ambient visual process. Neurologically, as was described previously, the central visual process is delivered primarily through the macula of the eye which is located on the retina at the central or posterior pole of the eye. The macula is composed primarily of cone cells which are especially dense in the fovea or central part of the macula and deliver the highest resolution or acuity. The nerve fibers from this area exit the eye through the optic nerve and emanate to central areas of the visual cortex. A primary function of cone cells is color detection as well as detail resolution.

The peripheral area of the retina is largely composed of rod cells. The further away from the macula, the fewer observable cone cells there are in the retina. The rods occupy a greater area than the cones and the density of rods is greater than the cone cells throughout much of the retina, but not in the macula and fovea. The rod cells are more important for scotopic vision, i.e., vision during lower threshold luminosity. They are also more sensitive to movement than are cone cells. Nerve fibers delivered from peripheral areas of the retina extend through the optic nerve and optic tract to the more peripheral area of the visual cortex.

Although it has been mentioned earlier that we are primarily concerned with the conscious visual image resulting from central vision function, it must be noted that many nerve cells exiting the eyes send collateral fibers to other areas of the brain before reaching the highly organized visual cortex of the brain. As noted above,

Trevarthen carried out research that was published in 1968[7] describing a bimodal process of the visual system. Trevarthen states in this early work that, "All vertebrates possessed direct projections from the eyes to a laminated cortex-like field in the anterior midbrain roof, the optic tectum. Other fibers, or collaterals, also passed to the pretectum and to the posterior diencephalon, the optic thalamus." He, along with Bishop,[8] concluded that the dorsal ganglion of the lateral geniculate body may function as an integrating center in addition to its role as a relay and distribution center. This means that the lateral geniculate is important in the relay of visual information to portions of the brain other than the visual cortex. The cells of the lateral geniculate body actively respond to diffuse retinal illumination whereas cortical cells respond much more reluctantly.

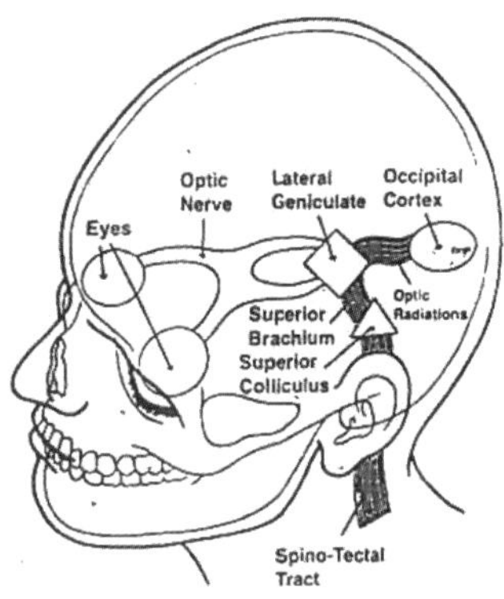

***Figure 1-1**. A Graphic Representation of Neurological Pathways of the Visual Process in the Cortex and Midbrain.*

Movement of light across the retina will cause active firing of geniculate cells regardless of the direction of movement, whereas response at the cortical level is often conditioned by the direction of movement. This was discovered by Hubel in 1960.[9] Many axons link up through the lateral geniculate with axons directed to the midbrain and with other areas that relate to motor and sensory functions. Retinal ganglion cells emanate from the retina of the eye, through the optic nerve, optic chiasm, and to the optic tract where they reach three major destinations. The first is the lateral geniculate body for relay to the visual cortex, the second is to the pretectal nucleus (pupillary constriction), and the third is to the superior colliculus which, importantly, is related to posture, movement and orientation to positional space. This has been described by Wolff.[10] The superior colliculus receives fibers from the optic tract via the superior brachium, from the occipital cortex via the optic radiations through the lateral geniculate, and from the spinal-tectal tract, thus connecting it with sensorimotor information from the spinal cord and medulla.

It is the ambient visual process that links up with and becomes part of the sensorimotor feedback loop at the level of midbrain (see Figure 1-1). The matching of information that occurs between the ambient visual process, kinesthetic, proprioceptive, vestibular, and tactile systems sets up a spatial framework that becomes the basis of higher sensory interpretation. The sensorimotor feedback loop provides a feedforward system to other areas of higher cortical functions. This has been described by Nelson.[11]

The midbrain receives as well as sends fiber tracts to all other areas of higher cortical function including the occipital cortex, temporal lobes, parietal lobes and the frontal lobes. The superior colliculus receives a large quantity of axons related to vision. This particular area of the midbrain is responsible for the primitive role of stabilizing the image from the peripheral retina. Without the matching of information that occurs between the ambient visual process and other portions of the sensorimotor feedback system, we would actually perceive an image as jumping and moving about each time we shifted our eyes or our body. This is an important fact that is frequently overlooked. Individuals who experience dizziness and vertigo are often diagnosed as having a vestibular problem. Many of these individuals will undergo vestibular therapy and not succeed in reducing or eliminating the vertigo or dizziness. It must be understood that the ambient aspect of the bimodal visual process has critical interactions with vestibular function and that often an imbalance in the ambient visual process can be misinterpreted as a vestibular dysfunction.

The midbrain is also responsible for providing information to the visual cortex about aligning and developing integration of the central images of both eyes.[12] The focal process of vision is attention oriented and is delivered primarily through the macula and para-macula areas of the retina, thus allowing us to center in on a detail. However, it is the ambient visual process which, in relaying information to the midbrain, matches information with other sensorimotor processes such as kinesthetic, proprioceptive and vestibular information. Organization of this information provides a context relating to where we are in our spatial world. This information is obtained through a feedforward mechanism to binocular coordination areas whose purpose it is to integrate the images from the right and left eyes. This occurs prior to the higher occipital cortex carrying out its role for defining detail. The information received from the midbrain, which is primarily from the ambient visual process, provides the spatial framework by which the binocular coordination cells develop the integration of the images from each eye.[10]

The emphasis on the neuroanatomy of the eyes and brain is provided to underscore the important relationship between the ambient visual process and the motor system, and the equally important relationship between the focal visual process and higher occipital cortical function. To summarize, the peripheral process of vision is ambient in function, expansive and more involved with spatial orientation and awareness than with detail detection. The focal-cortical relationship allows us to define and resolve information about the specifics of detail for higher cognitive processing associated with attention and concentration; the focal visual process develops with maturity. However, it is a fairly recent development in the millions of years it has taken our visual system to organize and evolve.

An example of lower order visual processing can be observed by studying organisms such as the frog. The frog has a visual process that is spatially oriented; it is designed to detect movement so that the frog can find food and avoid predators. Research[13] demonstrated that when a frog was placed into a box it was unable to detect a dead fly hanging from the ceiling; within a week it starved to death. In a similar experiment, the frog did not detect the dead fly for several days, but when a live fly was placed into the box movement was immediately detected and the frog caught the fly. This experiment demonstrates that the ambient role of the visual process is critical for survival. Without it our visual system would not have evolved.

Evolution has resulted in primates having a high level of visual function which combines the ambient visual process with the focal visual process. Humans have the highest level of visual function. Analyzing the relationship between the focal and ambient processes and human neurological development, we discover that nerve fibers from the central macula are not myelinated (sheathed) at birth. The signals received from the macula are not as distinct at birth as they are weeks later. Thus the visual process of the newborn is highly spatially oriented. It seems that the newborn infant's primary activity is to organize his motor function, and to gain control of limbs, head movements, etc. As was described, many of the nerve fibers from the eye are not delivered to higher cortical levels involving areas of imaging or seeing, but are oriented to midbrain, linking up with motor centers for balance, movement and coordination. Developmentally, the lack of a focal vision process enables the young infant to orient to the ambient process of vision and reinforces his efforts to organize motor control. Vision must lead motor. Research about development and vision by Arnold Gesell, MD[14] aptly stated that vision develops from an action system. While vision must lead motor, it cannot develop this function unless its basis and grounding occur in relationship to the motor system. The development of the child demonstrates that the ambient visual process is critical from the first moments of birth in establishing and grounding a relationship with the sensorimotor processes, thus establishing a spatial orientation that is based on motor and sensory relationships. This provides the platform by which higher focalization, perception, and even cognitive function develop.[15,16] The ambient visual process not only provides a feedforward system to binocular cortical cells and the occipital cortex, but it delivers information to all major areas of the cortex.

As has been stated, 20% of the peripheral retinal nerves relay information, through axons, to the thalamus or midbrain for spatial matching with kinesthetic, proprioceptive and vestibular information being received from other sensorimotor systems. Developmentally, this allows for organization of spatial information to orient more complex sensorimotor experiences affecting posture, movement and balance. Once this is established, information from the thalamus is sent to higher cortical levels.[10] The occipital cortex receives a major amount of spatial information in order to organize the detail process of focalization. The ambient visual process is not a conscious process as is the focal system. The ambient visual process is preconscious[17] and matches peripheral/spatial visual information to sensorimotor information for the purpose of establishing context for time and space prior to focalization on detail. This becomes the grounding or background relationship for the higher visual processes of perception and cognitive function. Without the ambient visual process, the visual world would become fragmented and isolated on detail. However, this critical bimodal process has been ignored and misunderstood clinically.[18]

To better understand the bimodal visual system, we can begin by examining the neurological substrate of the focal and ambient visual processes. Ganglion cells traveling from the retinas can be characterized based on physiology and function. There are three primary types of ganglion cells: P-cells (parvocellular), M-cells (magnocellular), and K-cells (koniocellular).The M-cells and the P-cells provide a physiological basis for the ambient and focal processes. M-cells transmit visual information about shape and movement which is more related to ambient visual processing. It is a rapid processing system and does not relay information about detail. P-cells transmit the detail information contained within shapes and are much slower in processing. The ganglion cells emanate from the retina primarily through two major brain pathways: the retino-geniculo-cortical and the retino-tectal pathways. The retino-geniculo-cortical pathway contains both P-cells and M-cells and is the most recent to evolve. This pathway provides a mechanism for focal processing and cortical function. The retinal-tectal pathway consists mainly of M-cells and is more primitive. It provides a basis for spatial information, especially for spatial orientation prior to focalization. For example, a saccadic eye movement (via the ambient pathway) first requires spatial orientation to establish the direction and correct trajectory of the eye movement prior to the focalization response. The retino-tectal pathway is most critical for the child during early development. It has been noted that some of these functions are taken over later in development by the retino-geniculo-cortical pathway.[19] The ambient system, however, remains important for spatial orientation and balance. It can be demonstrated clinically that children and adults with oculomotor dysfunction and aspects of dyslexia affecting reading ability will demonstrate a change in pursuit tracking and saccadic fixations as well as their ability to read a line of print when sensorimotor support, such as physically pointing to the words, is established.

The subsystem of P-cells is related to the focal visual process (ocipital-cortical) whereas the retino-tectal projection of M-cell subsystems (thalamus-colliculus) is a substrate for the ambient visual process. Neurons in the retino-tectal pathway are almost completely myelinated at birth. However, those of the retino-geniculo-cortical pathway are not.[20] Of interest, it is important to note that the superior colliculus has essentially a normal adult organization and neuronal activity at birth whereas the occipital cortex does not. This demonstrates that while the cerebral cortical processes have taken over much of the visual motor function, there are still massive innervations between cortical and midbrain functions.

By understanding the neurological substrates of the ambient and focal visual systems we can recognize that developmental experiences help to couple and balance the ambient and focal visual processes. As noted, the M-cell system is a component of the ambient visual process, but it must be understood that it is not inclusive of it. While balance between the spatial and detail components of the visual process provides a means by which time and space become organized, any neurological event such as a traumatic brain injury (TBI), multiple sclerosis (MS), cerebral palsy (CP), autism, or cerebrovascular accident (CVA) can affect that balance between these systems. This is often the result of a decoupling of the focal and ambient processes, including the M and P cellular systems, which affects function and performance. M-cells have larger diameter axons, and are more susceptible to damage. The damage may result from ischemia, space occupying lesions, etc.

Additionally, the decoupling of cerebral blood flow and cerebral glucose metabolism can be the basis for an ischemia-hyperemia resulting in metabolic imbalances that can derange neuronal energy production as well as affect cell membrane permeability causing potential cytotoxicity even in a minor whiplash accident.[21] This can often be the basis for visual problems following a TBI. MRIs and CT scans do not always show positive lesions yet individuals may continue to experience a wide range of visual dysfunctions affecting motor and even cognitive processes. This will be discussed later in this book in the chapter: "Post Trauma Vision Syndrome."

As motor function becomes organized, the focal process of vision develops and supports the refining of motor skills. These motor experiences later provide a base for higher level sensory discrimination. The ability to match information between the senses and the motor processes results in coordination of motor function. The limitation of one sense or motor process will alter the experience and affect how information can be matched. Thus a limitation to the visual process will alter the effects on the motor system and vice versa. The matching of information between these processes should be fluid at infancy. As the child develops, he will begin to organize movement such as of the arm or hand. At the same time, the child will begin to fixate on more focal components of the visual process such as the hand. This interchange between the focal and the ambient functions of vision continues throughout the child's development. It creates a habitual style of using vision that is unique for each person. This habitual style, utilizing the bimodal process of vision, further contributes to learning abilities, motor coordination, personality, etc.

The process of vision is established through the motor system, and through the motor system, the sensory system is organized. There is an intrinsic value established by the extraocular-motor system and its relationship to the kinesthetic and vestibular systems. The kinesthetic and vestibular systems are very important to ocular motor control.

The focal vision process isolates on detail, is stimulus bound and is conscious. This process alone is inefficient since it is reactive to stimuli (stimulus-response). The ambient vision process is spatial, not stimulus bound and is proactive (response-stimulus-response). It is the action system as described by Gesell[14] associated with motor and sensorimotor processes.

In order to shift the eyes from one position to another, we must spatially orient to the next destination before making the shift to fixate on the next detail.[15] The ambient process is critical for anticipating change. Without this process one would have difficulty shifting visual regard and would isolate on detail. Dysfunction of the ambient process can cause a lack of awareness of body position and spatial context. This, then, affects preconscious midline relationships supported by the visual process and may result in a shift in the concept of visual midline. Midline dysfunction occurs when there is a mismatch between the ambient visual process and kinesthetic, proprioceptive and vestibular input at the level of midbrain. It will be discussed later in relationship to Visual Midline Shift Syndrome.

Emphasis is often placed on the ability to fixate and attend without an adequate understanding of the fact that unless there is a release of focalization we cannot shift regard from one point to another. We must also release from focalization in order to advance the relationship of what we see and attend to, towards that to which we direct our higher thoughts and cognitive processes. The ambient visual process provides a gentle spatial support for the higher focalization system. The more imbalanced that relationship becomes towards focalization, the more difficult it is to release and anticipate change or to direct the visual process to the next point of fixation. For example, reading involves shifting one's eyes from point to point across a line of print. Good readers do not see all the letters, instead they spatially see the shape or framework of several words at one time. The focalization process allows them to see several letters from each word, and thus the concept of words and phrases is established. Children just learning to read often become over focalized on each letter. They attempt to try to work with groups of letters by sounding them out phonetically. The evolution of the visual process for reading enables the child to eventually release from that focalization and establish a greater role for ambient spatial organization while reading. The same is true for writing. We should not have to concentrate on the tip of the pen or pencil on the paper forming each letter. However, this is the way the young child will approach learning to control the pencil to form each letter. Eventually, the ambient visual process establishes a spatial context to permit a flow and anticipation of each letter and each word. This is combined and matched with a cognitive thought process that does not isolate to one thought, but becomes continuous.

The sensory function of vision ceases when the motor component of vision (namely the extraocular muscles) is paralyzed. There are minor flicks and tremors of the ocular muscles that cause the eyes to be in constant motion. These flicks and tremors never permit the image of the environment to remain stable on the retina. When the eye muscles are paralyzed with a drug such as curare, which stops the flicks and tremors, sensory imagery ceases. It is not until the effects of the drug wear off that seeing or imaging recurs. In addition, the spatial constricts of the visual environment are affected by the ocular motor relationship. It has been reported that when there is a tendency for the eyes to diverge (exophoria), there is a flattening effect on depth perception. A convergence tendency (esophoria) does not have this effect. Esophoria and exophoria are states of ocular motor imbalance. Some believe that these states are simple muscle imbalances. However, if one attempts to understand the dynamic interchange between the motor processing and sensory processing of vision throughout the child's development, additional questions must be addressed in order to learn what the presence of exophoria or esophoria really indicates.

These states may demonstrate the relationship between sensory and motor involvement. Amounts of exophoria or esophoria will vary during different developmental stages, and correlations between these ocular motor states and the stages of development do exist.

The purpose of this discussion is to establish a model for vision that will provide an approach to understanding that it is a dynamic process and that imbalances between the bimodal process and the sensorimotor systems can occur. By understanding that vision is a dynamic interactive process, we can also create a model for rehabilitation which can affect function and performance. This approach will go far beyond a sensory model that identifies only with a passive stimulus-response relationship of the eyes to the brain.

One's style of vision continues throughout life, and the patterns established by the way a person utilizes the focal and ambient functions of vision are reinforced through motor relationships. The perceptual aspects of vision are very much influenced by the motor functions of this process. This creates a dynamic interchange that is quite different from sensory models that are often used to describe sight. Sight, in those models, is a static concept of seeing that does not necessarily equate to performance and motor function. The model of vision that is now being presented can be applied to all aspects of performance and behavior and is developmentally influenced. This model will provide us with new insights into posture and movement which are important when considering the development of a child or of multihandicapped and traumatic brain injured individuals.

Time, Space and Movement

The development of concepts of spatial parameters and timing are very important to the overall development of the child. Depth perception has been studied by researchers for many years. Classical experiments have indicated that certain factors of depth perception are innate. In one study,[22] a kitten was placed on a table that was painted in a black and white checkerboard pattern. On the table was a cliff that was covered with a clear Plexiglas bridge. The kitten, when placed on the tabletop, demonstrated caution and refused to walk onto the Plexiglas covered cliff. The behavior suggested that, for this two-eyed animal, there was an understanding of depth perception; caution was demonstrated because the kitten saw the cliff.

In a classical experiment done by Richard Held, PhD,[23] a kitten was placed in a carousel; a second kitten was attached to a harness that pulled the carousel. The kitten in the carousel was denied motor movement from birth. The kitten that pulled the carousel was permitted to move. Both kittens were binocular. The results showed that the first kitten, after being taken from the carousel, did not have accurate depth perception for visually guided behavior, whereas the second kitten had a much greater ability to judge depth. Held's results supported his thesis that "self produced movement with its concurrent visual feedback is necessary for the development of visually guided behavior." Thus this study demonstrates that the visual process establishes organization of depth perception through the structure and reinforcement of the motor system.

Held's results raise some interesting implications regarding how we provide learning experiences for our children and even how we perform visual examinations for children and adults. As noted, his experiment demonstrates that our motor system is an important component for learning about our spatial environment. However, development of the visual process for the child should eventually lead the child to a level of skill where learning can occur by utilizing vision to more directly relate to past experiences. Unfortunately, there are many children who have difficulty learning this way. Some have been given labels such as learning disabled (LD), attention deficit disorder (ADD), and attention deficit hyperactive disorder (ADHD). While there can be many causes for the classification of symptoms related to these disorders, vision also can be considered a cause by understanding that the ambient aspect of the visual process establishes its base in sensorimotor function. For some individuals, this relationship is not established unless the motor system is actively involved. For others, the higher visual and cognitive processes become overfocalized unless the motor system engages the ambient visual process and, in a sense, grounds the visual process. For these individuals, constant movement may be the only means to maintain their orientation when using the visual and cognitive processes in time related space. This indicates that in order to use the visual process accurately for learning, we must be able to release from focalization and anticipate change. If we become bound by focalization we isolate to the present and cannot anticipate the future. This will directly affect learning experiences and will interfere in the classroom and elsewhere if movement is restricted.

If we think about the standard vision examination in our society, the doctor performs the exam while the child or adult is stationary, often in a chair. Both acuity assessment and corrective refraction, if needed, are carried out in this manner. However, we must ask ourselves what is really determined about the visual system from testing in this static manner. It has been noted that individuals with strabismus (an eye malalignment) who also demonstrate suppression (a lack of binocularity) have little or no depth perception when tested. However, it is in the author's experience that when individuals with no measurable depth perception (as measured on stereopsis tests) are permitted to reach up and touch a pencil, their ability to reach and locate the object is considerably reduced when the strabismic eye is covered. Why does this individual with no depth perception on a stereopsis test, and with central suppression of one eye, have difficulty localizing objects in space when the strabismic eye is covered? This leads to the possibility that such tests examine only one aspect of binocularity and depth perception. Further, it is likely that even individuals with a high angle strabismus turn of the eye can still utilize aspects of ambient visual processing in the strabismic eye to match enough information to have improved depth perception when using both eyes.

Present forms of vision testing permit limited interaction of motor and visual functions. Unless the visual system is examined as a dynamic process involving kinesthetic and proprioceptive reinforcement, findings from the examination will be limited leading to possible misinterpretation. This has direct implications in understanding the assessment of the neurologically challenged child or adult, as well as establishing rehabilitation of the visual process for these individuals. This will be discussed later in this book.

Ideally, the vision examination for individuals with sensory and/or motor disabilities should include both a perceptual motor evaluation and a detailed vision examination. These will enable the clinician to observe the behavior of the individual in an attempt to understand gross and fine motor abilities and their relationship to visual function. Basically, this means analyzing the behavior related to the bimodal visual process.

While movement is a critical component of the development of spatial-visual relationships, movement is also related to the development of time relationships.[24] Time and space experiences develop through an interchange of sensory and motor function. What does distance mean to the newborn infant who looks across the room without ever having had the opportunity to crawl or walk? It is through his motor system that the child first understands space by crawling across the floor, thus developing interaction between motor, visual and other sensory processes. The child may see, but does not have a meaningful experience until he is able to crawl or move about. The kitten crossing the Plexiglas bridge experiment demonstrates that depth perception is an innate observation. However, accurate object localization must be refined through sensorimotor interaction. This experience, once established, can be matched to new visual experiences allowing the child an understanding of depth perception even in new environmental surroundings.

Rudimentary time relationships are established at very early ages. Even in fetal development the child experiences the rhythm of his own heart, the beating of his mother's heart, and the rhythm of respiration. These rhythms are experienced early in fetal development through somatosensory stimulation and later, with the development of the auditory system, through audition. These rudimentary concepts of timing continue after the child is born and develop further as a spatial reference when movement is established. As the child moves through space, time is represented by how long it takes him to go from one point to the next. Once established, this information enables the child to match it with new auditory and/or visual information so he can judge how long it will take to move from one point to another. This process uses higher level sensory processing. However, it must be emphasized that the basis of this interpretation lies in the experiences that were matched between motor and sensory processes.

The focal and the ambient processes are very much involved in establishing temporal relationships to spatial perception.[25] The author has noted that this can be demonstrated by observing an interesting phenomenon. If one looks at a rotating drum of stripes, such as those presented on an optokinetic drum, the stripes will appear to slow down if the viewer focalizes intensively and concentrates. (Personal communication with Don Fong OD, 1978.) However, if the viewer relaxes and attempts to develop a more spatially oriented style of vision without concentrating and focalizing on the stripes, the stripes will actually appear to speed up. The focal and the ambient processes of vision allow one to manipulate temporal aspects of spatial perception. This usually occurs in an unconscious mode. However, any dysfunction of the ambient or focal processing systems will result not only in spatial mismatches, but also temporal misjudgments as well.

Understanding time and space relationships is important to the understanding of the concept of Neuro-optometric Rehabilitation. When a mismatch of information occurs between sensory and motor processing, particularly vision and motor processing, distortions in experience occur. One theory is that these distortions are represented in the visual process as anomalies, i.e., myopia, hyperopia, astigmatism, malalignment of the eyes such as in strabismus, and particularly in the measurements of phorias (tendencies of variations of eye alignment that do not result in strabismus or eye turns). This is not to say that there are no other reasons for these anomalies; there can be organic and pathological causes.[26] However, it is the author's clinical experience that all too often these anomalies, once diagnosed, are thought to be caused by an organic or pathological problem, and thus the visual/functional cause related to motor and perceptual processing is often misdiagnosed. The purpose here is to emphasize the relationships of motor and sensory processes to the anomaly so that it may be analyzed with a new and better understanding and thus be better treated by rehabilitative means.

When any type of impairment, especially a motor impairment, is involved the processing of information will be interfered with or distorted. Therefore, experience concerning time and space for a multi-handicapped child will be affected because he will not be able to match information appropriately between the motor and sensory processes, particularly vision. Once again we must question the appropriate mechanism for examination of a multi-handicapped child, as well as the normally sighted child or the visually impaired child, with regard to sensory and motor testing. It is the author's opinion that the various states of esophoria and exophoria, myopia, astigmatism and hyperopia represent distortion and imbalances in time and space relationships as they occur in early stages of development. Thus, if the child visually experiences distortions in space because of inaccurate sensorimotor matching, then these distortions can also affect oculomotor balances that will provide inaccurate information to the brain about spatial relationships. For example, this may be represented in the balance between the sensory component of the eyes and the ocular muscles, causing the eyes to over converge to a closer point in space than where the person is actually fixating (esophoria). This means that the person will perceive the object to be in a different and closer position than where it really is. In the state of exophoria, individuals tend to see objects further away in space than they really are. Clinically, these behaviors can be observed in patients diagnosed with a high state of esophoria or exophoria. If the person with high esophoria is given the opportunity to reach up and point to an object, he will often reach up and touch a closer point than where the object actually is located. However, a person with a high state of exophoria, when asked to reach up and touch an object will often attempt to touch beyond the object. Both situations indicate a distorted concept of space.

Myopia and hyperopia may be looked at in a similar manner. Rather than distortions of ocular motor position, these conditions result in distortions of focusing and sensory positions in space related to time concepts. For example, myopia is the tendency to focus at close points in space, blurring out distance. This pulls distance localization to near points in space.

Time and space relationships, established through sensorimotor matching of information with the visual process, become the basis for visual function. Any distortions that occur because of inaccurate matching may manifest as anomalies in the visual processing system. Over time, these distortions affect future judgments. The anomalies of visual development can be treated by changing perceptual and motor relationships affecting time and space judgments.[27] This will be discussed in a more practical manner in the chapters devoted to assessment and treatment.

Vision is a dynamic, interactive process of motor and sensory function mediated by the eyes for the purpose of simultaneous organization of posture, movement, spatial orientation, manipulation of the environment and, to its highest degree, perception and thought.

Through the remaining chapters of this book, emphasis will be placed on the role of vision not solely as a sensory process, but particularly as it is related to the sensorimotor feedback loop and to the motor system in general. This chapter sets the stage for the reader to examine relationships of development, posture and movement, and to then evaluate the effects on function and performance when the visual process is limited or compromised through a neurological event or vascular trauma.

Chapter 2

FACILITATING UNDERSTANDING THROUGH MANIPULATION OF THE VISUAL SYSTEM

Raquel Munitz

Visual impressions are so much a part of the world in which we live that it becomes impossible to completely separate what we see from what we experience, what we learn, and how we live. We move physically within a three-dimensional environment in which we anticipate certain responses, and plan actions in association with our feedforward mechanism (see Chapter I), which has a strong visual basis.

Our impression of the world that surrounds us enters our awareness through all our senses, creating for the viewer a "portrait" that is the interpretation made of the individually perceived world. The constructed portrait, or the object that is seen, has features that can be identified with each one of the human senses that have been used for learning about it through previous experiences. Form, color, size, position in space in relation to other objects, position in space in relation to the observer, as well as features of weight, texture, function or use are automatically taken into account by central nervous system processing. The object will have a name that identifies or classifies it in respect to everything else in one's personal world.[1]

The associated emotional reaction that occurs will vary in magnitude depending on the meaning that this object has for the person seeing it. It might give a sensation of secure familiarity in the case of something that is known or it might awaken pleasure, displeasure, fear or many other emotions. The meaning that any object has, according to the feelings that it evokes as something known or unknown, or based on what is understood about it, is the foundation for an immediate response.[2]

The experience of relating to or making contact with what surrounds us is very individual and must be represented in a multilevel experience model. All such experiences will tend to have a more dominant sensory characteristic, depending on the primary sensory organ activated and the consequent interpretation made by the subject. Vision most frequently emerges as the dominant sense in our modern society.

In the sighted individual, vision rapidly becomes the primary sense for discovering and understanding the surrounding world, and thus vision becomes the main means of relating to the external environment. Before the infant can move with any predictability, his vision begins to explore the persons, the toys, the room, the furniture and the changing light that make up the nearby world.

The information that the baby receives through the eyes is matched with impressions from the mouth and the tactile system as the physical body becomes more competent. This "knowing" that has been gained through association with the mouth, hands and feet, in addition to the eyes, enriches the developmental learning experience. The learning process evolves into a "knowing," eventually through vision alone, at which time it is no longer necessary to reconfirm the visual information with the tactile. The baby has learned to get meaning from what is seen and the reconfirmation of the other senses is superfluous because central nervous system integration has reached a new level. This level of integration sets the stage for anticipating the other sensory characteristics on the basis of visual information alone. This ability to anticipate information that is not directly available to the other sensory systems is the beginning of feedforward mechanisms that assist in correcting the postural set in order to develop adaptation. In this multi-level learning process vision becomes the basis for an internalized understanding of the environment and our orientation within it.

To reach its optimal level of efficiency, vision requires quality experiences in our relationship to our environment which, delivered over time, provide the opportunity for us to develop and mature. The visual system is representative of development since it reflects the double contributions of nature and nurture.

It is commonly known that the skill of sight is linked to the ability of the eye to focus on a stimulus and to see it clearly. This ability is referred to as sight with good acuity or "good vision," but such a definition limits itself to the reception of the stimulus. It is taken for granted that once there is a state of clear sight it happens automatically that the person will react properly to the stimulus with an appropriate behavioral change. In reality, the person first has to "understand" what he sees and the resulting understanding or interpretation of what is seen will initiate adequate performance in space. This might include moving with fluidity, knowing the limits of available space, and determining the speed and direction of the steps that are to be taken.

Such a sequence of events initially appears to be simple but it actually implies a complex neurological organization, the development of which requires about the first two years of life to complete. The young child must integrate the somato-proprioceptive-vestibular experience with the visual experience and be able to move in space securely using vision to lead motor function. He must also establish the relationship of his size in respect to the dimensions of the available free space and the limits created by the existing objects bordering that space. The child needs the experience of moving toward something and reaching the goal, of going up, down, under and around objects, avoiding crashes, etc. From this fundamental experiential base in development the child works to refine and combine visual and motor skills, constantly changing activities and orientation, and making the necessary adaptations according to the different dimensions that the spatial features present.

Visual development is important for orientation within our environment as well as for enabling one to develop concentration and attention. As described more completely in later chapters, the role of the ambient visual process, together with the focal process, creates both balance and impetus for development. This enables unconscious communion between ambient vision and sensorimotor input while permitting differentiation of the focal process to engage with higher perceptual/ cognitive processes. Eventually many of these tasks are managed without body movement and only by directing the eyes to a static or movable stimulus in order to know it. For example, the simple view of the side of a cup invites the mind to fill in the information related to use, shape and view from alternate perspectives.[3]

It is necessary to capture all of the pertinent features of the visual target to know the relative position of it in space and to learn its meaning. In this developmental process the child begins to give meaning to what is seen and to relate it to other stimuli, be they auditory, tactile or other visual stimuli until he is capable of responding in a differentiated way and is performing finer tasks at near space. Physical coordination and postural control are improved in a parallel developmental pattern to join the visual system in accomplishing the more refined tasks of reading and writing. Fine coordination skills mature as the postural system masters more upright positioning and the balance required for a smaller base of support.

The human being with an anatomically intact visual system and normal physiological function can use ambient and focal vision to deal with the world that surrounds him, paying attention to the peripheral or central stimulus according to the need of the moment. The ability to spot a sale sign in the store window while driving down Main Street is a practical example of this interaction.

For seeing and understanding to occur, the integrity of the anatomical system alone is insufficient. The importance of the opportunity to have experiences, and to learn from these experiences, cannot be underestimated. This "experiencing process" brings with it the opportunity for central integration and processing of visual information with all other intrinsic and extrinsic sensory information, each time creating a new pattern in the central nervous system. The way in which we integrate vision with other sensorimotor information creates a unique memory bank. We further elaborate visual images from our experiences.

A very important aspect of the early developmental period is the process of constantly comparing and matching stimuli in order to build a knowledge base that will permit not only the use of feedback information, which contributes to security in successful performance, but also to feedforward processes that permit accurate anticipation of and response to change. The brain activates the connections for carrying out a movement before the movement is actually initiated. That means that the "plan" for taking the coffee cup to the mouth exists before the reach starts. The complexity of this total process is such that it requires an ongoing fine tuning of the entire system that is gained with varied experiences and the mastery of new behaviors.

When a child has an intact physiological system and his development has proceeded without deviations or interferences, skills appear in a logical progression and within a predictable range of time. When there are manifestations of difficulties in the performance we become aware that there must be a deficit at some level of the process. It is important to identify the source of these difficulties, which may not be evident with simple observation of the child's initial responses. There may be an outward appearance of an intact system in that the eyes appear healthy and well aligned, and the movement and posture appear adequate for the age of the subject. Then it is important to question why this child who seems to have a healthy system is not using the system in the way that it was designed, or in the most efficient manner for the task. In some instances it is quite evident that identifiable deficiencies exist in the visual system or in the motor system or in the integration of the two. It may happen that the lack of very specific experiences has left learning gaps that create later problems.[4]

When professionals identify developmental problems that have the potential to respond to specific remediation or rehabilitation, it is essential to have the active participation of different specialists because such deficits have multi-modal manifestations. Each professional brings a unique background of education and experience that permits a specialized view of the problem as well as an individual fund of potential interventions. The most useful aspect of an evaluation is that it offers a place to start to solve the problem. Different views present more potential solutions.

In the case of an identified visual deficit, direct interventions have a much higher rate of success when consideration is given to all aspects of the personality and the previous development of the individual. That is why the neuro-optometric analysis takes on such importance. In this evaluation, visual acuity, accommodative function, ocular alignment, and binocular function are determined, along with how this person has learned to combine the incoming information. An assessment of peripheral and central skills is done and it is determined how these functions interact, how they are affected by and how they affect the posture/balance control. Such an evaluation leads directly to the priorities for intervention and the most effective way of carrying out a therapeutic program.

In order to give individuals the best possibility of developing to their optimum potential, there is a clear need for intervention at the physiological level through the prescription of the proper lenses that will not only optimize acuity but also permit comfort and efficiency in vision, with the possibility of functional change. This reduces physiological stress and lessens the need for compensatory measures on the part of the individual. When attempting to affect the relationship between vision and sensorimotor function, the optometrist who practices neuro-optometric rehabilitation is the professional best prepared to help with this initial intervention when there is any condition that involves the central nervous system. To complement the fitting of the proper lenses, a program of guided visual-motor activities or experiences can help many children to establish more efficient ways of making sense of visual stimuli in the everyday environment. Specific lenses and prisms can be used to lead the visual system to a functional level in its maturing process that will give a better understanding of the surrounding world. The use of prism lenses often creates a microcosm visuo-postural experience that has not previously been available. This is a direct manipulation of the immediate environment to provide a special learning opportunity.[5]

A very important aspect of the neuro-optometric intervention is the guided activities using specific lenses and prisms that will activate and develop the potential to learn through vision. Through neuro-optometric rehabilitation the appropriate lenses and/or prisms are to be used to create the different optical possibilities as the needs of the client evolve. Follow-up with feedback related to the individual's experiences is essential in this work. The concept of the total person must be given priority so it is important to provide opportunities to integrate responses that demand more and better function of the somatic-proprioceptive-vestibular experiences that can be linked to vision. Vision is not an isolated function.[6]

The clinician must carefully choose activities that will challenge the individual and offer the opportunity to experience space in relation to the moving body. The reaction must be elicited in such a way that the base of support is "seen" and "felt" by the subject, and matching of the "seeing" and "feeling" is accomplished. This type of experience may be carried out with the use of yoked prisms that create a shift of the midline, facilitating the body's ability to respond at a postural level. As the shift in the center of gravity occurs from the response to the prism orientation, the person reorients laterally and supports himself on the side that was previously neglected (see Chapter 7). Extension or flexion of the legs may be influenced as can be the inclination of the trunk and the orientation of the head in space. Support within the body structure is changing for the subject according to the way the floor is perceived, with inclination upward or downward. Adaptation of this initial posture determines to a large extent the quality of the movement to follow, so the intervention begins to affect the feedforward function. This type of guided experience with the prisms amplifies the person's knowledge base of spatial relationships and stimulates a new orientation of the body for movement in space and control of antigravity postures.

In giving the person a guided experience in which the body response to the base of support has to change in a brief time period, we are intensifying the visual-motor learning process. Each response is very individual and the clinician must be aware of the conditions of that response in relation to the previous ones. A change of postural orientation might occur to the right or left when the prism base is oriented laterally, or forward or backward if the prism base is up or down. We are challenging the adaptability of the balance and equilibrium systems that are integrated neurologically with the vision system at the midbrain level, taking them to a new level of refinement in timing of response and in quality. It is important that the clinician is aware of the adequacy of postural responses and that an ongoing reassessment permits anticipation of the subject's need for physical assistance. The clinician must continue to learn about quality differences in movement and posture control to be effective in this work.

In individuals who have adapted their previous movement in space according to a distortion in the appreciation of space, the experience of a new visual orientation is very strong. The process of changing from one extreme to the opposite, such as base-up to base-down yoked prisms, takes the individual away from the customary midline orientation or the individual compensatory adaptation that has been used. The experience of being "rocked" with different bases sets a new standard for the visual-motor orientation and generally creates a novel dimension that results in greater postural freedom and behavioral security.

Some children, who go through this experience while looking at their image reflected in a mirror, match what they see with what they feel. The spatial orientation labels of "up," "down," "left," and "right," discovered and identified by the child, help to generalize and internalize these concepts when the youngster is presented with a task to be done in a limited space, such as writing on a piece of paper, where there are fewer kinesthetic cues. There is less difficulty in the organization of the vertical tracings when a conceptual foundation has been established. The concept of left-right is difficult to establish at an internalized level for some children and they continue to look for outside cues. One example is the child who has learned the words "right" and "left" without having internalized the difference in the spatial orientation. Once such a child is "rocked" with the lateral yoked prisms and is guided to match the kinesthetic sensation with the transient visual distortion that is created, the ability to identify left from right without the need of the outside cues emerges as a verbalization of the displacement presented. This new certainty frees the child to move forward in cognitive development.

When the neuro-optometric rehabilitation is initiated it is very important to pay attention to the emotional environment in which the session is taking place. It would be absurd for the clinician to try to impose a "reality" that would be foreign to the subject because reality for each person is what the senses of that person dictate. Appreciation of space and objects depends on the individual way in which they are perceived. One only becomes aware of the existence of an internalized distortion when an unsuccessful response is made. For example, one might misjudge distance or depth in going up and down the stairs, or reach for an object apparently at a certain distance or walk between two objects and bump into them. It is the result of this behavior or the immediate feedback that indicates to the person that things are not where he sees them, that the dimensions and the relationship between him and other objects are not what was anticipated. This leads to feelings of insecurity and confusion. The feedforward and the consequent feedback are not corresponding. To remediate this situation it is not enough to tell the subject where the things are or to explain the distance between one thing and another, such as a chair and a table, etc. The person must have an opportunity to directly experience the objective dimensions of space in order to reduce the chronic mismatch that has existed between his appreciation of space and the physical reality. It must be kept in mind that these mismatches regarding larger space will be transferred to smaller spatial relationships and affect learning from printed material.

The benefits of this work for the person depend on the proper use of prisms in relation to the structured experiences, including choice of the prism strength and knowledge of the anticipated effects of the orientation of the prism base. Precautions have to be taken for the safety of the client using the prisms, and autonomic responses of the individual must be observed carefully. We can easily overload the system, creating greater disorganization or triggering adverse reactions of fear, anxiety and confusion. With an inadequate knowledge base or inattention to some of the factors discussed, it is possible for the clinician to establish even stronger distortions than the original, creating a visual warp or embedding the problem in the matrix of experience.

As it is true that one of the greatest concerns of the professionals who work with the individual with a central nervous system dysfunction is often quality of movement, the work of preparing for competency in the basic visual skills should not be neglected. An efficient visual system needs to be able to track, to make saccades (quick eye movements), to fixate and to sustain fixation. This security in visual function frees the postural system from having to participate in compensatory adaptations. *Problems in the execution of basic visual skills can result in the need for compensatory movements and postural patterns, and can add to the total stress placed on the comprehensive function of the individual.*

In providing meaningful intervention for visual problems, with normal development as a functional framework, we should remember the importance of the dissociation process. Individual body parts are able to move independently as another body part provides stability. The eyes have to be able to move from a stable base so the head needs to develop the ability to control its position, regardless of the orientation of the body in space. The head also has to be able to move in a variety of directions while the eyes maintain a point of fixation. In the visual system, as in the body, mobility depends upon stability, and effective stability relies on the refinement of the mobility that has been superimposed.

During the process of refining basic visual skills, one is confronted with many conditions that require accommodation. Through the ambient process we orient to the near space. Then the focal process provides the detail necessary to accommodate and associate attention and concentration. The release to far space involves the same process. In some cases this skill requires practice by the individual in order to enhance the performance. In a therapeutic situation we use the plus and minus lenses in order to intensify this practice effect. The plus and minus lenses alter ambient spatial information by changing the size and distance of the image. The focal system must then adapt by accommodating to this perceived change. As the ability emerges as a more consistent skill the amount of power in the lenses is increased, which permits work on the facility of the change and the amplitude of the accommodation. In this work the clinician must take care that both eyes have the same abilities of accommodation in order to balance the visual system function.

Through this work on improving basic visual skills and accommodation, we have an effect on the two major aspects of the visual system: one that matches information with the sensorimotor feedback loop for posture, movement, balance and orientation to space; the other to facilitate attention, concentration, interest, curiosity and cognition in general. To assure that the client is making positive change, the clinician continues to verify integrative responses that each time are more efficient and free of stress. In this way the client becomes capable of greater functional efficiency in everyday life, with reduced energy expenditure and increased success.[7]

Chapter 3

THE INTERACTION OF NEURAL SYSTEMS: HOW THE VISUAL, VESTIBULAR, AND SOMATOSENSORY SYSTEMS COLLABORATE FOR EFFICIENT FUNCTION

W. Michael Magrun

Introduction

Vision is the primary sensory system that organizes our world and provides a spatial framework for initiating, maintaining, and performing skilled activities. It has often been said that "vision leads movement." Vision allows us to initiate, anticipate, and react to our environmental world. Developmentally, vision is a major force in developing motor control. That said, it is also critical to understand how other systems, such as the somatosensory and vestibular systems, impact visual function. Understanding the collaboration and interaction of these systems is essential for planning effective rehabilitation strategies.

The foundation for skilled performance lies in the ability to match and integrate neural systems, particularly the visual, vestibular, and somatosensory systems. Within this triad,[1] the infinite possibilities of movement, posture, and skill acquisition exist. Each system has fundamental characteristics that provide us with knowledge of our external and internal world. These sensorimotor systems allow for the dynamic process of matching information, reweighting information, and integrating information that is task-specific and provides the foundation for learning through experience. Weighting and reweighting refers to how the sensorimotor systems are intra-organized and how functional tasks, movement, and learning are a complex interplay between systems, not only in anticipation of the functional task, but within and during the activation and process of the task. The sensorimotor systems have interchanging responsibilities and varying levels of influence during task-specific performance.

Function requires a foundation of musculoskeletal alignment, postural organization, biomechanical factors, and sensory processing to allow the initiation and the maintenance of a task-specific movement. Obviously we must always consider the acquisition of skilled function both from a volitional, or proactive learning process, as well as from a non-volitional, reactive supporting process. Both processes are simultaneously engaged in all performance and learning experiences. So it is fundamental to our clinical thinking to understand not only the success or difficulty of a functional process, but even more so to understand the underlying efficiencies or inefficiencies that contribute to, and are the ultimate reasons for, success or failure.

Neural System Organization

The acquisition of skills for learning and performance requires an organized central nervous system (CNS) that benefits from experience and can develop strategies for organizing sensorimotor information as well as initiating meaningful movement expressions. Shumway-Cook and Woollacott[2] define motor learning as involving the "learning of new strategies for sensing as well as moving." Emerging from "...a complex of perception-cognition-acquisition processes." But what are the underlying foundations for effectively utilizing perception, cognition, and acquisition?

Learning requires an awareness of time and space and the internal mapping of multiple sensory system information that is paired system to system, as well as with motor responses. Initially, learning occurs through feedback systems and then once learned becomes a more automatic feedforward process with anticipatory initiation. This learning most effectively takes place within the context of a meaningful activity and a spatiotemporal frame of reference. Skill acquisition requires sensorimotor consistency and matching along with practice. As Moore[3] points out, the term "motor learning" is somewhat misleading. Learning is a sensorimotor process.

It is also important to understand that movement can be reactive and proactive. Movement that is reactive relates to automatic reactions and responses to a change in the base of support and/or outside influences that unexpectedly challenge the body's center of gravity. These responses are more "hard-wired." They are "reactive" in nature and are based on a stimulus-response process, or sensory initiated motor response.

Proactive motor activity implies volitional activation of motor control for learning through cognitively-driven activity, and has an anticipatory component. This activity is more "soft-wired." It is response-driven in the sense that it is motor-sensory-motor in nature. The initial activation upon intent is internal and not initiated from an outside sensory influence. The initial proactive activation of movement further initiates sensory-motor processes. Interestingly, motor responses or movements are observed in the fetus before sensation is present.[4] Both reactive and proactive motor responses are required in all activities. They must work together for efficient motor control.

For example, walking from an even surface like concrete onto an uneven surface like sand requires righting and equilibrium adaptations to maintain a smooth progression of action. If the change in the surface is expected, (visual system initiates anticipatory readiness confirmed by the proprioceptive input of a different surface integrating with vestibular readiness) then the transition to the different surface requirements will be efficiently accomplished. If the change in the surface is not expected then the response will be completely reactive (hard-wired) and the righting and equilibrium reactions will be more abrupt as the postural mechanism adjusts without anticipation to the new surface requirements. The same is true when walking down steps. If an additional step is expected when in fact there is not an additional step, the pattern that is initiated through that anticipation is incorrect and we abruptly step unexpectedly onto the surface. In a more dynamic activity, suppose that we are running to catch a ball. Our ambient visual process orients us to space and initiates timing and rhythm anticipation to reach and catch the ball. Our vestibular system helps the eyes maintain gaze on the ball and focal attention. As we run toward the ball, our somatosensory system maintains postural control and dynamic balance. This is an interaction of volitional (soft-wired) proactive anticipatory initiation of praxis with background righting and equilibrium (hard-wired) support to adjust to the surface and speed of movement. If we unexpectedly step in a dip in the ground or onto an unexpected mound of dirt, then our anticipatory patterns and background cooperative control are interrupted. Our reactive balance responses become more dominant until we regain our balance and initiate an adjustment to our anticipatory motor activity to continue to attempt to reach the ball. If we anticipate the change in the surface, we adjust our anticipatory motor plan to avoid the obstacle or to prepare for an adjustment in background reactive demands. Sensorimotor control requires this intricate interplay that weaves back and forth between volitional motor activity and underlying righting and equilibrium control. The more complex the demand and the more complex the environment of the activity, the more intricately these systems interweave.

Postural Control

Postural control is essential for movement and serves as the background substrata for movement.[5] Without good postural control, movement efficiency is limited and compromised. Postural control involves alignment and postural tone (synergic muscle tone). Both alignment and tone must function dynamically throughout a movement task. Postural tone as well as alignment change during a movement performance. Starting alignment and tone are different than that required through the sequence or at the end point of the movement (task) experience.[6] Adler describes this process as a "ready tone," a "during tone" and a "termination tone."[7]

Resting postural tone is the automatic calibrated threshold muscle activity that provides tension against gravity to maintain basic upright control. Postural resting tension or tone is different than anticipatory tone that is initiated just prior to action as a preparation for movement. Muscle tensions increase to allow for stability required to initiate movement and then change throughout the range of the movement sequence. Postural tone changes as different sensory thresholds are reached depending on the demand of the movement or task that activates postural tone. These sensory influences include proprioception through weight bearing, vestibular processes to maintain head alignment and visual processes, particularly the ambient (peripheral) process that provides spatiotemporal orientation.

Within this process we also need to consider the musculoskeletal components of joint stability and mobility as well as specific muscle strength. Muscle strength and postural tone are different. For any movement to be efficient it needs to be initiated in the proper alignment. Kinesiologically, synergies can only be dynamic and efficient when movement is initiated in proper alignment so that the musculature is in proper orientation for synergistic co-activation.[8]

For example if sensory demands increase as in walking up a hill, postural tone increases to provide preparation for using more muscle strength in the legs and trunk. Strength relates to synergies of working muscles as opposed to postural muscles. Muscle strength relates to the skeletal integrity of the alignment of joints and joint mobility-stability factors. Young states that body segments held out of alignment for extended periods will result in adaptive shortening or lengthening and further result in postural deterioration. In addition, overused muscles may also cause adaptive muscle shortening and increase postural deficiencies.[9] Thus if the ankle has laxity, there will be less ability to increase strength of particular muscles due to less efficient muscle alignment. Or if the structure of the foot is not well developed, for example a flat arch with medial collapse of the foot, weight bearing will be affected and therefore this malalignment will cause inefficient interactions of muscle strength, joint proprioception in the foot and ankle, alignment, and postural tone. Likewise if the individual uses compensatory shoulder elevation and neck shortening for stability due to an inactive trunk, there will be consequential inefficiencies in trunk rotation and increasing postural misalignment. All of these musculoskeletal compensations due to developmental disability or as a result of a neurological disorder or trauma, impact the efficiency of the visual system.

Movement therefore is a complex process involving many systems that must interact in an organized cooperative and integrative manner. Sensory processes activate postural reactions. Volitional anticipatory postural preparation (initiated through cognitive intent) activates additional sensory processes. These relationships are constantly shifting and adjusting. As will be further examined, this type of process requires constant reweighting of sensory system influences and changing priorities, depending on which sensory system is the leading influence.

When we consider treatment approaches that purport to improve sensorimotor organization for learning and performance it is important to keep these concepts in mind. Treatment that deals primarily with equilibrium and righting reactions prepares one primarily for reactive motor responses. Treatment that emphasizes inhibition of "reflexes" does little for preparing or initiating activation of proactive motor performance or dynamic adaptation of equilibrium and righting reactions. Treatment that emphasizes practice prepares primarily for proactive motor responses but is dependent on the available postural organization. Failure to organize dynamic alignment and synergistic action of the musculoskeletal system will result in compensatory learning. Treatment that primarily provides sensory stimulation activates arousal (and in some cases inhibition) but may not be able to direct or organize postural activity for efficient motor control, either reactively or proactively. Treatment that emphasizes visual intervention, without understanding the dependence of the visual system on a dynamic postural base, results in compensatory visual function that lacks the ability to activate dynamic postural adjustments or efficient functional performance.

Without a dynamic neuropostural base, the risk is in training splinter skills.[10] Progressive treatment must address all these factors that cannot be integrated without a firm neuropostural base. They include normal distribution of postural tone, efficient distribution of weight, ability to grade weight shifts, diagonal and rotational movement components, ability to maintain dynamic postural alignment, and stability and mobility factors within both reactive and proactive responses. An organized neuropostural base allows for adaptive responses to new experiences and therefore is fundamental to learning and performance.

In order to achieve a learned adaptive response that can be developed into an automatic anticipatory learning foundation, the above-mentioned neural systems must be integrated. Organizing the visual-vestibular-cervical triad[1] (V-V-C) allows us to establish a neuropostural base with awareness of the body's relationship to itself, to gravity, and to space and time factors. Interactive integration allows for efficient learning. It is important to remember that all of these systems are proprioceptive systems.

Neural Systems Interaction

Shumway-Cook[2] cites research by Prechtl and others relating to the development of postural control that relates directly to the emergence of the V-V-C. For example, infants placed on a rocking board that tilted forward and back so the infant could be tipped up or down showed no antigravity responses up to 8-10 weeks of age. This indicated that regardless of whether the vestibular system received the information on perturbations there was no head reaction. Prechtl concluded this was the result of a lack of sufficient neck musculature due both to weakness and no experience in organizing muscle activity. Therefore the initial lack of stability of the rostral neck is shown at birth to be a limiting factor in integrating vestibular information.

In another cited study, researchers tested preterm infants born at 24-32 weeks gestation for the ability to keep the head in midline. They tested the response with and without visual information. When there was no visual information, the infant tended to turn his head to the right, but with visual information the infant was able to maintain midline orientation. When neonates were placed in a room with a pattern of stripes that moved forward and backward, the infants made head movements that corresponded to the visual information, such as moving the head back to the sensation of the stripes moving forward. It is the ambient visual process that orients to vertical boundaries.[11] These studies suggest the early and predominant role of ambient vision on postural adjustment and the importance of the interaction and organization of the visual system with the rostral neck as the first beginnings of the V-V-C triad.

Infants of 2.5 to 5 months were tested as to head tilt when tilted in a chair. Infants showed antigravity righting responses to the head tilt (indicating vestibular-cervical organization). However when a visual stimulus in the form of a woolen ball was presented with the chair tilt, the head tilt was less. This indicates visual dominance on grading the vestibular-cervical response to a shift in the base of support relative to the visual regard of the child. Therefore vision modifies vestibular reactions and moderates the more basic hard-wired balance reactions, thus allowing new internal mapping to take place on an experiential soft-wired basis that has adaptability potential for feedforward processes.

If we consider the child with functional vision difficulties, either in focusing at various distances or in ambient visual awareness, this visual control may not be activated sufficiently to prevent over-reactions in background righting and equilibrium responses. These children are often classified as "motor clumsy." Visual control contributes to smooth and adaptive motor control but if it does not modulate vestibular responses, over-reaction may occur. The above studies suggest the dominant role of vision in the V-V-C Triad. Vision is the primary sensory system[12] and the ambient visual process has been described as visual proprioception.[13]

Shumway-Cook[2] tested children under various sensory conflict conditions. She found that when visual and somatosensory information was reduced and the 4-6 year old had to rely mostly on vestibular information, all but one fell. Conversely no 7-9 year olds lost balance under the same conditions. This would seem to correspond to the dominant role of vision in the development of postural control up through 7 years of age. At around the age of seven the somatosensory system and vestibular system are able to maintain background control more efficiently without direct visual input. This switch from ambient visual dominance for managing posture, to a more somatosensory process, allows the visual system to more fully attend to other details for learning and indicates a complete integration of the ambient visual process with somatosensory-vestibular processes. In other words, there is a differentiation allowing focal vision for more cognitive learning as the ambient visual process integrates more efficiently with somatosensory and vestibular processes.[11] Thus, there is a more efficient V-V-C triad upon which learning, confirmation, correlation, internal mapping, body scheme and feedforward comparator circuits can develop dynamically to provide the infinite variability of movement, learning, and adaptation required for ongoing skilled performance.

Obviously, for maximum efficiency, the visual-vestibular-somatic systems must match consistently to develop the postural background for establishing the foundations of learning. Research has shown that when one system is unable to receive correct information, the other systems are able to compensate to a greater or lesser extent depending on circumstances. However, for the most efficient learning and performance to take place there needs to be accurate and consistent matching of all these systems.

The Importance of the Neck

As previously stated, the neck is critical in the organization of sensory processing for motor performance. According to systems theory[2] at about 2 months, coordinated neck musculature action for posture is present. This is followed by the mapping of the visual system to the neck musculature, followed by the mapping of the somatosensory system to the neck, followed by mapping of the vestibular system to the neck. This priority mapping is significant for understanding the influence and importance of each sensory system to postural control, visual organization, and each other.

A growing amount of research supports the critical importance of the neck in the integration of visual and vestibular information. Gdowski and McCrea[14] in a study of squirrel monkeys investigated signal processing in the vestibular nucleus by recording secondary horizontal canal-related neurons to neck rotation. They found that neck proprioception played an important role in shaping output of the vestibular nucleus. Most vestibular neurons were sensitive to neck rotation and the direction of the neck input was antagonistic with respect to vestibular sensitivity. In other words, neck proprioception reduced the vestibular response. We might surmise a similar relationship in man that might help explain vestibular hypersensitivity in the absence of good neck control.

Falla, et al.,[15] concluded that feedforward activation of the neck muscles was necessary to achieve stability for the visual and vestibular systems, as well as ensuring stabilization of the cervical spine. Normal healthy subjects were tested during rapid arm movements and EMG onsets were calculated for the sternocleidomastoid and cervical muscles. Flexor and extensor cervical muscles showed co-activation and during bilateral and unilateral perturbations the sternocleidomastoid and cervical extensor muscles demonstrated feedforward co-activation. When we think of some of the children with learning disabilities with low tone and inefficient stability of the neck, or adults who have sustained head injuries and cannot maintain head-neck-trunk midline orientation, it is not hard to understand how visual and vestibular processing can be affected.

Other authors[16] suggest a direct relationship between the alignment of the neck and vestibular function. Subjects who had suffered whiplash injuries and normal subjects were tested for postural control in a head-back position and it was found that the head extended position was more challenging for postural adaptation and that neck problems impair postural control. Further, the neck-back position may result in utricular malpositioning. Head extension has been suggested as a possible cause of physiological vertigo.[17] Neck fatigue affects posture by producing abnormal sensory input to the CNS, particularly without vision.[18] Considering children with both neck control /neck alignment problems, as well as functional vision problems, and adults who have suffered head-neck-shoulder trauma, it is clear that there would be a compounding influence on vestibular processing.

Bloudin, et al.[19] investigated whether accurate perception of body rotation required both vestibular and neck-body proprioception. The authors concluded that neck muscle proprioception contributes to vestibular calibration at a perceptual level necessary for body orientation and accuracy after rotations in the dark. We can infer from this that vestibular processing is not independent from neck and trunk proprioception.

Cohen conducted research on animals in the 1960's, and was one of the first researchers to understand the importance of the neck. He demonstrated that labyrinthectomized monkeys were able to initiate lateral lifting of the head with somatosensory input only. He demonstrated that when the dorsal roots of C1, C2, C3, of animals were anesthetized, they exhibited classical symptoms similar to labyrinthectomized animals. Cohen[20] concluded that even though the vestibular system is instrumental in orientation of the head in space, there is no possible way by which the semicircular canals or otoliths can inform the brain of the angle of the head to body. This can only be done by proprioceptors in the neck. Without this information there were still severe deficits in orientation and balance despite intact vestibular structures. He suggested that the preoccupation with the vestibular system led to errors in interpretation because the neck mechanisms were ignored, and further boldly suggested that there has been an overemphasis placed on the vestibular system; "it is incorrect to speak of the vestibular structures as the chief balancing or orienting organs of the body."

As previously discussed, Moore[1,12,21,22] considers the visual system as the primary sensory system. Padula considers the ambient visual process as the means to support and organize balance, posture, and an upright orientation against gravity. (See Chapter 1.)

These studies remind us that the control and organization of the neck has functional effects on vision and vestibular function and should be carefully considered before assuming that a balance problem has its origins in the vestibular system.

In treatment we need to keep these issues in mind if we are to be able to carefully analyze the results of the activities we choose, and if we are to anticipate readiness for an activity. Initial stimulus conditions must be viewed with respect to the rostral neck and its musculoskeletal readiness (stability) to allow vestibular-visual inputs to activate and/or reinforce the response. Understanding the quality of an individual's performance and therefore the potential system interactions, be they efficient or inefficient, is essential for clinical management of treatment needs and choice of intervention strategies.

The Importance of the Somatosensory System

The drive to be upright is an innate drive and is one of the primary achievements of the first year of life. The upright posture provides the most efficient alignment for the maximal integration of all sensory systems.[21] Postural control and organization against gravity is essential for sensory receptors to be in their most effective alignment for interacting and matching sensory information with each other and for maximizing sensorimotor experiences that establish foundations for learning and performance.

In addition to the importance of neck proprioception, somatosensory input from the rest of the body has also gained more attention. The somatosensory system is increasingly being suggested as a primary influence on vestibular function and balance maintenance. Crutchfield and Barnes[23] state: "the vestibular system is not as critical to maintaining certain conditions of balance as was once believed, that is, balance is not provided by the vestibular system alone."

Studies on muscle states, tension, Golgi tendon organs and muscle spindles, indicate that proprioceptive information shapes reflex responses and is the root of postural maintenance. Further, proprioception was seen as the most important factor in postural alignment.[24] Alignment is so critical to balance and the maintenance of posture that structural integrity of the musculoskeletal system is the first thing that should be evaluated in order to determine its effect on postural control[23]. Normal musculoskeletal alignment provides for kinesiological synergistic activation of muscle groups for stability in the core of the body and sustained activation of the musculature of the limbs to perform complex tasks.[8]

The base of support, namely the feet and ankles, plays a critical role in balance. Studies have identified the importance of the biomechanical constraints of the ankle and the importance of an ankle synergy in balance. Small perturbations do not challenge the center of mass and are easily handled by reactions at the ankle as long as there is a firm support surface and the outside force is not too intense.[23] Ankle strategies do not necessarily require vestibular input to maintain balance. This is important when we evaluate children with postural disorganization or adults with joint and soft tissue trauma, in terms of the structure and activity of the feet and ankles. Poor structure will result in a progressive compensation through the legs and pelvis and trunk, and contribute to a chain of inefficiencies in balance, movement, posture and functional vision.

Hip synergies are activated once the center of mass goes beyond the control of a stable base of support. Hip synergies assist in activating vestibular responses. Horak et al.[25] indicate that the cutaneous and joint somatosensory information from the feet and ankles play an important role in assuring postural control and monitoring appropriate biomechanical constraints, and once hip strategies are activated vestibular information along with somatosensory information contribute to the selection of postural movement strategies.

Shumway-Cook and Woollacott[2] describe neuroscience studies of postural control under various tilt conditions. In standing when the tilt was small and the surface firm, the primary balance reaction was initiated at the ankles (ankle strategy). In standing when the tilt was larger and the surface was a narrow balance beam, the primary reaction was initiated at the hips (hip strategy). When sitting on a surface without the feet on the floor, the primary response was initiated with the trunk (trunk strategy). These investigations were conducted without interfering with vision or vestibular conditions. In other words, different challenges require different postural responses. These responses require a flexible postural system in order to make the necessary adaptations to challenges in balance and equilibrium.

In the three above studies, the musculoskeletal system reacted differently to different environmental demands, suggesting that there is a selective process by which the somatosensory system reacts to balance challenges. These experiments involve hierarchical reactive conditions where balance is compromised from unexpected external forces. The ability to adapt to these postural changes is largely dependent on the integrity of postural tone, alignment, musculoskeletal strength, etc.

In addition, Mittelstaedt[26-28] has recently reported the discovery of graviceptors in the trunk. These receptors are important in the perception of body posture and according to Mittelstaedt, these somatic graviceptors equal or surpass the contribution of the otoliths and further contribute to the control of the posture of the eyes, neck and limbs. In order for the eyes and otoliths to know the spatial orientation of the body to vertical, the relationship of the position of the eyes to head to trunk must be known which is deduced through efferent copies measured by proprioception. Thus, proprioception mediates the perception of position that allows the sense organs in the head to orient to vertical.

We know clinically that establishing trunk stability and mobility in children and adults with both neuromotor and postural disorganization, positively affects the quality and adaptability of movement. Therefore, the importance of truncal proprioception to establishing alignment and sensory matching becomes more evident.

In other experiments it was found that somatosensory loss increased vestibular sensitivity.[25] The results suggested that under conditions of neuropathy or if the surface was unstable, the vestibular system was more sensitive to the control of posture. Interestingly however, this study reflects two different conditions, peripheral neuropathy or loss of proprioceptive information, and an unstable surface or proprioceptive disruption. Obviously proprioceptive disruption results in a reactive state and therefore a more reflexive process. Vestibular sensitivity is thus logically increased to initiate trunk and head and neck reactions to maintain balance. Conversely, vestibular responses are negated or dampened in self-generated (proactive) movement to allow adaptability and dynamic motor control and efferent feed-forward processes without disruption by constant vestibular weighting for balance reactions.[29] Dynamic movement is context dependent and the interaction of sensory systems is completely different than in reflexive activity. In neuropathy, however, this increase in vestibular sensitivity is compensatory, not reactive. There is a loss of proprioceptive information due to the disease state requiring the vestibular system to compensate. Compensation is an entirely different process than integration.

Because the upright vertical alignment places the receptors of these systems in their most favorable position for integrating and matching information,[21] it provides a significant clue as to how to provide effective treatment. Therapy needs to provide activity that enhances the interrelationship of the sensory systems and allows for accurate time-space information correlated with functional activity that helps build and sustain efficient sensorimotor mapping and programming. Essential to this accomplishment is the establishment of a stable neuropostural base of support and postural alignment. Any activity superimposed on inadequate postural control and organization will, in effect, provide a lack of integration of sensory information and create even more mismatches in the visual-vestibular-somatic proprioceptive systems leading to an increasing cycle of inefficient learning and lack of spatiotemporal constancy.

The following example was documented in the offices of Dr. William Padula. Figure 3-1 shows a young adult who suffered a head injury. We can appreciate the difficulty he has in maintaining dynamic and efficient balance during walking. Figure 3-2 shows the result on balance when he is fitted with prism lenses. There is less leaning to one side and the alignment of the body has improved; however, he still needs the assistance of the wall to support his balance.

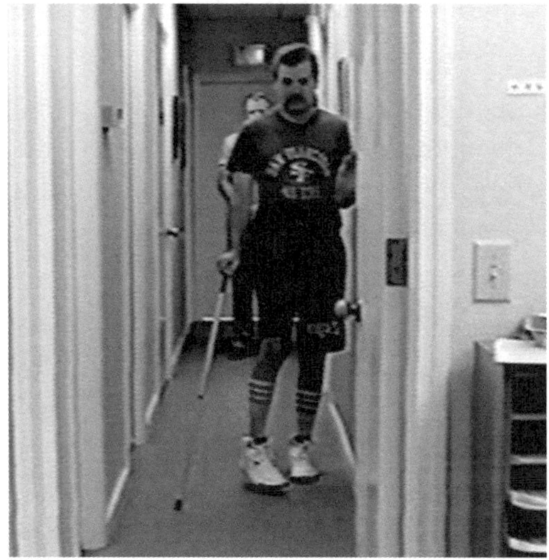

Figure 3-1. Initial gait pattern and balance difficulty.

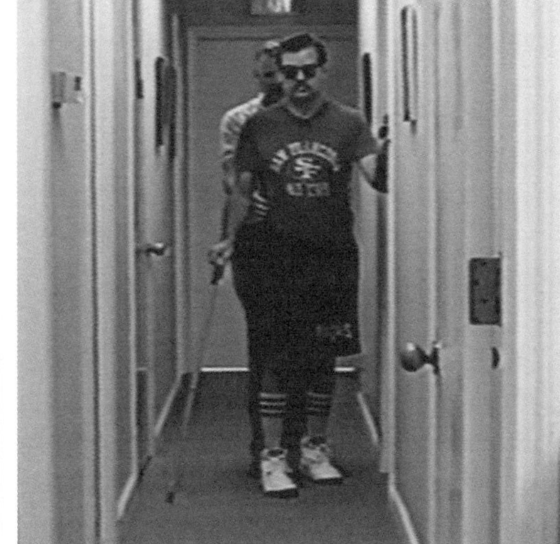

Figure 3-2. Gait pattern and balance difficulty #2.

After careful assessment by the therapist collaborating on this case, it was discovered that the right leg was not able to move over the foot. In figure 3-3 we can see that the right leg is back and the knee locked, with the foot in slight plantar flexion. The leg is not over the foot indicating ankle-foot malalignment. Additionally the body weight is displaced to the lateral border of the right foot. These factors result in the inability to bring the leg forward over the foot in gait, and the inability to pronate the forefoot during the step-off phase of gait. Figure 3-4 shows the use of a small foam wedge to help shift the weight more equally on the foot. We see in

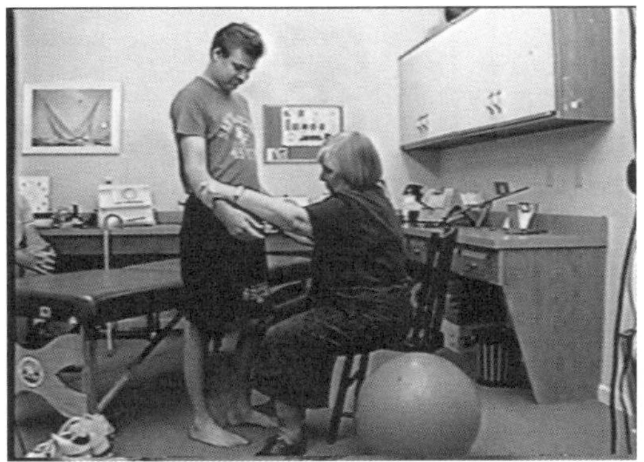

Figure 3-3. Standing alignment prior to mobilization.

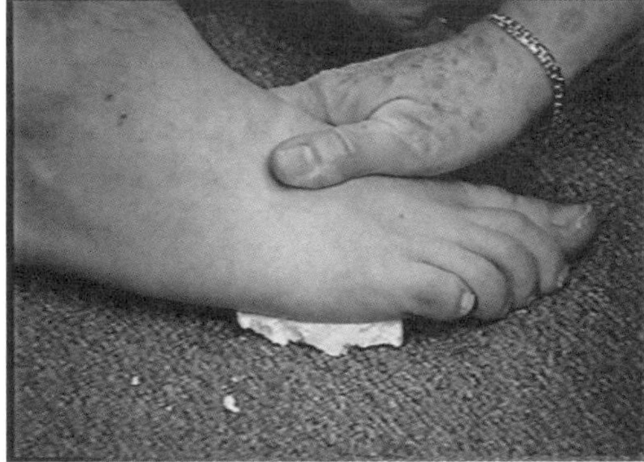

Figure 3-4. Metatarsal support..

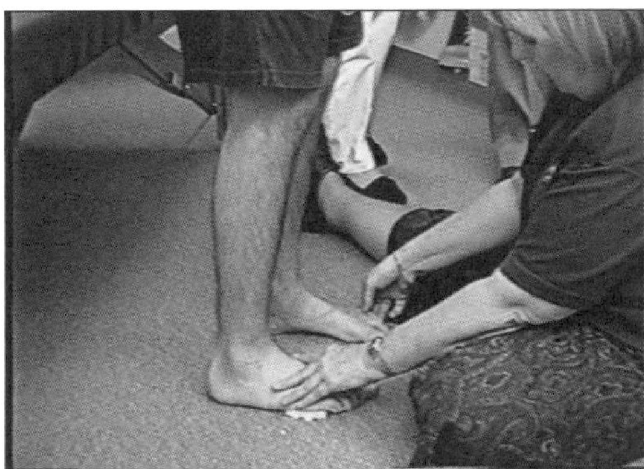

Figure 3-5. Standing with form wedge support.

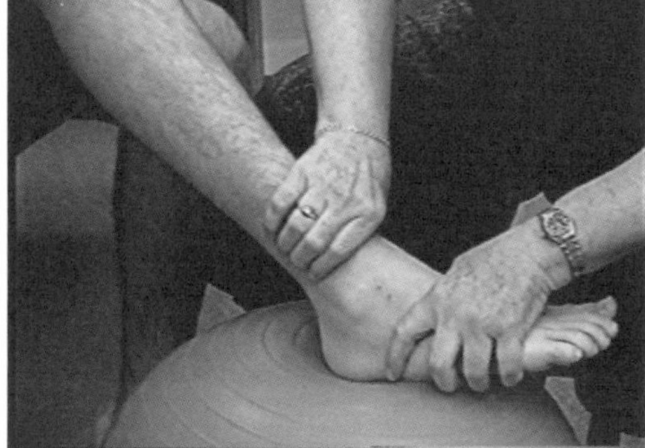

Figure 3-6. Mobilization of the ankle.

figure 3-5 that with the wedge, the patient is able to align his leg over his foot more normally and flex the knee slightly.

In addition to mobilizing the ankle as seen in Figure 3-6, the therapist provides experience in coming over the right side now that it is better aligned (figure 3-7). In figure 3-8 we see the therapist using physical handling to facilitate more pelvic mobility to assist in the subtle shifts needed in walking.

In Figure 3-9 with the foot insert and after mobilization and facilitation of adaptive movement, there is marked improvement in alignment of the right leg and more organized control of gait. He still needs a slight assist with his hand on the wall for support. In figure 3-9 when prism lenses are again provided we can appreciate the dramatic change in the quality of gait and postural alignment and control.

This example is a nice illustration of the importance of combining neuro-optometric intervention with physical handling and facilitation of alignment and motor adaptation to maximize the patient's potential.

It is important to remember that the variety and skill of "movement" and "vision" is soft-wired, or learned and refined upon a hard-wired base of sensorimotor activity

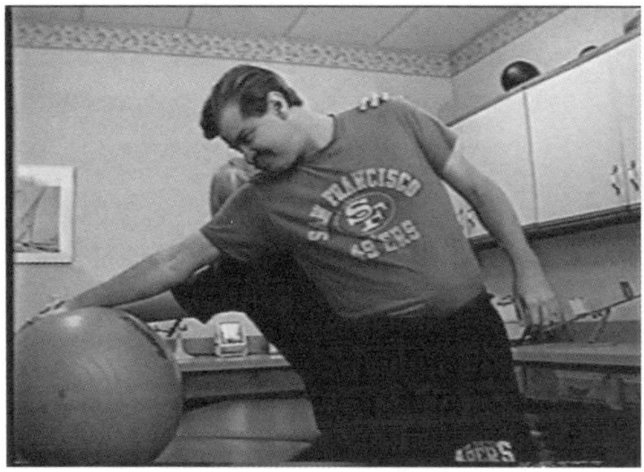

Figure 3-7. Facilitating lateral movements over the right side.

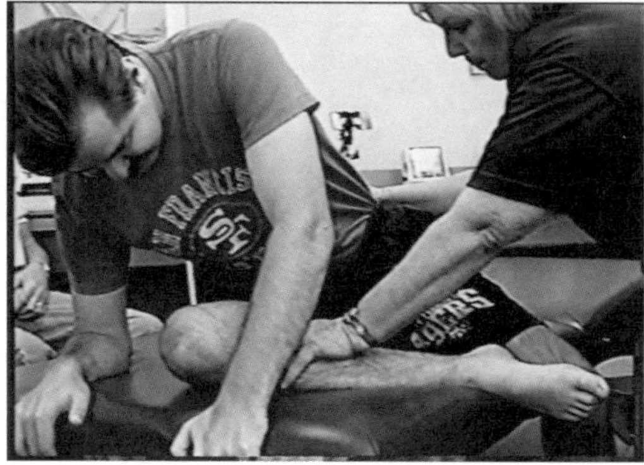

Figure 3-8. Moving the body over the right hip.

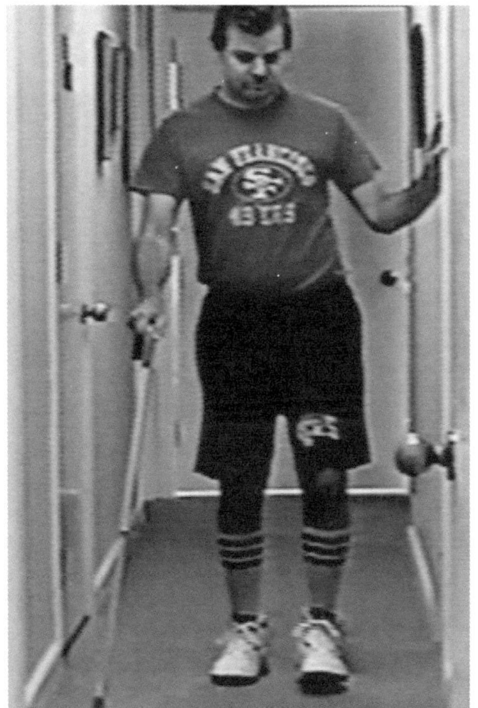

Figure 3-9. Walking after mobilization of ankle, hip, etc.

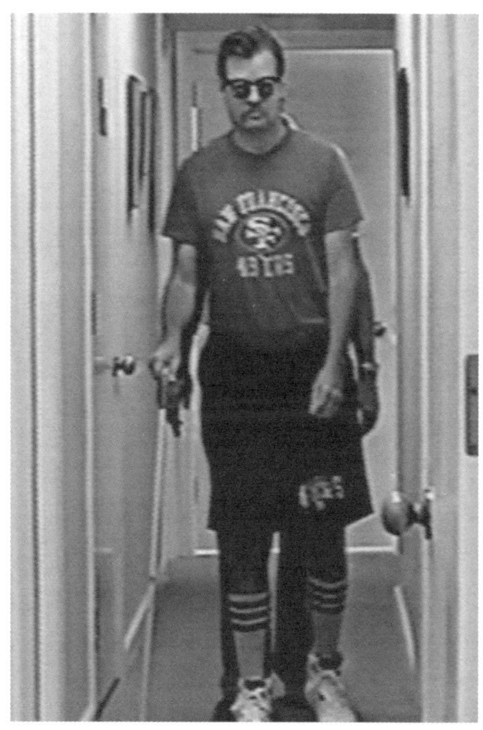

Figure 3-10. Further improvement through reintroduction of yoked prisms.

(automatic reactions and centrally generated spontaneous movements). Learned movement, when successful, is skilled integrated movement. As we develop our movement abilities we develop internal sensorimotor maps that provide for more feedforward initiation, anticipation, and instantaneous modification and correction (integration). How these maps are developed is critical to our concept of treatment. Faulty matches of incoming information result in inadequate performance due to inappropriate or inefficient learning. So learning can be positive or negative. We learn inefficiency in performance in the same way as we learn efficiency in performance.

Throughout the first months and on through the early years of development we are constantly "pruning and tuning" our nervous system.[30] The dendritic pathways most repeated (practiced) develop more automatic synaptic potential and lay down internal sensorimotor movement maps. These maps make no judgment as to quality as much as they do to repetition of use. So if a skill is developed, whether efficient or inefficient, and practiced enough, it will become a preferred process in the initiation and performance of function. It will either be a dynamic skill or a compensatory splinter skill, dependent on how and under what circumstances it was developed.

Practice as a means to gain performance skill has been researched primarily with normal adults in "motor learning" research. Success in this approach is dependent upon a normal postural and musculoskeletal foundation matched to normal visual and vestibular responses that can make organized motor adaptations to the cognitive demands for learning. "Motor learning" theories have demonstrated that practice which is self-initiated has positive effects on learning and, in fact, a self-initiated approach to learning new skills is the most effective way to learn new skills.[2] However, when we consider this research in terms of children and adults with neuromotor and neurological problems or movement disorganization, we need to understand that there is no clear a priori relationship.

Practice and self-initiated effort are important only if and when they are performed on a system prepared to respond adaptively. So there is a serious question as to what in fact is being learned, adaptive skills or compensatory skills?

In treatment we have two choices. We can treat within the range of dysfunction or we can expand the potential for more efficient adaptation. Treating within the range of dysfunction assists the individual in gaining compensatory splinter skills without dynamic adaptation. Treatment that expands the underlying foundations of skill acquisition provides a fundamental basis for the development and adaptation of skill. This type of treatment approach assists in integrating the various neural systems that learn through experience. New and organized experiences lead to adaptive responses and variations in skill acquisition that are not limited to compensations within disability parameters.

When only one system is treated, whether it be the visual system through neuro-optometric rehabilitation techniques, or the postural or vestibular systems through physical therapy and occupational therapy rehabilitation techniques, it most often leads to only partial improvement that plateaus and becomes another level of compensatory function. In some cases compensatory function may be the desired result for a more involved or damaged patient because it allows for some level of function not previously available to the individual. In other cases, and in most cases, isolated treatment of one system does not provide efficient reorganized matching of the neural processes.

Practice makes perfect if there is a normal neuropostural system. Practice leads to compensatory dysfunction if there is an inadequate neuropostural system. Both practice and a prepared musculoskeletal system are essential for success. The choice is not one or the other but the integration of both.

Visual distortion can also contribute to inefficient motor adaptation. Even if the individual's somatosensory-musculoskeletal systems are able to make adaptive responses to environmental demands, if the visual system does not orient in time and space through the ambient process and/or if there is not good interaction between focal and ambient processes, there will be a lack of organized motor control.

Because prism lenses can alter the individual's perception of space they can compensate for visual distortions. Once these distortions are modified the individual can initiate more normal alignment of the musculoskeletal system. This places the sensory receptors at their optimum vertical relationship and effectively allows initiation of more organized sensorimotor control. (See Chapter 7.)

Perhaps due to binocularity problems, an object appears blurred or double at a certain distance. The vestibular-proprioceptive systems are not able to react to perceived reality because the visual conflict cannot be resolved. Therefore the person ducks, or protects his face with his hands, or moves away from a ball being tossed to him. It is not simply an eye-hand coordination issue, but rather an ambient-focal visual relationship issue with possible visual misinterpretation or visual-somatic mismatching. Soft-wired comparator systems cannot be activated efficiently under such conflicts. Imbalanced developmental relationships between the ambient and focal processes and the sensorimotor processes create binocularity problems that further reinforce the imbalances in the ambient-focal relationship.[11]

The Importance of the Visual System

The visual system primarily drives the innate urge to move and explore the environment and be upright. However, even with this drive, if the postural system through musculoskeletal weakness or lack of development cannot respond properly, then there will be consequences not only to the development of ambient visual processes but also to the matching of visual-vestibular-cervical triad information. It follows then that the process of inefficient development between systems is a cycle. Without postural motor control to move through space, ambient visual processes are not as well developed. Without efficient matching of visual-motor information there is less initiative to move. The same cycle is true in the reverse. If there are visual distortions, lack of functional binocularity, or poor accommodation-convergence, then this will affect the level of accuracy and efficiency of motor development. The postural system may well be able to respond to the visual information received, and does so, thereby matching to the distortions or inaccuracies of the visual system. The result is less efficient motor skill development and reaching of a "plateau" where further improvement is inhibited.

The visual system, through the ambient process, is integral to balance, posture, and movement. (See Chapter 1.) Numerous studies of posturography and body sway experiments have demonstrated that vision is the most dominant system for maintaining balance when other sensory systems are either absent or distorted. Vision alone can compensate for vestibular loss.

Further, without visual organization of space, movement sensation is misleading. When subjects were blindfolded and rotated on a platform they were unable to accurately determine periods of constant acceleration or when they were being decelerated. When the vestibular system acted alone misinterpretations of movement resulted. Additionally, when the somatic and vestibular systems mismatched it caused visual misinterpretation. This is experienced when we think we are moving when we are actually not, such as in moving car or train scenarios.[23]

Anand et al.[31] concluded that refractive blur impacted postural stability, particularly if somatosensory or vestibular inputs were disrupted. This study reinforces the notion of the ability of a normal visual system to overcome differences or conflicts in other systems. It also suggests that in individuals who have postural somatosensory inefficiencies and functional vision problems, there would be posture, movement, and balance difficulties and the vestibular response would be heightened due to a lack of matching of vision and somatosensory information. This heightened response may be seen as an overreactive or hyperactive vestibular problem when, in effect, it indicates a need to normalize proprioceptive and visual input.

Vision has been downplayed as a contributor of postural control because early experiments in standing balance with eyes closed found no significant changes in postural control. However, more recent findings by Keshner[32] in virtual reality environments indicate that vision makes a far greater contribution, since studies of static balance reactions in the absence of or in substitution of inputs do not reflect the sensory processing required during dynamic movement. Thus, in natural environments visual information is constantly being received and therefore it is critical to the multi-model organization of sensory systems for postural control.

Visual flow impacts balance and posture and must be handled in respect to whether we are moving through the environment or whether an object in the environment is moving toward us, or both. Visual flow allows feedforward processing to avoid obstacles and handle uneven terrain. Visual flow is so closely related to movement that artificially generated optical flow can trigger locomotion.[33]

Both peripheral (ambient) and central (focal) vision contributes to postural control. In 6, 8, and 10 year-old children, it was found that central and peripheral vision had important regulatory impact on antero-posterior and medio-lateral oscillations. For the 6 and 10 year-olds, central and peripheral vision showed complimentary roles. In 8 year-olds, central vision provided greater postural stability in medio-lateral oscillations than peripheral vision, and after 6 years of age, peripheral vision was more efficient for regulating anterior-posterior oscillations.[34] The significance of these findings underlines the importance of the integration of central or focal vision and peripheral or ambient vision to the regulation of balance and posture. If these two processes are not integrated there will be postural imbalances.

Imbalances in the visual system and somatosensory system can cause a relative shift in the perception of space and time and the midline of the body. This is a powerful phenomenon, as the vestibular system accepts the understanding of this "midline shift." In fact, the individual will react as if there is a potential loss of balance if weight is shifted so that there is equal distribution of weight over the true anatomical "central midline." (See Chapter 7.)

Buchanan and Horak[35] concluded in experiments during sinusoidal support surface translations, that visual information stabilized posture by reducing the variability of the head's position in space and the position of the center of mass within the support surface defined by the feet, for all but the slowest translation frequencies. They suggested that visual information was important for maintaining a fixed position of the head and trunk in space, whereas proprioceptive information was sufficient to produce stable coordinative patterns between the support surface and legs. The visual system then is a critical component for organizing head/neck/trunk orientation necessary for maintaining alignment and matching of visual-vestibular-somatic information.

What can be easily misinterpreted as a motor impairment in the case of a patient who does not take weight well on the "involved side" or as a vestibular issue where a patient is fearful of movement and cannot maintain balance, may in fact be the result of visual distortions of space resulting in compensatory responses, or avoidance of certain responses.

In this example, again documented in Dr. Padula's office, we can appreciate the remarkable changes as a result of the use of prism lenses. This young man suffered a head, neck, and shoulder injury and as a result he experiences severe visual distortion and visual midline shift (figure 3-11). The remarkable change in balance with the use of prism lenses to reorganize his visual world can be seen in figure 3-12.

In this case there were no structural misalignment factors or joint or soft tissue restrictions, so the effect of the prism lenses immediately had a dramatic impact, because a more organized visual system was able to initiate appropriate motor adaptations. Again the importance of differential diagnosis is critical. Had this individual been considered to have a vestibular problem, without a thorough neuro-optometric exam, then vestibular therapy would probably have been initiated. In this case it would not have been effective and perhaps would even have exacerbated the visual-vestibular-somatosensory mismatch. It is clear that this individual had no vestibular issues, but was struggling to respond motorically to distortions of visual space.

The Importance of the Vestibular System

The vestibular system plays an important role in balance and postural control. The vestibular system, like the visual system and the somatosensory system, is a proprioceptive system. Integrating these three forms of proprioception is essential for efficient movement and posture.

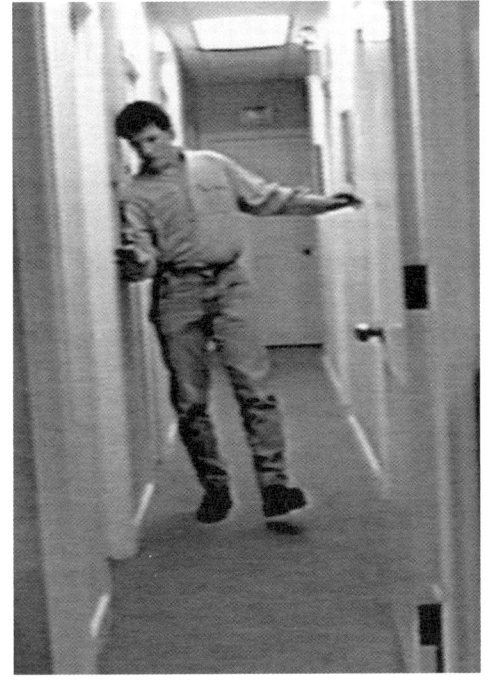

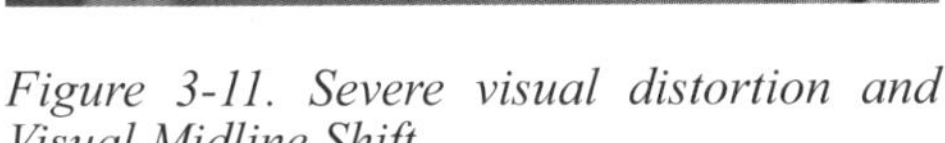

Figure 3-11. Severe visual distortion and Visual Midline Shift.

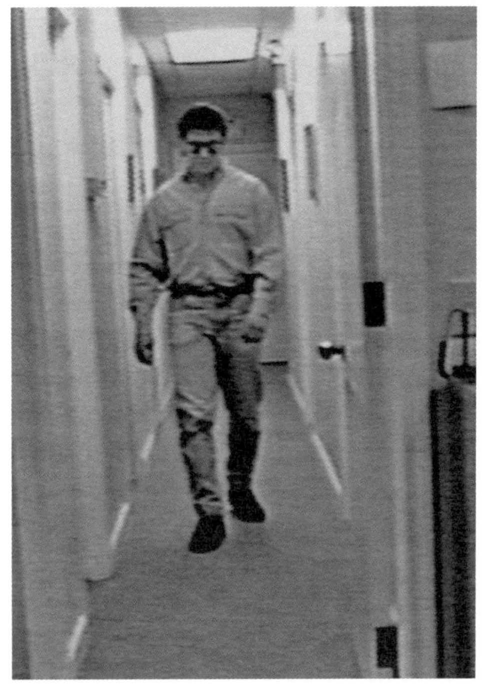

Figure 3-12. Change in balance with prism lenses.

Functionally the vestibular system consists of parallel structures, the semi-circular canals and the utricle and saccule. The three semicircular canals register rotational acceleration. Structurally each canal is located in a different plane such that rotational forces can be measured and integrated in all planes of movement. Within the semicircular canals is a receptor organ that reacts to rotational forces.

Within the utricle and saccule are the otoliths, which respond to the force of gravity and linear acceleration. The otolithic organ in the saccule functions to keep vertical orientation to gravity. It measures linear accelerations of up and down and back and forth. The otolithic organ in the utricle responds to lateral or horizontal forces and registers linear accelerations side to side.

These five individual motion sensors work dynamically in all planes of movement to maintain balance and equilibrium, monitor motion of the head and neck, and stabilize the eyes relative to the environment. Normal movement involves all aspects of these five motion sensors. We rotate as we bend diagonally forward or back. We accelerate forward and turn our head laterally. We stop, start, turn, and constantly tilt and sway laterally, forward, and back. Every movement we make combines some aspects of the five vestibular proprioceptive sensors. In order for this information to be relevant and efficiently used it must be matched with what is happening with the eyes, visual perception of space, the neck, and the body proprioceptors, both upper and lower body. So movement is an extremely complicated process and a harmonious dance between our proprioceptive senses. Each proprioceptive system is dependent on the other. Imbalances in any system will cause compensation by the others. In some cases compensatory responses maintain efficiency, particularly through the visual and somatosensory systems. However, many times compensations are inefficient and practice of inefficiency strengths the imbalances.

Understanding these interrelationships is important to observational assessment and treatment strategies. They must be appreciated in total. Much of our testing attempts to isolate specific aspects of our sensory systems, For example the vestibular-ocular-reflex (VOR) has historically received a large amount of interest as a way to determine vestibular dysfunction. And to some extent there has been an assumption of the dominant influence of the vestibular system to ocular control. Interestingly, the VOR is reflexive, while the visual system is responsive. The VOR is important for maintaining a fixed gaze on an object. This is critical when chasing an object like a baseball, or running after an animal or a person. Fixed gaze is important to maintain contact with an object of interest. Regardless of the bouncing of the head or effects of terrain on the movement, the eyes maintain stabilization. However, we do not always, nor constantly, move with a fixed gaze. We constantly shift our gaze, perhaps periodically returning to an object of interest but certainly we do not function through life with eyes fixed. Therefore the VOR is only helpful in certain situations. The VOR must be released or inhibited so that we can shift our gaze, scan our world, and attend to other stimuli within a task-oriented context.[35] So the visual system, through various pathways, can initiate feedforward processes that regulate the vestibular system's reflexive reactions, while at the same time these reflexive reactions can be instantaneously invoked when needed to maintain gaze, then regulated to release. In fact there are eight reflexes that are feedforward and feedback mechanisms between the eyes, vestibular system, and neck.[1] All of these influence the interaction and integration of sensorimotor processes and are task dependent. This dynamic interplay of volitional proactive movement intention, superimposed on underlying reflexive reactive responses, provides movement and postural control, intention, maintenance, recovery, adaptability and functional skill acquisition.[37]

Rotational movement around the body axis involves the horizontal semicircular canals. There are no standard tests that can totally isolate the superior or anterior canals, so rotational tests measure only one function in the absence of actual body movement through space or in consideration of visual and somatosensory influences. Thus when we test for vestibular function using rotation we are attempting to evaluate the horizontal semicircular canals.

Otolithic organs are important to the organization of body sway and therefore weight shifts, which are a part of all movement. When we move laterally, the otoliths in the utricle provide inertial mass through the movement of otolithic-gel. This provides for a reactive righting response to maintain verticality. The otolithic organs in the saccule respond to gravitational forces in body sway forward and back and up and down. So when we are tilted forward or back, for example, we respond with head righting to maintain vertical. The two otolithic receptors of the utricle and saccule give us all three planes of movement to which we can react.

Again these responses are reflexive but can be volitionally inhibited or dampened in context-dependent tasks. For instance we use forward flexion to get up from a chair, to pick up an object from the floor, to get up from a lying position, etc. In actuality, many if not most movements we make comprise an initial component of forward flexion. We don't stand up by thrusting backwards, for instance. Therefore in proactive volitional movements we must dampen the utricular otolithic response. Similar to dampening the VOR, it is context-dependent. When we intend to get up from a chair, we set up efferent copies throughout the CNS and anticipatory muscle activation of the trunk, neck and lower limbs precedes the movement. The head goes forward and that "controlled" proactive inertial force is used to increase musculoskeletal reactions to take weight over the feet to stand, and then return the head to vertical. This is completely different from having your chair unexpectedly tilted forward. Again there are proactive response initiated behaviors superimposed over reactive, reflexive support. In all movement there is interplay between these factors depending on the level of difficulty of the task.

The otoliths, like the semicircular canals, do not initiate movement but react to it. Volitional proactive movement is initiated through the visual system or through cognitive desire, and sets up potentials for activation of the somatosensory and vestibular systems.

To be organized in movement through space requires a complex mix of perceived space, predicting the expected visual environment, detecting image movement and/or movement of the body toward an image, and comparison as to self-motion and environmental motion. Jaekl et al.,[38] in a series of experiments with self-regulated motion in a virtual reality environment, determined that the vestibular contribution to the estimation of self-motion was subordinate to proprioceptive and efferent copy information. He suggested that the perception of gravity plays only a small role in determining perceptual stability during active head movement.

The possibility of "cervical vertigo" has previously been discussed, whereby the neck does not allow proper alignment of the otolithic organs in the utricle. Similarly "height vertigo" has been reported that is based not on utricular or vestibular disorder, but on visual destabilization.[39] Visual destabilization of free stance occurs when the distance between eye and object becomes too great. This is an interesting research finding particularly when we consider the responses of children on suspended equipment or large therapy balls. Consider the possibility of a child with low postural tone and poor neck co-contraction who cannot efficiently maintain a firm fixed head position. If the object of visual intent is too far away, there may be a "height vertigo" possibility. If, due to functional vision problems, objects appear blurred or perhaps are even perceived as double, depending on convergence inefficiency, the result would be fear and inability to maintain balance. The question to be asked while observing such phenomena is, whether we are seeing postural-visual inefficiencies causing an overreactive vestibular response due to mismatching of systems, or whether there is some primary vestibular deficiency. Is this a gravitational insecurity as described in sensory integration theory due to poor otolithic modulation, or is it proprioceptive-visual mismatching that causes the otoliths to have no accurate system with which to match?

Clinicians should always to be careful about causal assumptions, and should maintain objectivity and consider associations of various system interactions in order to better understand behavioral phenomena. When we place children or adults in high demand balance activities we are initiating reflexive reactions, reactive components of balance with visual surround demands. When there is any distortion, developmental immaturity, or deficiency in functional vision or somatosensory input, there will be a poor and inefficient outcome in maintaining balance, because the vestibular system is reactive and needs cooperation from at least one other system. Conversely, creating demands that require intentional responses completely changes the way the visual-vestibular-cervical/somatic systems interact.

The vestibular system is inhibited by self-generated head/neck movements[40] and this mechanism is directly tied to the internal prediction of sensory consequences and actual resultant feedback. This inhibition of vestibular responses during self-generated movement is important for the computation of spatial orientation. It is true that the vestibular system is sensitive to passive head/neck movements; however, these same neurons are not reliable encoders for head velocity during self-generated movements of the head and body. Clearly there are dynamic and parallel functions of our sensory systems, initiated as either reflexive when stimuli impact unexpectedly or at least with an unexpected outcome, and when there is intention or self-generation. This incredible interchange makes organized movement and posture possible. **Proactive intentional movement sets up conditions for dampening reflex patterns of our sensorimotor systems, allowing for adaptability. At the same time, the interaction of underlying reflexes with recovery and reactive components of movement provides the framework for volitional acts to maintain efficiency.**

Tests that measure control of posture have generally failed to provide useful information about vestibular function because postural control does not depend heavily on vestibular function, when vision and proprioceptive cues are available.[41] Vision and somatosensory proprioception can efficiently compensate for vestibular loss.

Reweighting and Dual Influences of Neural Systems

As previously discussed, reweighting of neural systems is important to efficient sensorimotor organization. Reweighting of neural systems during and throughout an activity may be more fully understood through a discussion of the dual nature of sensory systems. The visual system has two distinct processes, ambient and focal. The somatosensory system responds both to deep pressure and light touch. The vestibular system responds to linear as well as rotary stimulation, and can be reactive or supportive during movement. The relative influence of these systems and their respective dualities in a context-specific task will determine the intra-organization and matching of these systems. Primary influences of one system will affect how other systems relate, match, and react.

For example, if the ambient visual process is not efficient, there may be over-focalization and a lack of spontaneous awareness of spatial-temporal orientation. Feedforward processes may be compromised and the somatosensory and vestibular systems may function more reactively to outside influences without anticipation. This will make for clumsy, uncoordinated sensorimotor planning. The neural systems will match reactively and there will be limited reweighting of the neural systems within the task. Reactive functions of neural systems have limited adaptability. Proactive aspects of neural systems, i.e., anticipation, spatial-temporal awareness, and feedforward processes have maximal adaptability. That is why the vestibular system can react reflexively to maintain gaze on an object but then release supportively to allow a change in the direction of gaze. During any activity, the reactive functions of the neural systems and the proactive functions constantly interchange and reweight to deal with the demands of adaptability required for efficiency. Therefore, it becomes the purpose of intervention to facilitate dynamic matching of neural systems, rather than trying to stimulate or treat a neural system or a symptom in isolation.

Changing the perception of space changes the potentiality of neural systems matching. Changing the alignment or postural distribution of tone and weight changes the potentiality of neural systems matching. Incorporating vestibular responses as supportive within a context-specific task, rather than using stimulation of the vestibular system to initiate postural reactions, changes the potentiality of neural systems matching.

Hierarchical lower level automatic reactions (sometimes referred to as primitive postural reflexes; tonic reflexes, etc.) mature before higher adaptive sensorimotor processes.[42] At birth these reactions are stimulus driven and the infant reacts to the forces of gravity, vision, and somatosensory input. Adaptive responses can be influenced either by a lack of, or weakness of, primitive reflexes (low tone infants) or by hyperreactive tonic reflexes (high tone). Adaptive responses are learned through experience and intentional movement, incorporating feedforward mechanisms. This graded interplay between reactive and proactive sensorimotor mechanisms is critical to developing efficient and adaptable sensorimotor organization.

The potentiality of neural systems matching is dependent on the development of the adaptability of the sensorimotor system. Neural systems reweighting during context-dependent activity is, in turn, dependent on an adaptable sensorimotor system.

Difficulties in sensorimotor adaptation can cause inflexibility in sensory weighting.[2] For reasons previously discussed, there can be an over-reliance on a particular sensory system due to inefficiency in sensorimotor development and organization. Shumway-Cook[2] refers to these conditions as *dependence patterns*. There can be visual-dependence patterns, surface-dependence patterns, or non-dependence sensory selection problems.

Over-reliance on vision for postural control implies a lack of support from other proprioceptive processes such as somatosensory and vestibular proprioception. In other words, when vision is reduced or inaccurate, subjects experienced abnormal sway under experimental conditions. A strong reliance on vision is developmentally normal, as vision leads and initiates the development of postural control. However, at around seven years of age, this dominance reduces as the somatosensory system matures. Therefore at that age, as long as somatosensory information is accurate, there is no abnormal loss of balance or postural control when vision is reduced or inaccurate. This is an important process in sensory adaptation. It allows for the visual system to release background postural control, and at the same time, to become more anticipatory for activating postural reactions. It provides the sensory adaptation for shifting gaze and regaining gaze during movement, through the release and reactivation of the VOR. If over-reliance of the visual system persists past this point developmentally, it interferes with dynamic postural adaptation and becomes a visual-dependence pattern. Visual over-reliance will interfere with anticipation and therefore motor planning. The visual system will function more as a feedback system as opposed to a feedforward system, thereby, inhibiting dynamic sensorimotor anticipation necessary for efficient learning and performance.

This same condition is often observed in children and adults with neurological disorders. Individuals with closed head or brain injuries become subject to their visual distortions, and the somatosensory system is unable to make proper dynamic postural adjustments because the visual system signals a spatial orientation that is incorrect. Without intervening visually, through neuro-optometric rehabilitation and prism lenses, there can be no rebalancing for efficient sensory matching between visual, vestibular, and somatosensory systems. Reweighting will not take place, and balance and functional performance will deteriorate.

An over-reliance on somatosensory information leads to a *surface-dependence pattern*. This condition relates to an inability to adjust to changes in surface inputs. When the surface is more challenging, such as on sand, an incline, thick carpet etc., the individual is not able to adequately use ankle or leg proprioception to maintain dynamic postural verticality. This causes balance difficulties which activate reactive processes and inhibit feedforward anticipatory efficiency. This type of dependence is often related not only to sensory issues, but more likely to biomechanical and structural issues as has been previously discussed. Regardless of appropriate vestibular or visual function, sensorimotor performance will be limited due a lack of an adaptive and efficient somatosensory system. Intervention that does not address the fundamental underlying biomechanical structure and alignment of the body will not be effective in improving functional performance, regardless of the amount of vestibular stimulation or visual therapy that is performed. Reweighting of sensory systems, that must be dynamic and interchangeable throughout a functional performance, will not take place if the somatosensory system is limited in its ability to dynamically respond to the base of support.

When inaccurate information from one or more senses is experienced, individuals with *sensory selection* problems are unable to select a sense with accurate information to overcome the faulty sensory information. These individuals are best at maintaining balance and postural control when all sensory information is consistent and accurate. When there is conflict between sensory systems they are unable to maintain efficient postural control. The inability to make sensory selection under varying conditions inhibits the possibility for reweighting of sensory influences required for efficient sensorimotor function. Under this condition, sensorimotor function is primarily reactive. Since there is a lack of dynamic reweighting and sensory selection, feedforward anticipatory proactive sensorimotor function suffers. This condition is observed in patients with CVA, TBI, and developmental disorders. It would seem logical that a primary focus in therapy would be to establish one primary sensory system that can be relied upon for matching with other systems. The primary system most powerful for orientation in space is vision. Establishing good visual orientation can help provide the ability to organize the other systems around the accurate information of the visual system.

Summary

How the neural systems match within a functional context will determine the efficiency or inefficiency of learning. If they are matching reactively, then there is a constant feedback process of dealing with outside influences. It is less adaptive and more reactive, within a feedback dominated context. When they are matching proactively, there is a feedforward initiation of the adaptability of neural systems that is supported by the underlying reactive processes of the neural systems. The variations in the reactive and proactive nature of neural systems will assist in determining which sensory system may be "locked in" to a compensatory process that inefficiently matches with other systems, causing further inefficiencies. Changing the adaptability of that system leads to "unlocking" of the compensations of the other neural systems. Thus, a more dynamic matching can be gained through reorganizing how these neural systems relate, release, and reweight.

Sensorimotor control and sensorimotor learning are dependent on appropriate sensory system matching between visual-vestibular-cervical and somatic proprioception. Sensory system responses are both reflexive (reactive to outside forces) and proactive (self-initiated behaviors). These two unique but intricately intertwined processes must be supportive, integrative, and able to shift and reweight depending on the nature, demand, challenge or threat of an activity. To intervene effectively it is important to understand this dynamic interplay.

Preparation activities to establish musculoskeletal integrity may be necessary. Stimulation activities to arouse or activate systems may be necessary. Facilitating controlled equilibrium and righting reactions may be necessary. All these preparatory procedures, however, should be incorporated into meaningful transitions that allow the sensory systems to match effectively for efficient function. Physical handling that gradually allows spontaneous control by the child would appear superior in strategy than simply child-directed, stimulatory, compensatory practice, or other forms of intervention that do not specifically guide dynamic sensorimotor organization, and can often result in practicing and strengthening dysfunctional processes.

Neuro-optometric rehabilitation offers the essential possibility of establishing and rebalancing the focal and ambient visual systems. This alone will provide for better adaptation of motor control and to the extent there are no other somatosensory or musculoskeletal problems, this approach is very effective in reorganizing the world for a patient who has suffered trauma that resulted in visual distortions. To be most effective however, other treatment strategies must also be employed that deal with joint alignment issues, muscle paralysis or weakness, inaccurate initiation of coactivation of muscle synergies, soft tissue restrictions, postural stability and mobility factors, alignment and stabilization of the neck, etc. Neuro-optometric rehabilitation offers a powerful tool to deal with visual dysfunction. Physical handling and other specific physical techniques are essential to allow maximum adaptation and the ability to learn more efficient functional skills during the rehabilitation process.

Chapter 4

NEURO-OPTOMETRIC REHABILITATION EXAMINATION

William V. Padula

The neuro-optometric rehabilitation examination for a child or adult who has suffered a neurological event requires a thorough knowledge of vision including: ophthalmic health, medical health, neuroanatomy, and the science of optics and visual processing. It also requires considerable skill in and understanding of the examination techniques used to evaluate visual processing including the electro-diagnostic evaluation. These areas represent the scientific basis of optometry and the ability to adapt this science to clinically applicable assessment and treatment regimens. However, of equal importance is the need for compassion, patience and an ability to listen: to be patient-centered. Without these three components the neuro-optometric rehabilitation examination will lack the depth necessary to develop a truly effective vision rehabilitation model of treatment. This chapter will explore the necessary parameters of the examination. While the listing of techniques and procedures will be comprehensive, it is not meant to be complete since the examiner may require additional modes of testing and creativity to meet the individual needs of each patient.

History

Ideally, a comprehensive history form should be sent to the patient to be completed prior to the evaluation. However, at the time of the appointment, review of this information should always be preceded by a behavioral observation of the patient walking to and/or traveling via wheelchair to the examination room. This will provide the examiner with important information regarding balance, posture and movement in association with visual function. In many cases following a neurological event, patients will not have an adequate memory of other health issues, rehabilitative programs, or even an accurate assessment of their own needs. It is therefore important to request a full medical history for each patient who will be examined. This should also include a complete list of medications. As is sometimes the case with ophthalmic medications, other systemic medications may have been prescribed and placed on the list, but are not being taken according to the dosage schedule. It should be verified with the patient that all medications are being taken as prescribed.

The history of the time frame of the injury or neurological event should be reviewed and developed. When examining a child, a complete developmental history is also necessary, and should emphasize appropriate milestones and the effect that the neurological event has had on interrupting these milestones. The history should also include an account of any rehabilitation programs in which the patient has participated since the neurological event. These may include physical, occupational, speech/language, psychological and cognitive rehabilitative therapies. In addition, complimentary therapy approaches should also be determined including chiropractic, biofeedback, nutritional and other healing arts.

Background information concerning vision, both prior to the neurological event as well as following the event, is also important. Surgery affecting binocularity, injection therapies to reduce muscle tone, and a general ocular health history should be obtained. This should also include a time frame of previous prescriptions for glasses in order to attempt to determine if there were abrupt changes in the refractive state which may relate to such conditions as Post Trauma Vision Syndrome. A thorough discussion concerning visual problems should be developed with the patient, family members, and/or rehabilitation professionals. The visual problems may relate to issues of eye health, ability to see at distance, near visual function, eye-hand coordination, light sensitivity, symptoms of eye strain, headaches, and diplopia (double vision), as well as the tendency to turn or tilt the head which might provide a clue to binocular vision problems.

Questions related to balance, posture and movement should also be asked, and might suggest the need for specific examination procedures in order to understand components of a possible Visual Midline Shift Syndrome. In addition, the history should assess the use of peripheral vision and/or peripheral visual field loss, particularly when there has been a cerebrovascular accident or traumatic brain injury. This may yield information pertaining to types of hemianopsia or scotoma. The examiner should also take the opportunity during the history to ask some specific questions such as:

- Do you have difficulty in crowded or busy environments such as a supermarket during a busy period?
- Do you ever have panic attacks?
- Have you ever experienced claustrophobia?
- Do you ever have hallucinations?

Positive information received from these questions is frequently a red flag signaling the possibility of Post Trauma Vision Syndrome.

Ocular Health Assessment

It is imperative that a thorough ocular health assessment be performed as part of the neuro-optometric rehabilitation assessment. This should include a dilated fundus evaluation, and an anterior and media evaluation of the eyes. Biomicroscopy may be difficult to perform for physically disabled persons (especially children) due to the challenges of positioning the patient in the instrument and/or their fear of this or other instruments. Alternative means of assessment should be conducted by the examiner in order to be as thorough as possible.

Examination Procedures

An assessment of visual acuity is important and standard approaches using the Snellen chart and/or low vision acuity charts should be utilized, with the working distance adapted according to the abilities of the patient. In addition to the acuity test results, observations regarding the patient's responses and behavior during testing should be charted. Acuity should be measured first binocularly and then monocularly. Immediately following the standard assessment of distance acuity, the binocular acuity test should be repeated with binasal occlusion. If the patient is experiencing Post Trauma Vision Syndrome he frequently will not only report that the print on the chart becomes more clear and/or stops moving, but will also state that he "feels more comfortable."

Near visual acuity assessment should be carried out with either the standard Snellen near acuity chart and/or low vision acuity charts such as the Lighthouse near vision chart. Binocular testing and then monocular testing should be performed. Binasal occlusion should again be added and binocular testing repeated. Results and patient comments during unoccluded and occluded test procedures should be charted as was done during distance testing. A standard working distance of 40 centimeters is recommended. However, again the test should be adapted to the abilities of the patient, and his behavior. The distance the patient prefers when looking at the chart should be observed. This may be accomplished by simply handing the patient the chart and noting where he holds it. Best habitual distance and near correction should be worn during this phase of the assessment.

Sensorimotor Analysis

The sensorimotor examination should include binocular as well as monocular fixation pursuit tracking skills. Observations should be made as to any limitations of ocular motility or malalignment of the eyes, as well as the manner in which the person establishes pursuit tracking. A jerky quality to eye movements, and/or fixation losses, does not necessarily indicate weak extra ocular muscles but may signify high focal processing as is seen in the case of individuals with Post Trauma Vision Syndrome. The fixation losses or jerky quality to eye movements will often occur with individuals who cannot utilize the ambient process to anticipate spatial change of the targets. Testing should first be carried out binocularly and then monocularly. The convergence near point should be assessed by having the individual follow a target moved toward his face with both break and recovery points measured. A cover test should be utilized to assess states of binocular function indicating heterophoria and/or heterotropia. When appropriate, stereopsis testing should be performed to evaluate the ability to maintain binocularity at a near range. In addition, binocular tests such as the red lens test, the Maddox rod test, and other means to evaluate imbalances in the state of binocularity should be utilized by the clinician.

NOTE: Frequently when evaluating individuals who have had a neurological event, test results may provide information that is not always consistent. Therefore, test repetition and averaging of results should be conducted in order to give the clinician a better understanding of the state of the visual process. Behaviorally, it must be noted that inconsistency is often the result of over focalizing (or lack thereof), with limited balance of ambient visual function. In addition, different tests may produce different findings in states of binocularity. For example, a cover test performed in free space may result in a state of phoria that is different from that which is measured when the individual is placed behind the phoropter while using Risley prisms. The difference represents different forms of evaluation. The cover test yields more spatial information and active ambient visual processing, whereas the ambient visual system is interfered with when the phoropter is used.

Refractive Sequence

The refractive sequence should incorporate thorough and accurate retinoscopy of each eye as well as subjective refraction which should include binocular balancing of the visual process in an attempt to equalize prescriptions for each eye. Neurological events will often cause refractive imbalance. If the clinician is not careful and prescribes unequal refractive prescriptions, this will influence not only the refraction but may very well affect recovery from Post Trauma Vision Syndrome. In addition, it can reinforce abnormal states of visual midline, thereby interfering with rehabilitation for posture, balance and ambulation.

Next, the full 21-point optometric evaluation should be performed when possible. This is indicated for those individuals who can utilize a phoropter. This will include phoria testing at distance and near, as well as assessment of lateral and vertical muscle balance. In addition, distance and near duction testing should be performed to analyze visual balance in relationship to functioning on near-far (Z-axis) planes.

The refraction and refractive sequence should be performed by the examiner with sensitivity to the patient's behavior. Throughout the examination, and particularly during the refractive sequence, the examiner should pay attention to any statements of discomfort expressed by the patient. Often patients will discuss their intolerance to lights such as from the retinoscope or ophthalmoscope. Patients may also describe sensitivity to the background illumination from projected acuity charts. Observe the patient for discomfort about the neck and shoulders. Frequently, patients who are having difficulties with binocular vision will also experience discomfort in the neck and during the examination will often reach up and touch or massage their own neck muscles.

The examiner should also pay close attention to the responses of the individual. By using directions for each test that are consistent from patient to patient, the examiner may find differences in individuals who are suffering from Post Trauma Vision Syndrome and the way in which they perform the tests. Symptoms such as not being able to follow verbal directions, asking the examiner to repeat directions, having difficulty discerning relationships during the tests and requiring the examiner to repeat the tests, may give clues concerning the nature of the visual processing difficulties. The refractive sequence can often cause persons with Post Trauma Vision Syndrome (see Chapter 5) to lose the ability to organize spatial information through the ambient process. This causes the person to work harder and harder in an attempt to focalize on the individual letters or numbers presented on the acuity chart. This, in turn, may cause significant variations in phoria measurements and duction measurements.

Posture is also critical in relationship to the evaluation. Phoropter use may not be appropriate with persons who are physically challenged. A trial frame and trial lenses may be necessary in order to perform the refractive portion of the examination. When working with children with physical disabilities, the examination may need to be performed in a manner that is more physically comfortable and appropriate for the child (see Chapter 10). The examiner should pay close attention to head tilts and turns as well as body position, since these may be associated with visual field loss, oculomotor difficulties including strabismus and visual midline shift (see Chapter 7), as well as variations in muscle tone produced during increased visual demand activities. The examiner should particularly note positions of the head and neck, such as capital extension (head projected forward and rotated upward) as well as capital flexion (head rolled down with chin to the chest). These positions of the head and neck may be related to strabismus, oculomotor and binocular difficulties, as well as to Visual Midline Shift Syndrome.

The refraction should analyze asymmetry in power between the two eyes. The examiner is cautioned that simply measuring the power of each eye does not yield a final prescription, even if each eye is corrected to its best visual acuity. Asymmetry (anisometropia) found on refraction is often the result of dysfunction of the ambient visual process in relationship to neuromotor processing. Upon monocular analysis of the refraction, the examiner should attempt to develop a binocular balance between the two eyes refractively. This means one must either utilize Polaroid filters or work with binocular balancing of the prescription. The effects of a more balanced prescription can often induce balance between the ambient process and neuromotor function.

Individuals who suffer from Post Trauma Vision Syndrome frequently will have an increase in myopia. It has been the author's experience that individuals who may have been stable with their prescription may demonstrate a myopic shift even at 50 or 60 years of age. For individuals who are hyperopic, there may be a considerable variation in the prescription and/or a decrease in hyperopia. For individuals who are myopic, the examiner is cautioned about prescribing the full extent of the refractive state measured during the examination when an increase has been determined. By increasing a minus (concave) lens power for individuals who have Post Trauma Vision Syndrome, the greater compression of peripheral space this can cause may result in an increase in the individual's PTVS symptoms.

When individuals have characteristics of Post Trauma Vision Syndrome (see Chapter 5), the examiner should follow the refractive sequence by introducing low amounts of base-in prism (ranging from ½ prism diopter to 2 prism diopters) before both eyes. The patient may respond that the print on the acuity chart appears to stabilize if it was moving, or that the print appears larger and the patient is more comfortable in looking at it. Binasal occlusion may again be used to probe the ambient visual system in relationship to focal processing.

Accommodative tests should include amplitude testing as well as dynamic testing, such as Bell retinoscopy, MEM retinoscopy, and book retinoscopy. Bell retinoscopy is performed with the examiner facing the patient and holding a wand with a small (½") diameter steel ball at the end of the wand. With the retinoscope before the examiner's eyes, the examiner moves the wand toward the patient while the patient fixates on the silver ball target. The point at which the motion changes from "with" to "against" is recorded as the *"grasp"* of the accommodative response in inches or centimeters from the patient's face to the position of the target. The examiner then continues moving the ball toward the patient's face and back out again until the "against" motion changes back to "with." This is recorded as the *"release"* in inches or centimeters. Probing with plus lenses is then carried out to determine if the range increases or decreases.

Book retinoscopy is performed with the examiner holding the retinoscope to his eye, positioned behind the plane of a book that the patient is reading. A determination is made as to whether there is "with" or "against" motion. "With" motion indicates a tendency to focus *beyond* the plane of fixation, whereas "against" motion indicates a tendency to focus *within* the plane of fixation. Plus lenses are then used to probe the visual process in an attempt to bring about a "neutral" or slight "against" motion while reading. Prisms and binasal occlusion should also be used at this time in the examination.

Neuromotor Assessment

Visual midline assessment should be made by having the person follow a wand and respond when it appears to be directly in front of the person's nose, as well as at eye level (see Chapter 7). Consistent responses as well as variable responses should be noted. A stable response may indicate more consistency in the shift of visual midline affecting posture and balance. However, instability in the visual midline will offer information about spatial disorientation and projection of visual midline in its relationship to fixation changes. The latter might be behaviorally observed by finding an individual who seems to lose balance in the direction of a fixation change while walking. For example, if the person looks to the right he will tend to lean or drift to the right, while looking to the left might cause him to lean or drift to the left. The visual midline testing should be performed in a seated position and then, if possible, in a standing position. It has been found that the standing position may be more accurate in predicting effects on ambulation. However, in both cases repeated testing should be done in order to average information.

Visual Evoked Potential Testing

Persons who demonstrate the characteristics of Post Trauma Vision Syndrome should be scheduled for a visual evoked potential examination. Visual evoked potential testing can provide the examiner with important diagnostic information regarding the functional integrity of the visual system. The cross-pattern reversal analysis is recommended and standard monocular testing procedures[1] should be performed to rule out afferent sensory nerve dysfunction. This testing should be followed by binocular testing, first with best correction and then with low amounts of base-in prism in conjunction with binasal occlusion. This modification can provide very useful information regarding dysfunction of the focal/ambient aspects of the visual process.[2]

An analysis of the VEP should include more than just latencies. Amplitude differences are also critical in determining if an individual may have Post Trauma Vision Syndrome. An increase in amplitude under binocular conditions after base-in prism and binasal occlusion have been positioned before the person's eyes is considered a positive test for Post Trauma Vision Syndrome (see Chapter 5). The examiner should be cautioned, however, to watch for the changes in N1 (N75) the negative wave potential preceding the P1 (P100) positive wave potential. Sometimes, individuals with Post Trauma Vision Syndrome may show a decrease in the amplitude of the P1 potential because the N1 potential decreases. This decrease in negative wave potential following base-in prism and binasal occlusion is also considered to be a positive sign for Post Trauma Vision Syndrome. It indicates that by utilizing prism and binasal occlusion there is increased ambient visual processing, thereby affecting states of binocularity and thus spatial organization.[2]

If the examiner is not equipped to assess visual evoked potentials, the patient should be referred elsewhere for this testing. However, the examiner must request that the visual evoked potential testing be performed binocularly: first without base-in prism and binasal occlusion, and then with both. It is often challenging for the examiner to request this information from technicians and/or doctors who are not familiar with these procedures. It is therefore recommended that the examiner accompany the patient for the visual evoked potential exam if possible.

The VEP results can provide the examiner with an unparalleled demonstration of the existence of changes in the visual process. Together with a detailed refractive sequence, sensorimotor analysis, and neuromotor assessment, the VEP can help the examiner understand visual dysfunction and its relationship to the patient's symptoms beyond that which can be determined by standard optometric/ophthalmological examinations alone.

Other Tests

Additional tests, such as central threshold visual field, arc perimetry, eccentric fixation analysis, and other binocular tests, should be performed during the neuro-optometric rehabilitation analysis as considered necessary by the examiner. Color vision testing is also an important test for determining dysfunction in the processing of color. Frequently, individuals with Post Trauma Vision Syndrome will show a diminution of color vision function. After treatment for Post Trauma Vision Syndrome, the color vision response will frequently improve.

Chapter 5

POST TRAUMA VISION SYNDROME CAUSED BY HEAD INJURY

William V. Padula

Traumatic Brain Injury

Traumatic brain injury (TBI) is devastating to an individual and to the family. Family members and loved ones have great difficulty dealing with the suddenness of an injury which can result in a deep coma or multiple problems with motor function, speech, and cognition. Many survivors of traumatic brain injury will have an understanding or recollection of normalcy but will experience bewilderment in their present situation. Psychologically, this state can cause severe depression, anger, frustration and a feeling of helplessness.

In traumatic brain injury cases immediate attention is to the emergency medical needs of the victim. The medical team involved in primary treatment will cope with the survival needs of the patient. At the hospital new teams of physicians and paramedical professionals will continue to address the emergency of the physical trauma. If the individual is in a coma, special medical treatment programs will be initiated.

Decisions will be made quickly by medical teams. Their treatment directions may often require decision making by family and loved ones regarding surgical and/or medical interventions. The immediate family often struggles to understand medical terms and treatment regimens so that appropriate decisions can be made.

Once an individual recovers from a coma or other medical conditions, the hard realities of physical limitations and cognitive function must be addressed. While medical treatment programs and surgical intervention may still need to be carried out and decisions made to enable continued recovery from the trauma, now the family and medical teams must also deal with the rehabilitation. During this period, family members must cope with the realization that life styles will change and that treatment programs for rehabilitation will continue for long periods of time, if not indefinitely. Many will experience denial, depression, and psychological states that will also need treatment from the appropriate professionals.

As an individual recovers from a coma, testing is done to determine levels of function. The testing may involve neuropsychiatric test batteries, medical tests, imaging studies, and electro-physiological tests to determine states of brain function and central nervous system involvement. From these tests physicians, physical therapists, occupational therapists and other professionals will determine appropriate modes of rehabilitation. The team might also include psychologists, cognitive rehabilitation specialists, speech-language pathologists, and neurologists, all of whom will decide on particular forms of therapy necessary to attempt to bring the patient to his maximum level of rehabilitation.

The purpose of this brief discussion is to orient the reader to the immediate and long-term care directions that are required for many persons who have had a traumatic brain injury. Treatment programs begin with emergency procedures and then slowly blend into various rehabilitative therapy programs.

If there are any concerns regarding possible ocular problems, an ophthalmologist will be called to join the emergency team early on in the treatment program. The ophthalmological evaluation will attempt to determine if the trauma has caused damage to the patient's sight. If no ocular problems exist and the patient is placed into a rehabilitative program, professionals may find that certain aspects of performance do not meet the expectations of the therapist. At this time a vision examination should be recommended.

Unfortunately, it has been observed that little regard is given to an individual's level of visual function throughout most medical and rehabilitative treatment programs. Even in the later stages of rehabilitation, if a question is raised with regard to a visual problem that may be a result of the traumatic brain injury, the eye examination may emphasize treatment of sight as opposed to visual function.

For many persons with a TBI, past experiences that occurred when vision and motor processes were intact have little meaning when compared to new levels of motor and cognitive dysfunction. The therapist, in an attempt to provide an appropriate medium for the matching and transferring of past experiences to new situations, will encounter great difficulties when the visual system cannot achieve a balance to enable past experiences to be matched appropriately. Due to the critical importance of the visual system in cognitive and motor function, the visual rehabilitative needs of a person with TBI must be addressed as early as possible and integrated into all aspects of the rehabilitation program.

The Visual Sequelae of a TBI

Following a TBI as a result of direct trauma to the head or from whiplash, the majority of individuals will have binocular function difficulties.[1,2] There are often specific characteristics of binocular dysfunction that will be demonstrated in the form of strabismus, oculomotor dysfunction, divergence excess, and convergence and accommodative abnormalities. The visual symptoms that may be experienced include reduced acuity, horror fusionalis (an inability to integrate the images from each eye), diplopia (double vision), seeing print appearing to move, difficulty shifting gaze, inability to adapt to environmental changes when there is movement in the periphery, and photophobia.[3] (See table 5-1.) When these conditions occur, the individual will have to develop either compensations or avoidance measures. For a person who has had a traumatic brain injury, compensating for a binocular function problem may be quite difficult. If some of the above described conditions occur in childhood, for example strabismus, the brain will adapt by suppressing central vision in the strabismic eye. However, when the condition occurs abruptly, as in TBI, the brain will not have a chance to adapt gradually, and in many cases it is quite possible that the individual will be left with serious vision problems.

When there is extreme dysfunction the ambient visual process is decoupled from the focal visual process. This can result in high amounts of exophoria (a tendency for the eyes to deviate outward), or strabismus such as exotropia (an eye turned outward). While exophoria is more common, vertical tropias, esotropia (an eye turned inward) and/or esophoria (a tendency to deviate inward) have also been noted. In the case of esophoria and esotropia, this can often be the result of over-compensation or an imbedded tendency towards over focalization.

As described above, one of the visual sequelae of traumatic brain injury is diplopia. An eye deviation such as is seen in strabismus (e.g., exotropia) can cause diplopia and, along with reduced acuity, it is prevalent among those who have TBI.[4] This condition can severely affect recovery from the TBI. All past experiences were based on a single visual world. However, double vision interferes with depth perception and object localization, and the ability to match visual information with kinesthetic, proprioceptive and vestibular experiences becomes greatly compromised. In turn, balance, coordination and movement become affected; movements will often appear clumsy. Fixations, as well as eye movements, may appear to be quite varied. The varied fixations as well as strabismus can also affect motor function. It can often be observed that the person experiencing this condition will demonstrate a limitation of ocular movements. In some individuals, intermittent diplopia will be experienced in certain gaze positions.[3] Behaviorally, Soden and Cohen, [5] and Benabib and Nelson[6] have found postural adaptations of the body, as the individual attempts to compensate for the visual dysfunction and diplopia that often occur during certain positions of gaze.

The severe spatial distortion that occurs from horror fusionalis may also cause varying states of increased muscle tone and extension patterns. Thus the person may show extension of the head and neck, and high muscle tone, particularly about the head, neck and shoulders, as well as in other areas of the body. In most cases suppression will not develop since the brain has not adapted to the strabismus; therefore these individuals, too, may develop abnormalities in head posture in an attempt to compensate for the strabismus.

Unfortunately, after traumatic injury to the brain there is a very high prevalence of exotropia and exophoria.[7-9] As described above, exotropia is defined as an eye deviated outward. With exophoria the eyes will have a tendency to turn outward in the absence of a visual stimulus (e.g., during a cover test), and there is also a tendency for the eyes to align on a point in space further than the object of regard. While studies have emphasized the high prevalence of exotropia following a TBI, it is commonly suggested that this eye alignment imbalance is attributed to nerve palsy.[10] However the mechanism for the cause of binocular dysfunction, including exotropia and exophoria, appears to be more complex and related to the effect of the insult to the cortex and/or midbrain resulting in disruption of the bimodal visual process.

In normally sighted patients who have not had traumatic brain injury but have exophoria or exotropia, behavioral observations reveal symptoms of staring, frequent daydreaming, loss of comprehension when reading, having to reread to understand context, a lack of attention and concentration abilities particularly during near vision activities, peripheral distractibility, spatial disorientation and generally poor organizational abilities. It is interesting to observe that many of these symptoms become manifested in those TBI patients who also have a high amount of exophoria or exotropia. *The condition of exophoria is not just a muscle imbalance. It is the barometer of the status of motor and sensory organization for the individual.*

The effect on vision as a result of an insult to the ambient/focal relationship primarily involves peripheral fusion and spatial organization. This dysfunction appears to occur in the ability of the ambient visual process to match information with other sensorimotor systems at the level of midbrain. The result is that the person loses the ability to organize spatial information. As was noted in Chapter One, the spatial information from the ambient visual process is provided to midbrain to match up with information from the kinesthetic, proprioceptive and vestibular processes. The spatial information being matched is provided as a sensorimotor feedforward to binocular coordination cells which, in a series of consecutive matching organizational processes, begin to establish integration of the images from each eye through the process of fusion. When this matching process is disrupted then spatial organization is also disrupted, and the visual process is left with a very unstable and highly focal processing system. Focalization becomes an attempt to isolate detail and in so doing causes problems with binocular integration, or fusion, of the images received from each eye, and may cause the person to experience fragmentation of the visual world.

When disrupted, the spatial binding provided by the ambient system will not only interfere with binocularity, it will also result in a lack of stabilization of the visual system that is provided back to the ambient visual process as part of the sensorimotor feedback loop. The ambient visual process is also responsible for grounding the visual system through sensorimotor processes of matching information. Dysfunction of the ambient visual process will also interfere with this grounding. Without the ambient support and grounding, isolation on individual details occurs through over focalization. This will often cause the person to project his own movements onto the stationary objects on which he has fixated, resulting in a perception of seeing stationary objects appearing to move. This can occur not only during ambulation but also during attempts to read so that the individual may see print on the page appearing to move. When an individual who has instability in the ambient visual process is exposed to busy, crowded environments with movement, such as shopping malls, airports, etc., the over focalization and isolation on detail will be highly overstimulating to the person. The experience can be extremely confusing and spatially disorienting to those with this visual dysfunction.

Visual Evoked Potential (VEP) Analysis in the TBI Patient

In the 1994 study by Padula, Argyris and Ray[11] the authors measured visual evoked potentials using binocular cross-pattern reversal testing to elicit the VEP response. Testing was carried out on a control group of persons who did not have traumatic brain injury, and an experimental group composed of persons who had experienced a traumatic brain injury. Cross-pattern reversal evoked potentials are measured by attaching electrodes to the scalp over specific areas of the head while the subject watches a black and white reversing checkerboard pattern on a monitor. For most clinical purposes pattern reversal is the preferred technique since results are less variable in waveform and timing than is the case using other stimuli.[12] It is also considered more sensitive in the detection of minimal visual pathway lesions.[11,13]

It was theorized that, as described previously, the ambient visual process, upon matching information with other sensory systems, acts as a feedforward system on afferent focal processing by first stabilizing the visual field and then permitting binocular integration of the foveas. It was therefore hypothesized that disturbance of the ambient visual process would interfere with the amplitude of the VEP under binocular conditions and that an increase in binocular VEP amplitude would occur if the ambient visual process resumed its role in stabilizing the peripheral field and in enhancing foveation. Previous work with TBI patients had shown improvement in stabilization of the ambient process when using binasal occlusion and base-in prisms, as described elsewhere.

In this study the experimental group initially demonstrated reduced binocular VEP amplitudes compared to the control group. However, when binasal occlusion was provided and base-in prisms were introduced before both eyes, the experimental group demonstrated statistically significant increased amplitudes (N1-P1) while members of the control group showed a statistical decrease in the binocular amplitudes (see Figures 5-1 and 5-2). The study documented the fact that persons with traumatic brain injury may have reduced binocular visual-evoked potential amplitudes. Our interpretation of this is that the binocular cortical cells in the TBI group have been compromised in function so that they are unable to fuse or integrate the images of both eyes as well as those in the control group.

The fact that the introduction of binasal occlusion and base-in prisms resulted in an increase in VEP amplitudes for the TBI subjects suggests that the visual system dysfunction of the subjects was not an oculomotor (eye muscle) problem, nor was it simply an oculomotor palsy. This study, in conjunction with that of Sarno et al.,[13] documented that after a TBI there are significant changes in binocular function that can be better explained by visual processing dysfunction. These findings are also consistent with our hypothesis that as a result of the binasal occlusion which helps

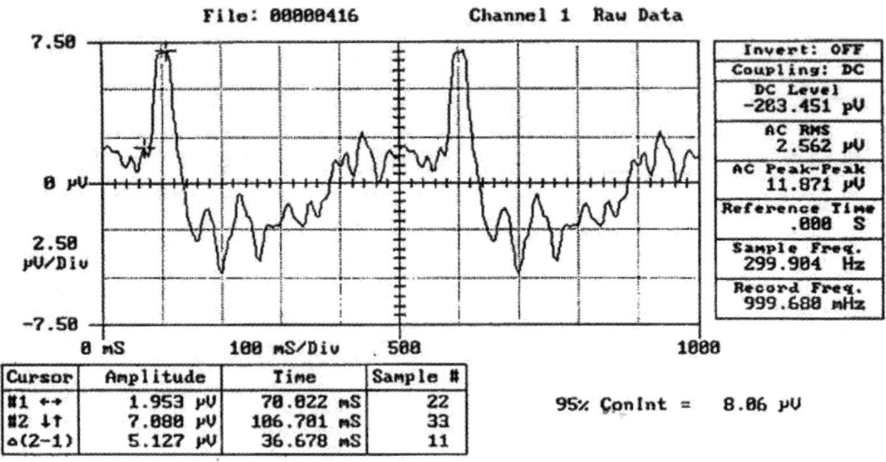

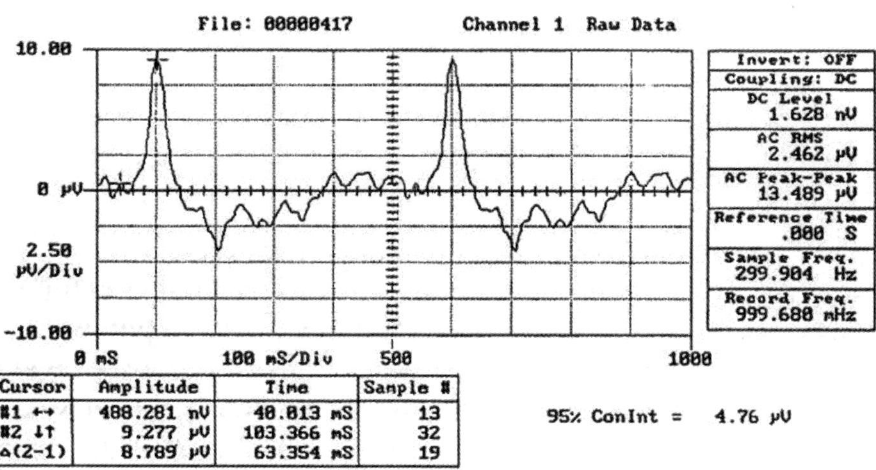

Figure 5.1. Visual evoked potentials demonstrating increased amplitudes (N1-P1) following treatment for Post Trauma Vision Syndrome.

to structure the peripheral field, and the base-in prisms which expand the field, there is an improvement in ambient visual function which results in an increase in binocular cortical function. The latter correlated with the reports of subjects during other parts of the study that with base-in prisms and binasal occlusion, the perceived movement of the floor or letters on the chart had stabilized. They also reported that it was easier to fixate with two eyes, and, for some, the diplopia was eliminated.

The previously described results are also consistent with our interpretation that in the TBI subjects the feedforward system was not successful in stabilizing the retinal images developed in the visual cortex causing an interference with the integration of visual images. This dysfunction produces the common characteristics and symptoms shown in Table 5-1 and has been termed *Post Trauma Vision Syndrome* (PTVS). It has been named this to emphasize that this multifaceted condition is caused by a disruption to the ambient process of vision, and that the disassociation

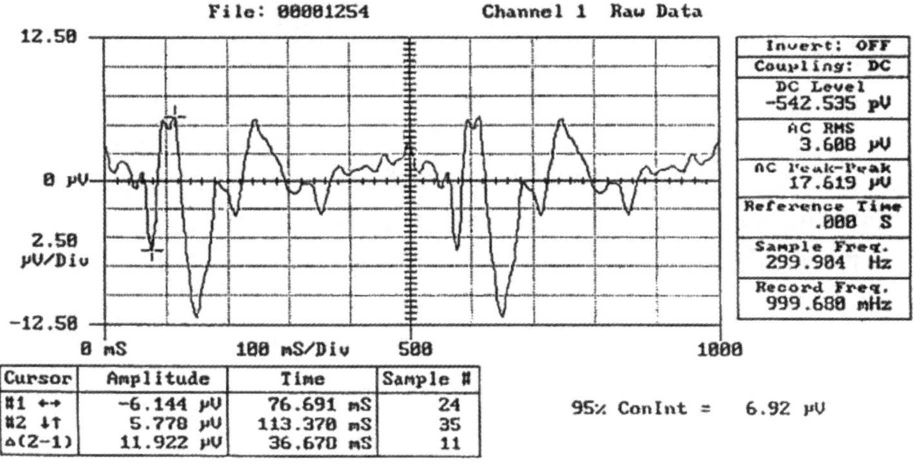

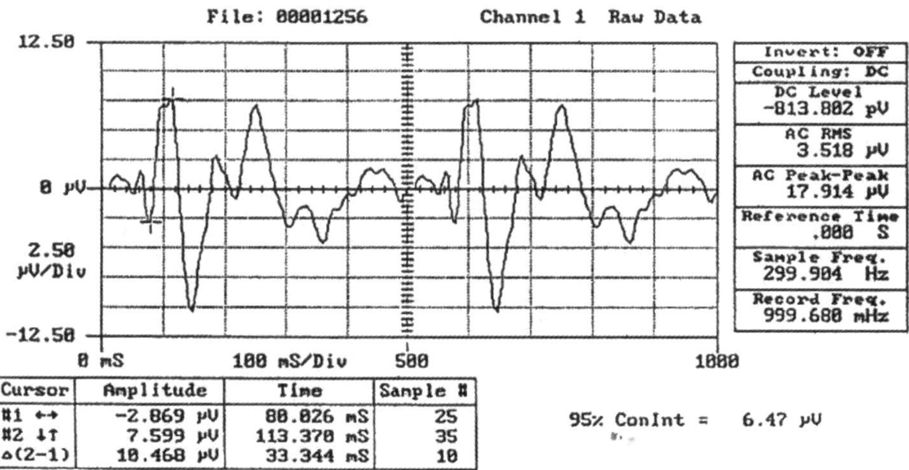

Figure 5.2. Visual evoked potentials demonstrating a decrease in negative wave potential following treatment for Post Trauma Vision Syndrome.

of the ambient process from the focal process leaves the visual system compromised and with an orientation toward high focalization without spatial grounding. This often results in the exotropia or high exophoria as a result of the greater visual problems involving the ambient processing dysfunction, as previously described and supported by the VEP study.

The result is that the higher focal process cannot maintain states of binocularity in a dynamic environment. This in turn interferes with spatial context in three dimensional space. It collapses spatially affecting planes of the X, Y, and Z axes. I propose that the development of binocular dysfunction, particularly the collapse of the Z or near/far axis, will result in the individual having more difficulty shifting from near to far fixation. The exophoria that results appears to be more related to the spatial flattening of the Z axis than it is related to an oculomotor disturbance in and of itself. The extreme collapse of the Z axis is demonstrated in the development of strabismus such as exotropia. Therefore, the binocular dysfunctions of exotropia, exophoria, accommodative dysfunction, or convergence insufficiency should be recognized by the clinician as spatial dysfunctions affecting the Z axis or near-far planes of fixation, rather than as only an oculomotor problem.

Post Trauma Vision Syndrome

While discussion in this chapter has been focused on the studies related to traumatic brain injury it must be understood that any neurological event such as a cerebro-vascular accident, Parkinson's disease, multiple sclerosis, cerebral palsy, autism, etc., can have the effect of causing dysfunction of the ambient visual process. Any disturbance neurologically, that interferes with the ambient visual process, can cause Post Trauma Vision Syndrome (PTVS). Therefore, a binocular problem that occurs with any neurological event can be, and most likely is, the result of this dysfunction of the ambient visual process thereby causing Post Trauma Vision Syndrome.

TABLE 5-1.
Common characteristics and symptoms associated with Post Trauma Vision Syndrome.

Characteristics:

- Exotropia or High Exophoria
- Accommodative Dysfunction
- Convergence Insufficiency
- Low Blink Rate
- Spatial Disorientation
- Poor Fixations and Pursuits
- Unstable Ambient Vision

Symptoms:

- Possible Diplopia
- Objects Appear to Move
- Poor Concentration and Attention
- Staring Behavior
- Poor Visual Memory
- Photophobia (glare sensitivity)
- Asthenopic Symptoms
- Associated Neuromotor Difficulties
- Balance
- Coordination
- Posture

As noted above, the visual condition which we call PTVS is multifaceted and thus the neuro-optometric rehabilitation evaluation of the traumatic brain injured patient, particularly the low functioning patient, may have to be averaged over a series of examinations. This means that, if at all possible, the examiner should see the patient over several days. When therapists are available, the examiner may recommend the use of special prisms to be used over the course of the examination period with detailed notes made with regard to motor capabilities or other functions so that the therapists can report back to the clinician. The result will be a more detailed understanding of the effects of lenses and prisms and how behaviors may be changed.

For these low-functioning TBI patients, the examiner must use objective means of testing and analyze behavioral changes that relate to the visual and neuromotor processes. Behavioral observations should include the state of muscle tone, particularly in the head, neck and shoulder areas. For example, spasticity in the temporomandibular joint can sometimes be related to stress from the visual process. Upon the introduction of appropriate lenses and/or prisms, a release of motor spasticity can often be seen. Therefore, the examiner must take time to observe postures, movements and motor functions in general. When possible, the examiner should invite other therapists and relatives to the examination, since they have had more experience in observing the patterns of function for that individual. Videotaping the patient during the examination is also very helpful. Changes that were not immediately recognizable often become apparent when reviewing the tape.

For higher functioning TBI patients who may be able to sit, stand, walk, and respond either motorically and/or verbally, testing should proceed beyond the examination chair. It is very important to observe postural adaptations and compensations while sitting in different seats, walking and also standing. Speech patterns may also be affected by the Post Trauma Vision Syndrome and a speech pathologist may be helpful in determining the effects of lenses and prisms on speech and language.

Many patients who can respond verbally will discuss their resulting visual instability. One patient explained that everything he looked at moved, and often objects or persons would appear distorted. He described it as:

> *"...a world that visually makes no sense. It constantly changes—but I will not be fooled—I know that it cannot be this way even though there is no order to things...."*

He said that faces would stretch in different directions, and when he walked, the walls moved and the floor appeared to bend and bow before him. Obviously, for this individual mobility was very difficult. He also had high muscle tone in his head, neck and shoulder areas which restricted upper body movements.

When previous optical lens prescriptions are available, the examiner should utilize them to determine changes that have resulted from the traumatic brain injury. The examiner must never assume that a prescription used successfully prior to the TBI will remain the same. The Post Trauma Vision Syndrome is the result of dysfunction and stress in the central and autonomic nervous systems. This in turn causes imbalanced states of neuromotor function. While affecting the ambient visual process, it is likely that these neuromotor imbalances will also cause imbalances in refractive and accommodative states of function as well as in ocular alignment. The clinician should consider that vision treatment programs for the traumatic brain-injured person affect the neuromotor system and vice versa. When the clinician prescribes lenses for the TBI patient, the emphasis should be to balance the visual system, which will in turn affect neuromotor function. When possible, lens prescriptions should be balanced between the two eyes. Initially, if it is not possible to prescribe equal powers of lenses, prescription changes should be directed toward balancing the prescriptions for the two eyes as the visual system becomes more flexible in adapting to changes in the process of vision.

Considering that the visual process plays a primary role in neuromotor organization and cognitive development, as previously noted, it is important, that the visual process be examined early in the rehabilitation of persons with traumatic brain injury. The visual system will demonstrate changes that are a direct result of the insult to the cortex or midbrain. These changes will be in both refractive imbalances and oculomotor states affecting fusional abilities, eye teaming responses, fixation, saccades and other sensorimotor relationships. It is the author's experience that the earlier neuro-optometric rehabilitation can be established, the faster and more complete the recovery.

When developing a rehabilitation program for vision, the examiner must keep in mind the several visual characteristics that seem to typify those patients who have had a traumatic brain injury (See Table 5-1), especially the very high incidence of exotropia and exophoria described previously.[11]

In treating patients with Post Trauma Vision Syndrome, it has been found that a low amount of base-in prism can be very effective in reducing stress in the ambient visual system. Two prism diopters base-in before each eye (in addition to the distance refractive prescription) can very often reduce or even eliminate many of these bizarre symptoms that are experienced by the patient. The base-in prisms reduce peripheral fusion demand on the ambient process, thereby relieving stress on the oculomotor system. Additionally, it helps establish a new relationship to the sensorimotor aspect of the visual process, thus affecting spatial and temporal relationships. As visual stress primarily in the ambient system is relieved, the focal visual function improves, thereby affecting the higher perceptual processes. Attention and concentration are also affected. The author has found that most individuals will respond quickly to the base-in prism prescription, reporting that they feel more comfortable or that their vision seems more stable. In addition, walking patterns and posture can also change.

For the individual discussed in a previous paragraph, who had an unstable visual system, the base-in prisms enabled him to walk without experiencing movement of the walls and floor, and he no longer experienced the distortion of his visual world.

He explained that the effect of the base-in prisms was to allow him to "understand" his visual world. This statement of understanding the visual world underscores the important but delicate balance between cognitive function and sensorimotor processing.

This same patient, when attempting to read, would hold his hand up to block off peripheral information from the page. He explained that when he tried to look at a word on the page, everything else on the page became an extreme distraction, and he had to physically block off all other areas of the page. With the low amount of base-in prism, he felt more comfortable as he read and he had better control over the peripheral areas of his vision.

An explanation for this is that this patient's visual system was highly ambient in function, and that he could not suspend peripheral visual information in order to organize focal vision processing. The base-in prisms alone were not enough for developing reading abilities. It was found that patching in the temporal area of his reading lenses was very important to help him limit peripheral areas of vision. Occluding the peripheral vision limited his visual field[14] and provided a structural boundary for the ambient visual process to help organize spatial information. The base-in prisms also relieved this patient's high muscle tone in the neck and shoulder areas. This enabled the physical and occupational therapists to increase the range of motion of the head and neck, and to improve fine motor capabilities.

Initially, when this patient was examined, questions about his visual function had to be directed to his wife because he appeared to be severely confused and disoriented. Once the treatment program had been established with prescriptive lenses and associated movement therapy it was interesting to note that the patient responded directly to the examiner. In a team meeting with his physiatrist, neurologist, therapists and psychologist, significant improvement in cognitive function was reported. The psychologist noted that the patient now had much greater ability to establish time continuity in both speech and motor organizational patterns. In addition he had more normal conversational patterns than were expected based on earlier testing.

Most persons with a TBI do not require temporal occlusion. Often binasal occlusion will be effective in providing structure to their visual fields. However, the examiner must be sensitive to the importance of the ambient component of the visual dysfunction causing PTVS. For some individuals, if base-in prisms are not enough to balance the ambient process, then temporal or nasal occlusion may assist further in helping to organize peripheral information.

Again, it must be emphasized that the visual system relates to motor function as well as to cognitive organizational abilities. Speech patterns, thought patterns and perceptual abilities are all going to be affected when the visual system, as a processing system, is disrupted. If visual rehabilitation for a person with a TBI can be provided in a behavioral way, to attempt to reestablish visual organization, then functional capabilities in other areas will also be affected.

For many individuals, including those who are very low functioning, prism therapy regimens can be very productive in attempting to reestablish balances in the oculomotor and sensory components of vision. Yoked prisms (the base end of the prism placed in the same orientation for both eyes) can be very effective in making changes in visual processing affecting oculomotor function which thereby affects sensory function. Yoked prisms provide preconscious change between the ambient visual process and the sensorimotor systems. Change offers the opportunity to adapt. Adaptation creates the dynamic interaction and differentiation between focal and ambient visual processes.

Ambient visual adaptation provides the vehicle for change in the relationship between flexion and extension against gravity. This shift in orientation to space may at first seem quite simplistic. One might believe that if the person shifts his weight in one direction or the other as an adaptation to the prisms, once the shift is made everything will appear the same. In reality, the effect of making a postural adaptation occurs as a problem-solving attempt by the individual to deal with his spatial environment through a vision-neuro-motor relationship. If the person is successful in making this shift in motor orientation, it occurs not simply because of the eye muscles change in position, but because information is matched and reestablished between the sensory component of vision, the motor component of vision, the vestibular process, and the kinesthetic and proprioceptive inputs to the brain. The visual system should act to reestablish the balances between these systems when yoked prisms are utilized. Therefore, the use of vertically yoked prisms can be an important element of rehabilitation for persons showing problems with flexion or extension.

Lateral yoked prisms or vertical yoked prisms are effective by offering spatial change depending upon the type of prism used. Wearing yoked bases left or right prisms while attempting to walk will produce some interesting motoric changes. Very often posture will change due to the fact that the person will experience the environment as slanted to the left or right, depending upon the type of prism. This orientation to space will cause the person to experience a weight shift to the left or the right because the perception of his midline is shifted. Utilizing base-left or a base-right prisms can be very effective in attempting to orient a patient to the left or right side of his body, particularly in cases involving a hemiplegia. (See Chapter Seven.)

For the treatment of strabismus and phorias, it has been the author's experience that it is not necessary to prescribe high amounts of base-in prism to correct for exotropia or exophoria. Many traumatic brain-injured patients will actually show avoidance of high amounts of base-in prism. The examiner should approach the prescription of prism in a conservative manner, starting with low amounts and increasing the prism to the point where positive changes begin to occur. As a general rule, only two prism diopters before each eye are necessary for the majority of patients.

Neuro-visual postural therapy (NVPT) can also be developed for the TBI patient suffering from Post-Trauma Vision Syndrome. However, the clinician should be cautioned not to emphasize fusion which will cause over-focalization and embed the condition of PTVS. Significant changes in performance have been observed with the utilization of various types of lenses and prisms in repeated weekly therapy sessions, particularly with higher-functioning TBI patients. For the patient discussed in this chapter who expressed extreme spatial distortion and disorientation in his visual environment, the examiner provided weekly sessions. The NVPT therapy utilized many different lenses and prism combinations, and a variety of perceptual motor activities including general walking and orientation, reaching, touching and movement activities.

Generally, NVPT in most optometric offices is developed through specific activities. It is not necessarily the activity that makes the change for the patient whether the patient is traumatically brain injured or not. Rather, it is the lens or prism that establishes the change in the visual-motor relationship. Therefore, if therapy is developed for TBI patients, the procedural activity is not as important as the lenses or prisms that the patient wears during that activity. The most effective NVPT treatment program is simply to utilize varying types of yoked prisms and enable the person time to experience each through active involvement of the motor system. Initially, for patients who have dysfunction within the bimodal visual process, very low amounts of plus lenses in addition to low amounts of yoked prisms should be used, and the amount of prism increased as adaptability is observed.

The purpose of this book is to provide a greater understanding of the process of vision; it is not intended to be a cookbook for dealing with visual problems. However, it is hoped that the reader will be able to begin using more behavioral methods of analysis for neurologically challenged patients and that the optometrists' and ophthalmologists' awareness of the indications for neuro-optometric rehabilitation or neuro-visual postural therapy will be enhanced.

Post Trauma Vision Syndrome is often a major obstacle in rehabilitation after a TBI. It can occur even with a minor rear-end collision causing only a whiplash. Persons with this condition require an aggressive neuro-optometric rehabilitation approach, first to reduce stress in the ambient visual process, and second to establish basic visual skills necessary for complete rehabilitation. PTVS is treatable, and the results of treatment emphasize that vision affects neuro-motor functions as well as cognitive abilities.

Chapter 6

POSTURAL DEVELOPMENT AND VISION

Christine Nelson

As has been previously discussed, the visual process has an intimate relationship with posture, movement, balance and spatial orientation, neurologically as well as developmentally. It is the author's opinion that there has been minimal attention paid to these important developmental relationships because many professions emphasize the sensory aspects of vision. The visual system is thus often relegated to learning experiences that are sight related and highly cognitive in function. This chapter will examine the relationships of vision to postural development in greater depth.

At birth an infant enters a gravity-based environment. In order to cope with this new existence the baby must develop an ability to right his body in space. Righting responses occur at an automatic level of the central nervous system and start with the lifting of the head off the surface. This is a life-saving reaction to keep the air passages of the infant open when he is in the prone position. Its importance to our understanding of the interrelationship between postural control and vision is that the weight of the head on the nose and mouth causes a reaction in the extensor musculature of the neck, which in turn causes the infant to lift his head off the surface.

The early and automatic turning of the face to one side already offers the newborn infant a change of visual environment. That postural response also creates an opportunity for the visual system to begin to organize the three-dimensional world parallel to the postural reactions to gravity.

Although there is some light perception in utero, we might think of the discriminative features of vision as beginning at birth. During the first few weeks of life the normal infant makes a systematic effort to develop extension of the body that moves him away from the physiological flexion with which he was born. In the prone, or face down, position he stretches his legs out one at a time as his pelvis shifts from one side to another. His center of gravity is forward at this stage of development, with the body weight sustained over the sternum and chest. Early arm support is characterized by the elbows being at the level of the chest. The long extensor muscles of the back lift the head and shoulders as a unit away from the surface, which in turn permits the arms to move forward gradually in a more versatile support of the torso. Each of these changes brings the face a little closer to a perpendicular alignment in relation to the base of support, in what Arnold Gesell identified as a "level three" head lift. Visual interest contributes significantly to the maintenance of uprightness, which is sustained a little longer each time.

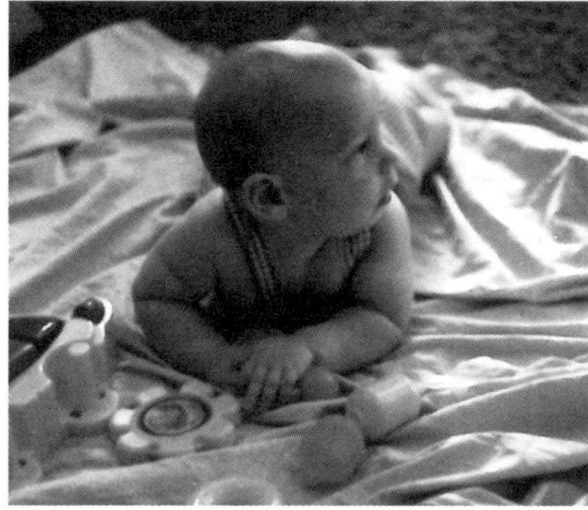

Figure 6.1. Vision and posture. Normal postural control supports visual exploration.

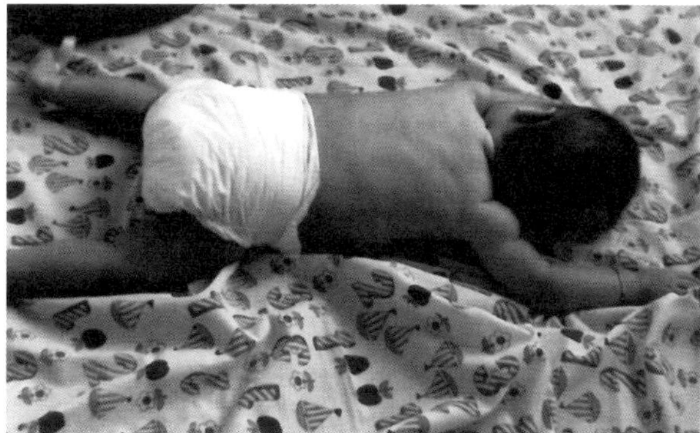

Figure 6.2. Prone without extension. Lack of back extension and inactive legs are causes for concern in baby development.

It is characteristic of normal development that movement occurs away from the surface, that is, against gravity, which is perceived by the organism as a pleasant challenge and acts as a stimulus for normal reflexive movements. The child with a neuromotor dysfunction can be identified as the infant who fails to accept the challenge of gravity, and is seen to be caught in its pull instead of moving away from its influence. The involved baby will have difficulty lifting his head and shifting over the longitudinal midline of the body.

A lateral shift of weight is essential to organize the musculature of the trunk for postural control. The baby prepares himself with many subtle weight changes to support his body on one side while he reaches for a toy with the opposite hand. Initially, he overbalances just as he visually misjudges the distance to an object. By seven months, however, the active baby is able to pivot in the prone position to obtain a toy placed at his side, an accomplishment that represents a significant level of integration of vision and posture. It is also an important step in the establishment of bilaterality, which is essential for the sensory organization of vision, and audition and for motor learning by the central nervous system.

Early changes in postural orientation, from one side of the body to the other, begin to integrate the longitudinal midline as one arm is used to reach and the other to support body weight. This early turning of the body is accomplished by a lengthening of the side that maintains the body weight and a shortening of the moving side. It reflects the interaction of stability and mobility so essential for smooth movement reactions. Although this maneuver is already seen in the baby of 6 or 7 months of age, it is a sign of developmental preparation for the distant ability of taking a step forward with one side of the body while the opposite side maintains the upright alignment.

The second half of the first year of development is filled with movements that permit the normal baby to refine this initial contrast between stability and mobility and combine it with a myriad of developmental movements motivated by interest in the environment and the sheer joy of moving.

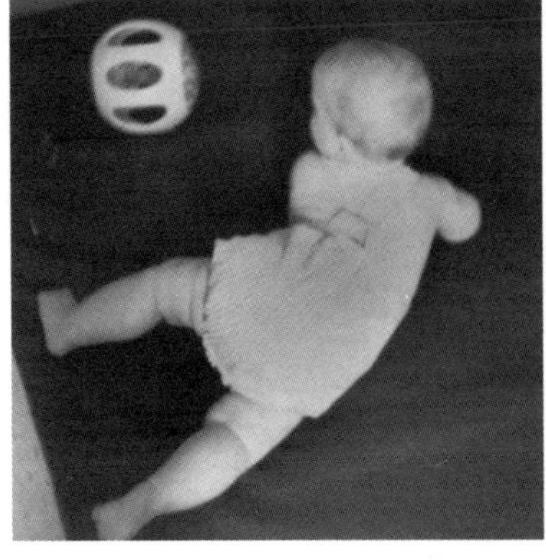

Figure 6.3. Pivot prone. Lateral flexion of the trunk in the "pivot prone" response corresponds with lateral eye movement.

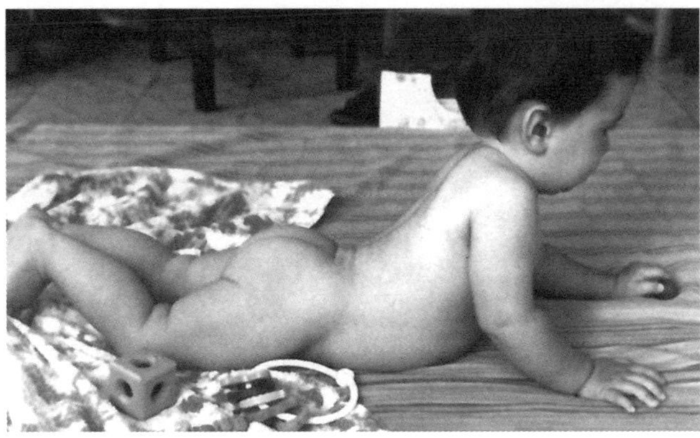

Figure 6.4. Baby extension. Extension in prone at 8 months has served to move the center of gravity back toward the pelvis.

The gradual mastery of flexion, or folding together of the trunk, head and limbs in the supine, or face-up position, develops parallel to the body extension. Lifting the head often occurs in response to a visual stimulus from the adult who stands nearby. It becomes a communication that indicates "I want to come with you" or "I want to be picked up." The infant has previously shown a cessation of postural activity in order to focalize vision, and is now able to move while maintaining visual contact. The intriguing experience of moving feet encourages the baby to reach with his arms and lift the pelvis or the hips to bring his feet closer for visual and tactile examination. This lifting of the lower trunk by the musculature of the ventral surface at this stage of development insures later mobility of the pelvis so essential to sitting and standing. Mobility within the trunk itself prepares the child for the barely perceptible adjustments of position made by an adult who can sit or stand while keeping the eyes focused on an interesting target or while involved in an activity or just lost in thought. It is an error to think of the development of postural orientation of the infant without recognizing the influence of the ambient visual process.

The reader is reminded of the direct neurological relationship of the ambient visual process to the midbrain and its intimate association with nerve fibers that are both afferent, as well as efferent (sensory as well as motor) from the neck, trunk, arms and legs. The focal process of vision is interwoven at various stages permitting the direction of interest and curiosity for the development of higher cognitive and perceptual functions.

In viewing the dynamic interaction of the visual and postural systems during early development, we can note that the body has developed its extremes of movement in both extension and flexion. At the same time that the infant is mastering balance while sitting, which requires a subtle combination of flexion and extension influence, he is also enjoying rocking forward and back on his abdomen. This action often terminates in a sudden landing on the hands and directing of the gaze down-

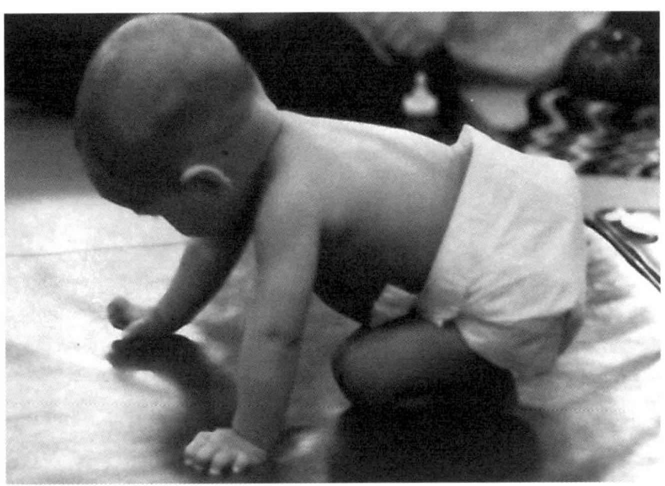

Figure 6.5. Baby flexion. By 9 months the baby is moving along the floor in a combination of flexion and extension.

ward. Especially during the second half of the first year, babies expend great quantities of energy in physical exploration of their environment. They are guided by visual, auditory and tactile novelties and the pleasure of smooth, ever-adapting kinesthetic feedback. The proprioceptive system is clear about its need for change, and the baby openly seeks a new toy or play experience and temporarily rejects the familiar. At this stage one observes a difference in the development of blind infants who cannot rely on visual interest to draw them to further exploration of their surroundings.

The righting and equilibrium reactions that serve to sustain us against gravity have been well described by Karel Bobath[1,2] as he studied the absence or partial expression of these reactions in children affected by cerebral palsy, a central nervous system dysfunction. His concepts are helpful in gaining an understanding of the integrative nature of postural stability. Postural reactions form the base for normal movement control and permit predictable relationships to develop between different parts of the body. As the baby masters extension of the body against gravity in the prone position, he is aided by the coordinated antigravity movement of the limbs, as seen in the 4-month-old who pulls his elbows back symmetrically to stabilize his shoulders while he rocks to and fro. Due to the head-righting reaction in relation to the trunk, the head position becomes more vertical relative to the supporting surface. The visual system also seeks an upright alignment from which to view the world, while the vestibular system confirms this useful head position.

The righting or repositioning of the head in relation to the body position and, conversely, the body in relation to the head, are two of the primary righting reactions that follow lifting the head relative to the support. These righting responses of the head and body, which are based on the perception of body weight in contact with the surface, influence all of the baby's early postural changes. The ambient visual process first facilitates postural information matching with kinesthetic, proprioceptive and vestibular information. The focal visual process then offers higher sensory reinforcement together with vestibular orientation. The blind child without motor impairment will also show many of these early automatic responses in the adjustment of his posture in space. The blind baby who has his position changed by his caregivers has the opportunity to more effectively use the important cue of proprioceptive experience of the body weight to change the alignment of body parts.

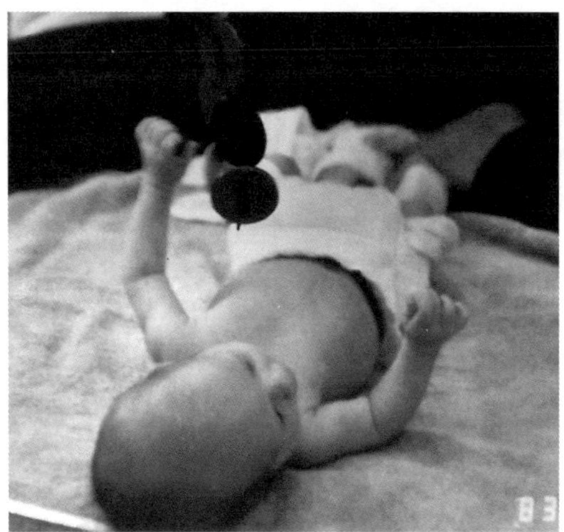

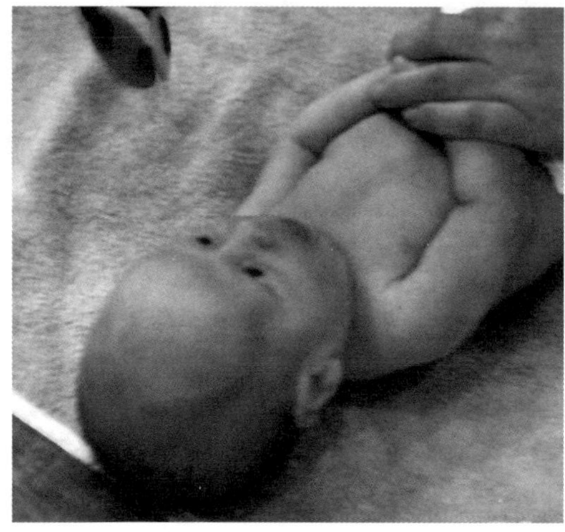

Figure 6.6. Infant stabilizing to direct gaze. This 1-month-old baby tracks the visual stimulus much more readily when her limb movement is controlled for her.

The righting reactions essentially respond to proprioceptive deep-pressure awareness of gravity and are then integrated with the proprioceptive and vestibular-based equilibrium reactions. This combination of sensory input gives impulse to the antigravity stability of the trunk, permitting the limbs to move freely. The righting reactions provide central organization and security through the initial deep-pressure proprioceptive experiences. This is the beginning of interplay between stability and mobility which stays with us throughout life.

In order for the eyes to develop good-quality movement, they also need a stable base which is provided by graded motoric control of the neck in all positions in space. The growing ability of the baby to monitor the position of the head permits more consistent visual examination of interesting objects in the environment. As adults we adapt the head position to meet our visual needs by means of change in the neck alignment. Skilled gymnastic performers must consciously control their automatic reactions in order to accomplish their elaborate flips and turns. Otherwise, the head would tend to automatically maintain itself in a position perpendicular to the base or the floor. Dancers must control visual responses by fixing their gaze on a distant point in order to perform a smooth pirouette. The average person pushes his way through a crowd to meet a friend or walks across a footbridge without losing equilibrium by keeping visual contact with his goal and depending on his automatic equilibrium reactions.

During the early months of life when the child lifts his head and moves more in free space, the activity of the vestibular and proprioceptive systems begins its influence. This is another aspect of the postural reflex mechanism described by Bobath[1,2]. The vestibular system initially integrates its activity with that of the deep-pressure proprioceptors. As the infant is more upright in space, vestibular reactions begin to lead the balance or equilibrium together with the ambient visual process. The equilibrium responses of the human body are automatic and total in nature; the legs and arms move, the trunk curves and the head assumes an alignment related to that of the trunk to shift the center of gravity. All this happens without the central nervous system giving a single conscious command to individual body parts. The maintenance of balance in space is automatic and is a function of our preconscious behavior.

As the young child still lacks the fluidity of movement necessary to maintain his balance consistently in a coordinated way, he resorts to stepping to avoid a fall. With increased maturity of the postural responses, the trunk will be activated when the balance is threatened, and only in the last moment will protective extension of the limbs be activated.

The child with marked visual impairment is not able to use the optical righting response to reinforce the head righting that is seen in the Landau reaction, or in the prone position while exhibiting extension. The baby who suffers injury to the optic nerve or some other crucial part of the visual system, and lacks even general light sensitivity, will soon diminish his postural responses and be content with postural adaptations to the immediate surface. Movement responses will be of reduced amplitude and will lack the joy and spontaneity of the normally sighted child. There will tend to be a lack of security and a greater reliance on the righting reactions that depend on deep-pressure proprioceptive information rather than on the vestibular and proprioceptive reactions. Partial vision, or distorted functional vision, may create fear of new situations that lack predictability for the child and may reduce significantly the experimentation with postural control that is a part of normal development. The world does not automatically beckon such children to participate. There is no reason for them to maintain balance while striving to reach an object of visual interest. In order to develop a functional postural system, these children need to be given vestibular and proprioceptive experiences in play that stimulate their interest in movement and build confidence in their own body. They need to be introduced to the environmental space that they miss through lack of an active visual system.

The postural system is not only useful as a means of dealing with a gravity environment, but it also unites with visual responses to create the first communication system known to the infant. The child still being fed in a highchair vehemently turns his head away to indicate that he wants no more dinner. A moment later he points clearly to the plate of his father to request a more interesting menu. Small children are accomplished in managing adults with a mere glance and the simplest of gestures. While this is an interesting and useful development that precedes the organization of spoken language, it also sets the stage for vision and movement to work together as when the child in school must copy information from the chalkboard or whiteboard. It reflects the fact that the younger infant has spent much time comparing kinesthetic and tactile feedback with visual feedback to correlate the varied information.

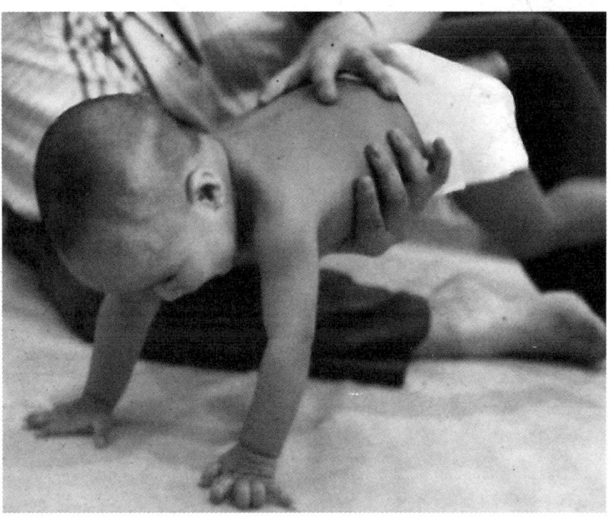

Figure 6.7. Protective extension. Protective extension is one of several automatic responses that reflect the integrity of the postural systems.

Without an organized postural system, the sensorimotor data acquired by the child from his environment remains fragmented and comparatively disorganized. It lacks a consistent base or frame of reference, and compensatory systems tend to come into play to permit functional independence. The problem is seen clearly in children with learning problems who demonstrate postural disorganization. Their central nervous systems have never succeeded in relegating postural reactions to the automatic level. Such youngsters are constantly distracted from an immediate task by their need to concentrate on maintaining body balance on the chair or moving themselves across the room. Therapy directed to the organization of postural responses results in positive behavioral changes as well as improved fine coordination. Quality of handwriting control improves, and better organization of school work is noted with no direct practice on the specific task.

Careful observation of a baby's most important first steps reveals that the body responds to the child's visual interest in someone or something across the room, or perhaps to the feel of an unexpected shift in the child's center of gravity. Initially, the forward progression is dominated by lateral movement that creates an impression of a toppling forward. As with reaching and other physical activity, the baby

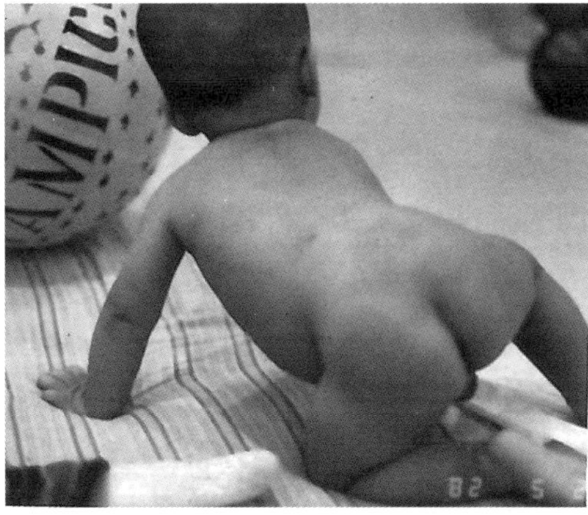

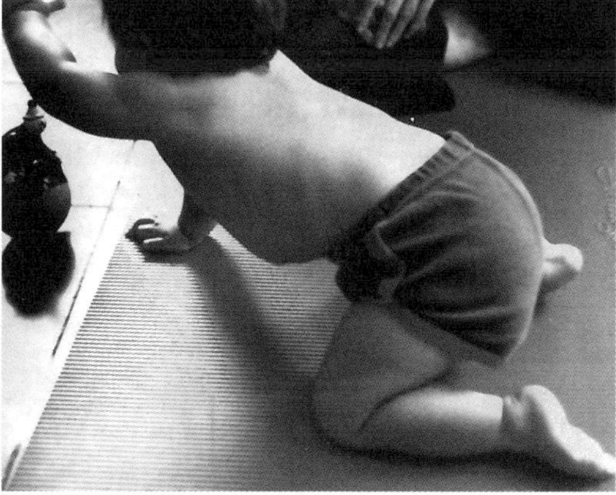

Figure 6.8 Movement on the floor. The baby on the left easily shifts to one side to sit. The same transition is an effort for the child on the right because of his wide base of support and poor trunk control.

does not seem to monitor this forward movement directly, but appears to use a trial-and-error approach followed by self-correction until a more sophisticated movement pattern emerges. The two visual processes are now functioning. The ambient process serves to anticipate needed movement in a feedforward mode for posture, balance and orientation to space. At this level of development the focal process of vision becomes subservient to the child's interests and interaction with the environment. Now the possibility exists to explore the visual environment, locate sound sources and match sensory information. The postural and visual systems have developed in a parallel fashion, periodically intertwining their respective contributions into an integrated functional organism.

Chapter 7

VISUAL MIDLINE SHIFT SYNDROME

William V. Padula

Persons with neurological dysfunctions, including cerebrovascular accidents (CVA), traumatic brain injury (TBI), multiple sclerosis (MS), cerebral palsy (CP), etc., frequently will have postural problems resulting in displacement of the body mass. Thus the person may lean to one side (commonly observed with a hemiparesis or hemiplegia), or exhibit an anterior (flexion) or posterior (extension) malalignment. At one time neurological dysfunctions that interfered with posture, balance and mobility were thought to affect only specific limbs or neuromotor groups. Rehabilitation was attempted by medical or surgical means, or through the use of adaptive aids and physical and/or occupational therapies. The role of the visual system in establishing posture, movement and balance was taken into consideration to a limited extent. However, a clinical model of treating posture and balance disorders through the visual system was, for the most part, lacking.

Our research[1] working with subjects who had a CVA (experimental group) and subjects with no neurological dysfunction (control group) resulted in the following findings:

1. There is a statistical correlation with shift in visual midline and direction of lean.
2. Yoked prisms can shift the visual midline to a centered position.
3. The direction of lean correlates with the shift of visual midline.
4. Proper positioning of yoked prisms not only realigns the visual midline, but also improves posture and balance, and increases weight bearing on the affected side.

In the case of a CVA or TBI, the prevalence of a hemiparesis or hemiplegia is common. However, even after undergoing rehabilitation many of these courageous survivors still tend to lean away from the hemiparetic side. The author recalls countless situations in which therapists would position a mirror in front of the patient to provide an orientation for the person to "straighten up." When the mirror was removed after the therapy session, the person would return to his abnormal posture.

Could the visual system somehow be involved in creating distortion of space affecting the person's perception of his own erect posture? While taking the history of a patient referred to me for a neuro-optometric rehabilitation evaluation, I questioned him about his visual problems and asked how I could help him. The patient said, in an unassuming manner, "Well, you can straighten this floor out." When asked what he meant, he said that the floor was tilting down on the right side. It was observed that even while seated in the chair, he was leaning to the right. When standing, he also leaned to the right, placing most of his weight on his right leg. His left side was hemiparetic, the result of a cerebrovascular accident two and one-half years prior to the examination. Other patients have reported similar types of distortions. However, not all patients seem consciously aware of these distortions of space.

With an understanding of the visual process and its uncompromising relationship to the neuromotor system, the possibilities of developing a theory as to why visual space might become distorted following a neurological event becomes plausible. In studying the possibilities, I became interested in the primitive yet obscure portion of the visual process called the *ambient system*. As reported in Chapter One, it becomes part of the sensorimotor feedback loop at the level of midbrain. Many of the visual fibers emanating from the two eyes do not go to the occipital cortex, but instead are delivered to various areas of midbrain, including rostral midbrain and the superior colliculus. At these levels visual information is matched with other sensorimotor information being delivered from kinesthetic, proprioceptive, vestibular, and tactile systems.

The cerebellum monitors this information closely, amplifies or minifies it, and formats the information before a feedforward system delivers input to other higher organizational centers in the cortex for stabilization and anticipation of action. Specifically, a feedforward system to the occipital cortex provides for the stabilization of the peripheral retina, for the control of the spatial environment, and also for the fusion or integration of the images from both eyes. Without this sensorimotor feedback loop and the feedforward system to the occipital cortex we would be left with a sensory message that provided no spatial meaning or understanding. Instead, detail would be seen without spatial representation. An example of this is trying to recognize a person's face when you stand on your head. The information is the same; however, the spatial representation of the person's face is lost in the details of the eyes, nose, mouth, lips, hair, etc. If, for example, a person has spent his entire life matching his ambient visual information with balance and sensorimotor information from the two sides of the body, a relative level of equality is created from that experience. The person then relies on this information for orientation in space. If, however, after a neurological event such as a cerebrovascular accident a person has a neurologically affected side such as a hemiparesis or a hemiplegia, the information received from the kinesthetic and proprioceptive systems from one side of the body is different from that of the other.

The ambient visual process serves as a master preconscious regulator attempting to balance information in an effort to establish a meaningful interpretation of higher order sensory input. Following a neurological impairment, the ambient visual process creates a relative balance between the mismatch of information received at midbrain, and thus expands and contracts space internally in its attempt to manage the dysfunction. This expansion and contraction of space in persons who have a neurological dysfunction can be observed in their own posture (see photo, Figure

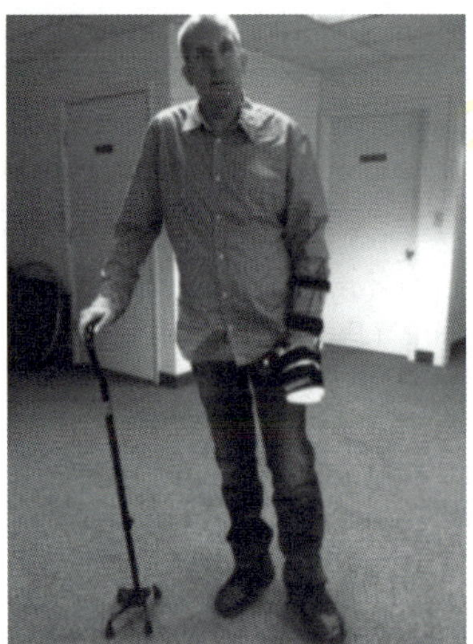

Figure 7-1. Person with a left hemiparesis and visual midline shift to the right.

7-1). The contracted side reflects a compression of space internally, whereas the extended side reflects an expansion of internal space.

The ambient process, through a feedforward mechanism to the occipital cortex, then projects this expansion and contraction of space externally and causes distortion of the higher sensory spatial environment. In some individuals this distortion can be observed and they will actually report a tilting of the floor in one direction or the other. For the majority of persons this distortion appears to become the norm, and since they have no other means to judge the spatial environment they are cognitively unaware of the change. This mismatch of information and resulting distortion of space has been termed the Visual Midline Shift Syndrome. Tables 7-1 and 7-2 describe the common characteristics and symptoms of Visual Midline Shift Syndrome. On the following pages a method of analyzing this distortion and a means to affect it utilizing yoked prisms will be discussed.

VISUAL MIDLINE SHIFT SYNDROME Associated Neuromotor Characteristics
• Hemiplegia
• Hemiparesis
• Flexion
• Extension
• Side Neglect

Table 7-1. Characteristics of Visual Midline Shift Syndrome.

VISUAL MIDLINE SHIFT SYNDROME Associated Symptoms
• Floor May Appear Tilted
• Walls and/or Floor May Appear to Shift and Move
• Person Leans and/or Increases Weight Bearing to the Unaffected Side

Table 7-2. Symptoms of Visual Midline Shift Syndrome.

Testing for Visual Midline Shift Syndrome

Evaluating patients for the presence of a visual midline shift can be done in several ways. The most effective way to assess VMSS is to combine techniques of observation of posture and balance and a simple test for VMSS which will be described below. The difficulty with clinical observation is that it is a subjective assessment and requires that the examiner must be skilled in understanding posture, biomechanics and the dynamics of neuromotor function associated with movement.

The VMSS test is also a subjective test and often results in variable responses. If the responses are averaged over several trials, the results will in most cases provide the clinician with a direction of visual midline shift. However, the VMSS Test must be combined with an observation of posture and balance.

A more objective and accurate means of VMSS is through instrumentation such as the *NeurOpTrek*™. This instrument assesses dynamic weight bearing and provides an objective mathematical analysis of gait and balance associated with VMSS. The results provide the examiner with an accurate assessment of the VMSS as well as a treatment protocol.

For those who have suffered a traumatic brain injury, cerebrovascular accident, or have cerebral palsy, multiple sclerosis, etc., a simple test may determine the relationship of the visual midline shift to neuromotor dysfunction. It is important that the patient have the necessary cognitive function to respond to the examiner's questions. The test may be performed using a wand or pencil. The vertical target is held approximately 40 centimeters in front of a patient's face and is moved from left to right across his visual field. The patient should be instructed to track the wand as it is moved, but to do so without moving his head. He should tell the examiner when the wand appears to be directly in front of his nose. A patient who is binocular and has no shifts in his visual midline should report the object to be directly in front of his nose, i.e., his structural midline, when it is actually in this position. The test should be repeated by bringing the object from right to left across his visual field. (The examiner should be positioned off to the side of the patient, not directly in front of him, so that the patient will not use the examiner's features to determine his own midline.)

If the patient consistently stops the wand when it is either to the right or left side of his structural midline, it is an indication that he has shifted his concept of visual midline in that direction. To record the findings, the examiner should draw a vertical line to correspond to the patient's responses (see Figure 7-2). An arrow should

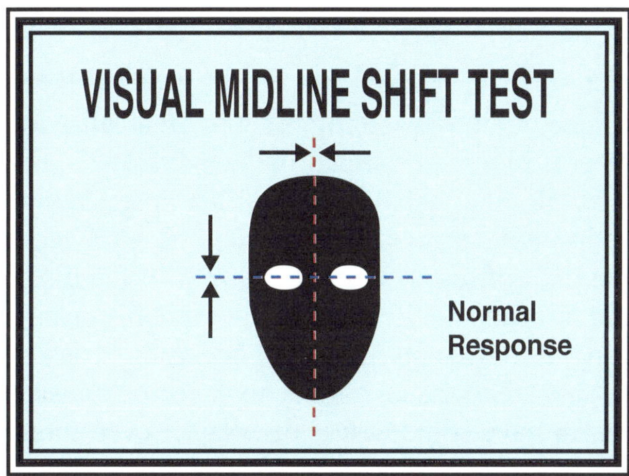

Figure 7-2. Graphic Representation of Visual Midline Shift Test.

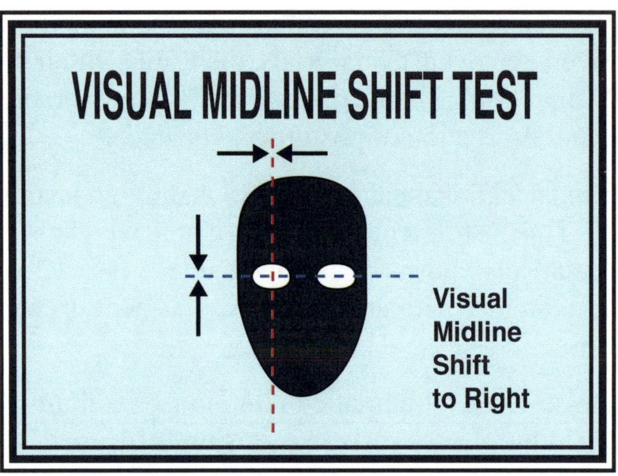

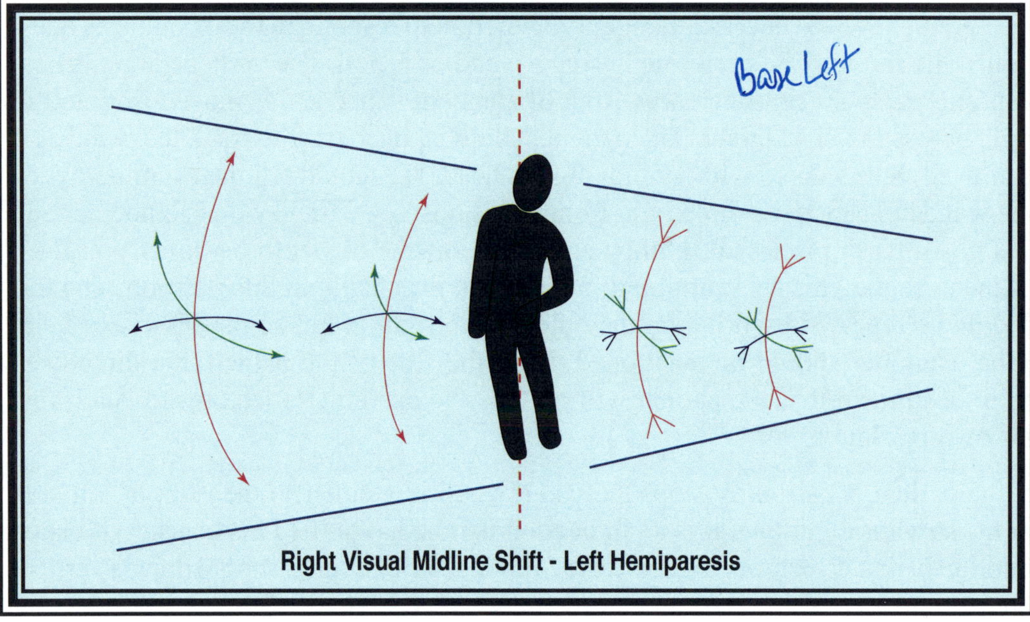

Figure 7-3. Visual Midline Shift to the Right with Left Hemiparesis. Inward pointing arrows indicate compression; outward pointing arrows indicate expansion.

be drawn adjacent to that line indicating the direction of the wand's movement. Frequently, the position of the visual midline shift will localize to one side, showing a correlation between vision and the neuromotor dysfunctions of hemiparesis or hemiplegia. For example, if a patient has a left hemiparesis (left sided weakness) the visual midline shift will frequently be found to have moved away from his left side and toward the right of his nose. In effect, by shifting his concept of a visual midline to the right, the patient will actually reinforce his own hemiparesis. When standing and walking, it may be observed that he has difficulty transferring weight to his left side. The shift in his visual midline to the right is a reinforcement mechanism to enable him to have some aspect of balance even though it is abnormal. Figure 7-3 demonstrates a schematic representation of a visual midline shift to the right as is frequently observed in persons with a left hemiparesis.

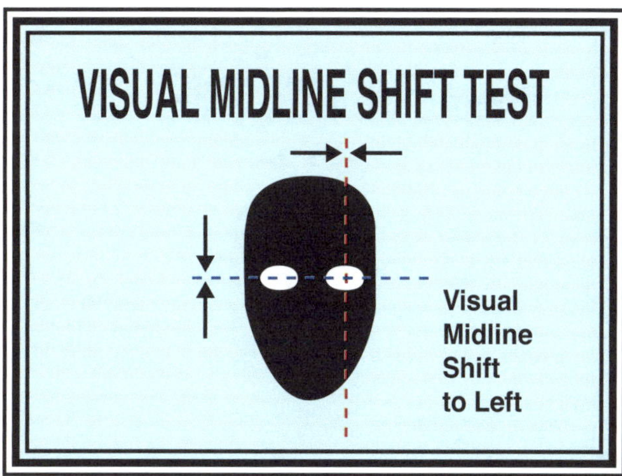

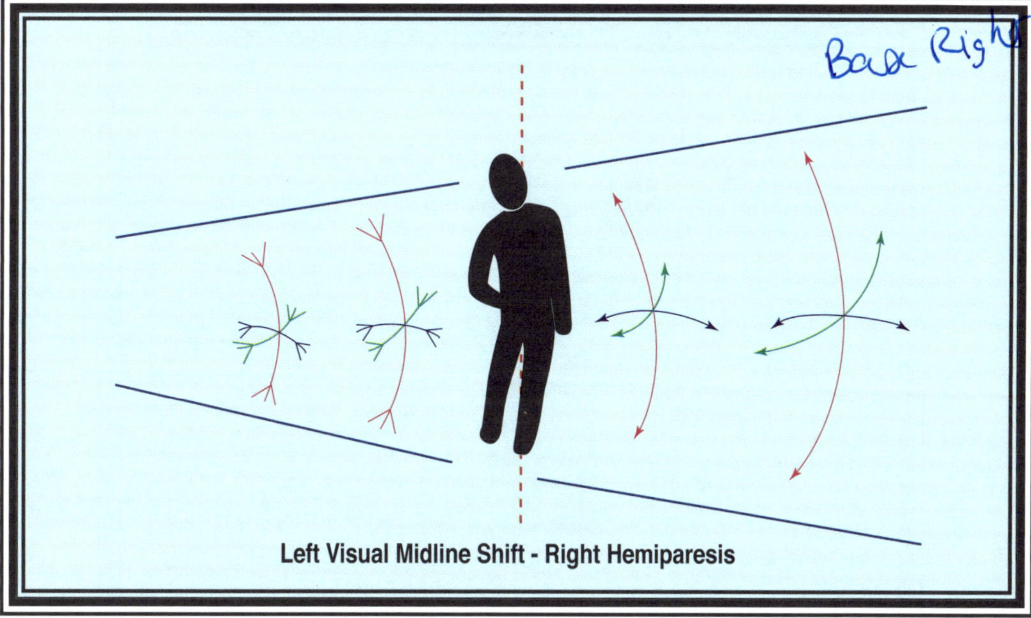

Figure7-4. Visual Midline Shift to the Left with Right Hemiparesis. Inward pointing arrows indicate compression; outward pointing arrows indicate expansion.

The second phase of the testing may be done by holding the wand horizontally and passing it vertically in front of the patient's face. The patient should be instructed to tell the examiner when the wand appears to be at eye level. First, hold the wand horizontally above the patient's face and have him look upward toward the wand. Bring the wand from this position downward and tell the patient to instruct you when the wand appears to be at eye level. Draw a line horizontally on the graphic drawing to represent his response. Also, draw an arrow downward to the horizontal line indicating the direction of the wand's movement. Next, hold the wand below the face and move it upward asking the patient to respond when the wand appears to be directly at eye level. Draw a corresponding line on the graphic representation with an arrow directed upward. If the wand was reported at eye level when it was actually above his eye level it indicates a shift in his visual midline poste-

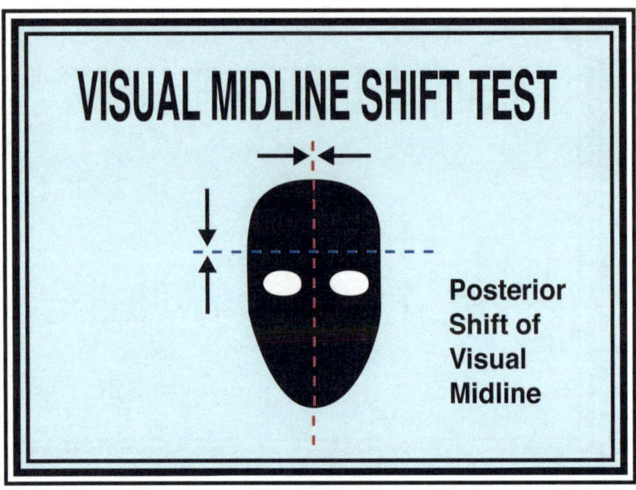

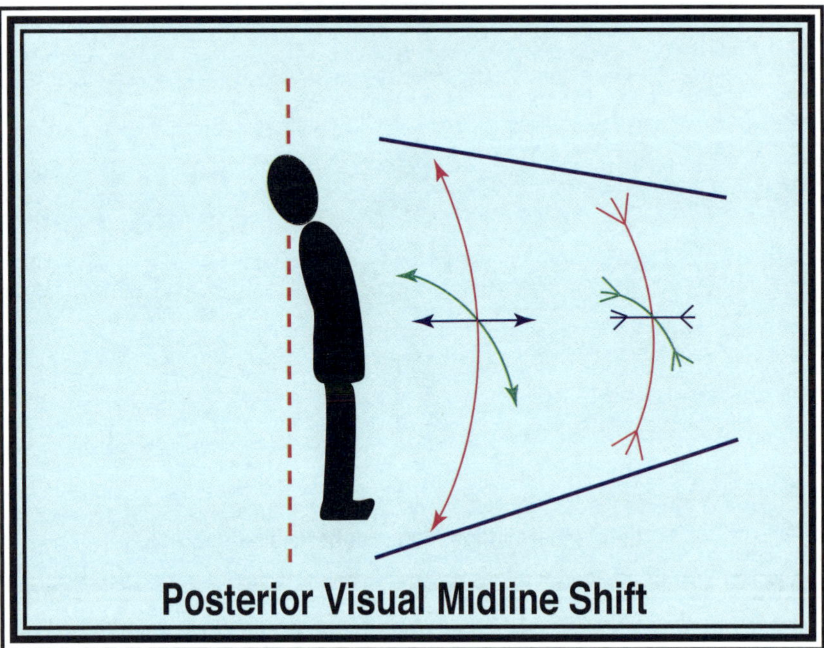

Figure 7-5. Posterior Visual Midline Shift. Inward pointing arrows indicate compression; outward pointing arrows indicate expansion.

riorly (Figure 7-5). Frequently patients with this shift in visual midline will show extension in posture and thrust their weight backward when walking or seated in a chair. Figure 7-6 represents a shift in concept of visual midline anteriorly causing a flexion posture. If the wand was reported at eye level when it was actually positioned below the eye level, it indicates an anterior shift in the perception of visual midline. Patients with this distortion will show a flexion posture or a tendency to lean forward while seated or walking.

The shift in concept of visual midline occurs from a mismatch of information in the sensorimotor feedback loop between the ambient visual process and other sensory and motor systems. Averaging information causes a shift in the visual midline and in

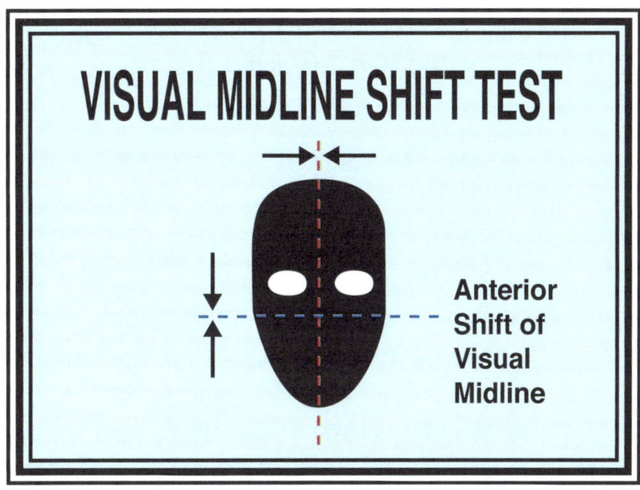

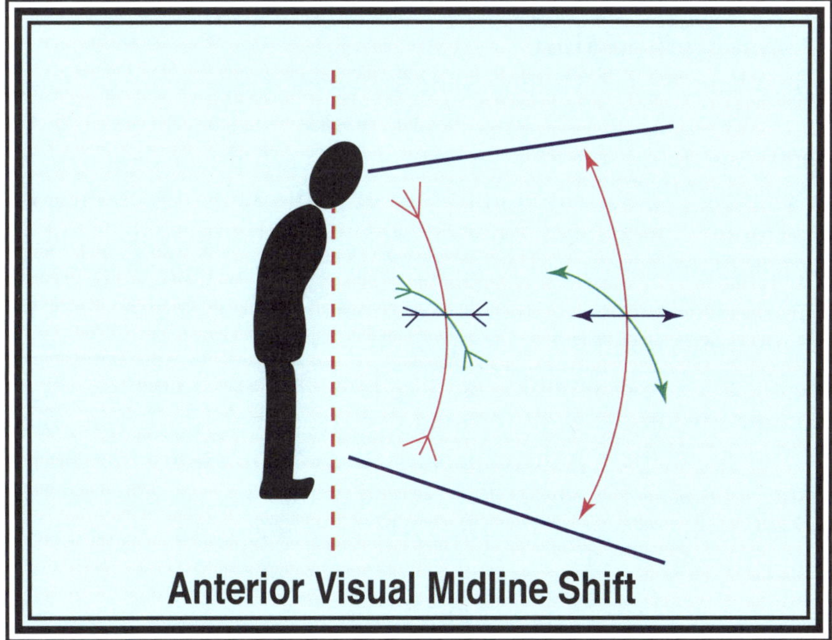

Figure 7-6. Anterior Visual Midline Shift. Inward pointing arrows indicate compression; outward pointing arrows indicate expansion.

turn a distortion of space. This distortion occurs by establishing a relative compression and expansion of space which can be noted in the schematic figures. In most cases the shift is away from the affected side as has been described. However, in some instances, a paradoxical effect may be noted when the midline shifts toward the affected side (see Table 7-3).

Initially following a TBI, CVA, etc., the person will lean into the hemiparetic side. This is the visual uncompensated state. Within several days the brain will attempt to reorganize ambient visual and sensorimotor information for survival purposes. The visual midline then shifts away from the affected or hemiparetic side. This

PARADOXICAL VISUAL MIDLINE SHIFT SYNDROME Associated Characteristics • Person Leans Into the Affected Side • Visual Midline Shifted Toward the Affected Side or Variable

Table 7-3. Paradoxical Visual Midline Shift.

is termed the compensated state. For some individuals, the compensated state is never achieved, causing what we have termed the Paradoxical VMSS (effect).

Determining the Appropriate Type of Yoked Prisms to be Utilized with Visual Midline Shift Syndrome

Lateral Visual Midline Shift

The majority of the Visual Midline Shift Syndrome cases involve a lateral deviation of the midline. As noted, typically the visual midline moves away from the side of the paresis. In these cases the base end of each prism should be positioned opposite the side of the visual midline shift or in the same direction as the paretic side. For example, if the patient shows a visual midline shift to the right, it is likely this person has a left hemiparesis or hemiplegia. The base ends of the yoked prisms should be positioned on the left in order to move the visual midline back toward the left side. Conversely, if there is a visual midline shift to the left, with an associated right hemiparesis or right hemiplegia, the clinician should position the base ends of the yoked prisms on the right for both eyes (see Table 7-4). The yoked prisms have the effect of countering the expansion and compression of space.[2] The apex of the prism expands space while the base end of the prism compresses space. ***The following table is for "typical" CVA or TBI, etc., patients who have a hemiparesis and associated VMS.***

AREA OF INSULT	PHYSICAL STATUS	DIRECTION OF VMS	PRISM ORIENTATION
Right brain lesion	Left hemiparesis	Right VMS	Base Left
Left brain lesion	Right hemiparesis	Left VMS	Base Right

Table 7-4. THERAPEUTIC Rx OF YOKED PRISMS (Right and Left VMS)

While fitting prisms would seem to be a straight forward procedure, and is so in many cases, there are always exceptions to the recommendations noted above. That is one of the reasons why we stress throughout the book that patients must be observed in a variety of situations such as walking, moving with the help of an assistive device, sitting (with and without support, if needed), standing, etc. You may also note references to prism use in other chapters describing specific cases.

Anterior/Posterior Visual Midline Shift

When there is an anterior or posterior shift in the visual midline, prisms are utilized in a different manner. They are placed vertically and have the effect of compressing and expanding space around a near/far axis (Z axis). If the midline is shifted *posteriorly,* observation of the patient's posture will show that he is leaning posteriorly with increased weight bearing on the heel(s). The patient will report the wand at eye level when the examiner has positioned it above the line of sight. The base of the yoked prisms should be placed in the *base-up* position. The base-up yoked prisms *compress near space while expanding far space*, thereby altering the distortion frequently observed in patients who lean backwards in extension and who will sometimes observe that the floor appears tilted upwards.

If there is an *anterior shift* of the visual midline, observation of the patient's posture will show that he is leaning forward with increasing weight bearing on the toe(s) or even "toe walking" as in the case of many autistic and spectrum disorder children and adults**.** He will respond that the wand is at eye level when it is actually below the level of their eyes. The yoked prisms should be positioned base-down before both eyes. The base-down yoked prisms will *expand near space and compress far space* countering the distortion of the downward tilt of the floor seen with patients who lean forward in flexion.

PHYSICAL STATUS	DIRECTION OF VMS	PRISM ORIENTATION
Flexion	Anterior VMS	Base Down
Extension	Posterior VMS	Base Up

Table 7-5. THERAPEUTIC Rx OF YOKED PRISMS (Anterior and Posterior VMS)

While vertical prisms may be useful in dealing with VMS in various age groups, they are often also helpful in working with children with cerebral palsy, autism, and other neurologically based disorders. Again, careful observation of the child during various activities is very important in determining which prism paradigm is most appropriate. For example, while some children in a flexion posture may benefit from base down prisms, others with different postural tone may do better with base up vertical prisms.

Visual Midline Shift Syndrome has also been identified in the so-called "normal" population. It has been the author's experience that athletes, in particular, may frequently have a disturbance affecting the concept of visual midline which can dramatically affect their performance. Simply because there is a dysfunction of the visual midline in the normal population does not necessitate treatment of it. Rehabilitation using the neuro-optometric approach should only be carried out when performance is affected and function is compromised.

Other Observations of Posture Associated with VMSS

Lateral shift of the visual midline will affect the relative position of the shoulders to the trunk or pelvis. In most circumstances a VMSS shift away from the affected side will cause the non-affected shoulder to appear elevated and the non-affected side of the pelvis to be depressed, causing lateral extension or expansion on the non-affected side, and lateral flexion or compression on the affected side of the body. While this posture will be observed by the clinician in the majority of cases, a reverse posture is possible causing a lowering of the shoulder opposite the affected side.

Posture for the patient with an anterior or posterior shift of the VMSS depends on the dynamics of movement and compensations associated with this. A typical anterior shift of VMSS causes a flexion forward with weight bearing on the toes or balls of the feet. However, the clinician should be cautioned not to misidentify a posterior VMSS with weight shift on the heels but with the compensatory posture of positioning head, neck and even shoulders forward as "ballast" to reduce the risk of falling backwards. The opposite situation may also occur. An anterior shift will sometimes be represented with head, neck and shoulders extended backwards (capital extension) while the weight bearing is shifted forward on the toes.

Confusion about VMSS

Understanding VMSS requires an understanding of the bimodal visual process. There have been a number of publications[3-6,] written by authors who have demonstrated that although they have attempted to assess and treat VMSS with yoked prisms, their understanding of the bimodal visual process and the effect of a neurological event such as a CVA or an acquired brain injury (ABI) is limited. They have described VMSS in terms of a conscious awareness of the egocenter or what the person consciously interprets as the perceived location of the projected center of his own personal space. This has led some to mistake a shift in attention delivered through the focal visual process for the preconscious shift of the ambient visual process. This is a critical point.

The ambient preconscious visual process is a component of awareness, but it is responsible for establishing an accurate relationship between the sensorimotor process and the spatial visual process. This in turn becomes the foundation for the focal process to match conscious egocenter with the preconscious percept of visual midline. When the ambient process becomes affected through a neurological event, the postural orientation becomes compromised, thereby affecting the ability to remain upright against gravity. This does not occur because of a misinterpretation of conscious space and conscious egocenter. It occurs because of an altered percept between the sensorimotor system and the ambient visual process that is preconscious in nature.

Unfortunately, some clinicians[4,5] have misunderstood the visual process and, as noted, have attempted to explain the VMSS in terms of the conscious focal awareness of egocentcr and its localization. This lack of understanding about the bimodal visual process will always lead to misdiagnosis and ultimately to yoked prism prescriptions in the wrong direction. It will cause a misinterpretation of egocentric visual midline shift, or the perception of "straight ahead," being in the opposite direction for patients with unilateral spatial inattention compared to those with homonymous hemianopsia. The misinterpretation is the result of not understanding that VMSS is a visuo-spatial-postural phenomenon, and that when this visuo-spatial-postural relationship is disturbed it can create distortion in the focal visual process due to the lack of fundamental spatial support from the ambient and sensorimotor processes

The VMSS will always result in a shift away from the affected side. This is true whether there is a hemiparesis, homonymous hemianopsia or a spatial neglect. The only exception to this is in the case of a paradoxical VMSS which develops because the compensation for the neurologically affected side does not occur during the early stage of recovery and adaptation. This leaves the person in an uncompensated state and causes him to initially lean into the affected side rather than away from it.

The confusion about visual processing has led some clinicians to create a dichotomy between cortical processing of vision (termed "top-down") and sensorimotor/visuo-spatial visual processing (termed "bottom-up"). Some emphasize that conscious top-down visual processing leads function. The reality is that both top-down and bottom-up processing occur simultaneously. One provides a "feedforward" of spatial information and the other gives "feedback" to refine and filter information.

Summary

The Visual Midline Shift Syndrome represents another perspective on viewing posture, balance and movement, particularly for patients with neurological dysfunction. It is obvious that there is a neurological basis for the postural disorientations in those with traumatic brain injury or cerebrovascular accidents. Treating a person with Visual Midline Shift Syndrome is not a cure for the neurological dysfunction. Rather, when undertaken by those with a thorough knowledge of the visual process, it is a means of rehabilitation that can often influence and maximize potentials beyond the more conventional approaches for treating these disorders.

Chapter 8

PERCEPTUAL DEVELOPMENT OF THE SIGHTED CHILD

William V. Padula

To perceive, an individual must first be able to discern differences. If there are no differences resolved, perceptual experience will be lacking or inappropriate.

The sighted infant can experience visual differences. He fixates on objects, pursues movement, and displays general visual attention. Different visual stimuli demand his attention. He may notice differences in brightness, color and movement. He may not, however, experience a perceptual difference in distances of two objects. Perceptual discrimination develops along with physical abilities, intelligence levels and environmental influences.

The infant's earliest visual attention is fixation on a light source.[1] As the infant matures, he will fixate on objects and forms. Fixation represents a type of perception. He has discriminated a figure from the ground. He has recognized a contrast between two visual stimuli. The development of figure-ground perception is important because it marks the ability to discern visual relationships. With maturity and physical development, the infant utilizes figure-ground perception as a basis for developing other forms of perception.

As his motor coordination improves, the child will become intrigued by his extremities and his ability to control movement. Fixation on the hand is first noted during the asymmetric tonic neck reflex. The head turns in the direction of the extended arm. When an alternation of asymmetric tonic neck reflex occurs, so does the fixation. The reinforcement of the kinesthetic awareness of arm extension with visual fixation gives the infant an awareness of his near-space world. As he gains greater control of his extremities and is able to manipulate objects, he begins to develop form perception and object constancy. The tactile sense is a concrete experience for the child and will be used to reinforce the experience of vision. In turn, the child begins to transfer information from one sensory modality to another, ultimately building various perceptual experiences.

The child develops perceptual experience by extracting and analyzing information from the environment through his senses. The more able he is to extract information and discriminate similarities and differences in information received, the easier it will be for the child to build his perceptual experience. Many factors influence the development of the perceptual experience. Physical factors can interfere with the reception of information; emotional and psychological factors may interfere with the ability to both extract and analyze information. The analysis of information, of course, deals with meaning. Therefore, perception involves discerning relationships about information received in order to establish meaning.

Development of the Sighted Child

As the normally sighted infant develops, he shows increasing alertness and makes contact with the world through his vision. The infant learns to use his vision to guide his developing motor system. This is the most efficient and effective means for the infant to deal with his environment.

In 1906 Sherrington published a monograph[2] with his well known "second law" the law of reciprocal innervation, which states that the inhibition of one set of muscles while opposing muscles are in excitation is a condition of coordinated movement. He asserted that the structural basis for this physiological mechanism is gradually built up by ontogenetic maturation (the life cycle and biological development of a single organism). There are two types of muscle groups: flexor and extensors. These are opposing muscle groups which, through growth, are brought into reciprocity. The maturation process tends to be rhythmic and for a given period of development emphasis on the flexor component of a behavior pattern is preceded by an extensor period. The flexors emphasize compression and may be linked with visual attention (i.e., focal behavior). The extensor periods relate to an expansion of the perception of both internal and external space, and may be associated with a more general awareness of the visual field (i.e., ambient behavior). The relationship between reciprocal innervation associated with flexor and extensor tone, and a visual process emphasizing focal and ambient function are quite similar. The neurological interweaving which brings together opposing motor components is also responsible for changes in visual function relating to the focal and ambient visual processes.

This reciprocal interweaving relationship involves not only gross posture and locomotion but can also be related to vision, as has been mentioned. Gesell, Ilg and Bullis[3] discuss this relationship in depth: "It operates in sensory-motor aspects of vision, where a host of double alternatives calls for harmonization and modulation: monocular versus binocular fixation; near versus far focus; central versus peripheral awareness; incoming versus outgoing fusion; abductive versus adductive eye movements; skeletal versus visual components; left versus right ocular dominance."

The following description of development of the normally sighted child is a review of the noteworthy work of Gesell et al.[3] studying the relationship of vision to development. Adaptation of this material has been made to provide greater emphasis on focal versus ambient function.

The functioning of the newborn's physiological and perceptual vision is peripheral, or ambient, in nature. The child will track an object as long as the movement of the object is beyond his central fixation. According to Trevarthen and Sperry[4] there are two mechanisms of visual functioning: focal visual function and ambient visual function (as discussed in Chapter 1). For the infant the visual system functions primarily as a signal detection system. The evolution of such a process is, of course, for survival. Lower-order animals, which have not developed a focal ability, respond to movement as either a signal of impending danger or a food source.

The ambient visual process, through matching information in the sensorimotor feedback loop, provides a spatial orientation that enables the child to then develop a focalization on the outstretched hand. This is the first time that he is able to match information received through one sensory modality (vision) with another (kinesthesia and proprioception). In the asymmetric tonic neck reflex the child begins the process of restricting his visual awareness to a particular aspect of time and space rather than operating in the state of sensory scan. Over time, an ability to control the ambient and focal states will develop.

When the child has an ability to focalize and release with equal control, development will appear balanced and symmetrical. Increased focal ability will develop reciprocally during stages of asymmetry, i.e., a tonic neck reflex. Table 8-1 summarizes the chronological visual development of the sighted child.

TABLE 8-1. DEVELOPMENT OF THE NORMALLY SIGHTED CHILD

Age	Visual Development
0-8 weeks	• Monocular visual fixations in asymmetric tonic neck reflex • Spatially oriented ambient function • World segmented
8 weeks	• Begins to develop binocular control • Able to converge the eyes • Near-to-far fixations demonstrated • More focal in attention • Unable to fixate at midline
16 weeks	• Shows general awareness of environment • Stimulated by peripheral movement to direct central vision toward an object • Fixations across midline show delay
20 weeks	• Intensified focal visual behavior with fixations on objects at near range • Fixations at midline improve • Eye-hand orientation control improves
24 weeks	• Able to team eye-hand responses • When seizing object with hand, child will bring it to his mouth (refining form and substance perception)
28 weeks	• Immediately releases object after touching lips (Evidence of developing perceptual constancy) • Demonstrates general awareness of surroundings
32 weeks	• Able to localize auditory sounds by directing visual fixation on sound source • Focalization extends to more distant environment • Seems unable to deal with tri-dimensionality of space; instead, segments space and seems to look at an object moved from one position to another as a completely new object

40 weeks	• Deals with the world as a whole • Rises to hands and knees and begins to creep • Visual attention diminishes as child explores new balance and visual-motor relationships
12 months	• Rises to feet and begins to walk • Focalization that began to appear for short period disappears as child explores visual-motor relationships • After balance improves, the child will again develop interest in detail and will focalize visual function • Looks back and forth between hand and object when attempting to grasp object
15 months	• Becomes more aware of relationship between sight and sound • Visually focuses on the object he intends to grasp rather than between hand and object
18 months	• Driven by motor movement • Ambient visual function • Attention fleeting • Able to build blocks vertically
21 months	• Visual focal behavior • Actively looking and visually intense • Visually cautious • Balance falters • Gives thought to visual situations and appears to ponder a situation before becoming involved
2 years	• Predilection for small objects • Focal behavior continues • Develops dimensions of language to visual-spatial dimensions • Increased eye-hand coordination
2 ½ years	• Easily distractible • Very peripheral • Increased ability to discern relationships between other senses and vision (using past experiences)
3 years	• Plans in advance • More attentive to eye-hand coordination • Central in attention • Able to confine to boundaries and draw rather than scribble
3 ½ years	• Becomes uncertain and anxious about abilities • Clings for protection • Fear of high places
4 years	• Understands symmetry • Very assertive • Sees part-to-whole relationship • Seems to shift from one thing to another
5 years	• Greater stability and much more in charge of situation • Deals with one thing at a time • Greater ability to make vertical strokes than horizontal • Able to match according to size and shape

6 years	• Appears clumsy • Becomes unsure of himself • Attempts oblique stroke • Eruptive behavior
7 years	• Withdrawn and pensive • Lacks self-limits • Easily frustrated • Prints smaller
8 years	• Expansive • Increased social behavior • Grasps totality

In the first 8 weeks the visual system of the sighted infant has not developed coordination of binocular fixations. Just as his motor movements are erratic and show lack of control, so are his eye movements. Fixation is monocular, and unilateral divergence and convergence movements are seldom observed. Because the infant is still exhibiting the asymmetric neck reflex, monocular eye fixation to his outstretched hand may occur. As the infant shifts from the left to the right side, fixation often changes from one eye to the other. His visual world is segmented.

At 8 weeks of age the sighted infant begins to develop enough control to binocularly align his eyes to fixate and converge. This establishes new spatial relationships since there is a transition from near to far through the convergence and divergence of the eyes. The infant at this age is intrigued by bright objects like candle flames, and increases his attention to the object when it is moved.

By 16 weeks the infant begins to respond to his visual world as if he were experiencing a new setting. He shifts his attention, showing increased awareness. Fixation changes are easier for the infant when he is in the supine position.

At 20 weeks fixation intensifies and the infant focuses on objects placed within a near range at chest-high level. He watches objects at his midline with increasing efficiency. Before this period, visual fixations across the midline showed delays of eye movements or loss of fixations. The coordination of binocular fixations on the midline permits the child to improve head manipulations, and by 24 weeks he is able to team eye-hand responses.

When the infant seizes an object with his hands, it is drawn immediately to his mouth. This response indicates that he is developing perception of form and substance. The infant is using tactile information to reinforce vision. As his visual perceptual experiences are reinforced by other senses, he will no longer need this added input to derive meaningful information about an object. By 24 weeks the infant immediately releases the object upon touching it to his lips. He relies on his visual interpretation of the object and has less need for other sensory reinforcement. The infant is more inspectional.

By the age of 32 weeks the infant is able to localize sounds beyond his reach. This ability reinforces the infant's visual projections into his space environment. He is still unable to conceive of the tri-dimensionality of his environment. He needs additional experiences to develop depth perception. However, the 36-week-old infant shows better orientation in space.

At 40 weeks the infant responds to the totality of a situation. He views the world as a whole rather than as isolated or segmented portions. Development continues in a series of cycles. When a cycle is repeated, the infant uses his newly acquired abilities to examine his environment in a new way. New perceptual experiences are developed. In contrast to the 32-week-old infant, the cycles of development have brought the 40-week-old to a more focalized regard of his environment. At this age the infant can be observed to shift objects obliquely. This is a method of exploiting and reorganizing his perceptions of space. Spatial exploration through motor movement and visual organization progressively constructs a perceptual model or an interpretation of the three-dimensional domain. By the age of 40 weeks the infant begins to explore the relationships of three dimensions.

The 1-year-old child shows a basic understanding of his three-dimensional domain. At this age he shows auditory perception of distant objects. It appears that the basic understanding of three-dimensional space develops through an interweaving of multi-sensory experiences. The child is able to sight an object visually, reinforce the sighting with motor movement involving tactile and kinesthetic input, and also integrate the auditory perception of sounds with visual and motor perception of distance. Spatial perception is also observed with the child's ability to move objects alongside or above another object.

By the age of 1 year the child shows increased interest in small objects such as buttons and buckles. At this age he appears intrigued with the permeability of his space world and shows interest in placing objects through holes. There is also an awareness of emotions perceived through facial expressions. The child may begin to imitate these expressions.

At 15 months the child becomes more acutely aware of the relationships between sights and sounds. He demonstrates interest in following moving objects or people, particularly if there are accompanying sounds. The child's motor movement and hand manipulations have continued to improve. At 1 year of age, when the child wanted to place an object in something else, he picked up the object and watched his hand move toward the final position. As the hand approached the final position, correctional movements would then be made to bring the object into the desired position. The 15-month-old child grasps the object but looks at the point toward which he is directing his movement.

The child's development proceeds with a purpose to maximize efficiency within his environment. Vision as the dominant sense allows the child maximum efficiency and a conservation of energy. Because of this, the child allows vision to lead motor movement.

By 18 months the child is strongly driven by motor movement. This drive is so strong that it appears as if motor function is leading vision. The child is occupied by the present, and his attention appears to flit from one activity or thing to another. At this age he is able to build blocks vertically but has difficulty arranging them horizontally.

Growth is rapid during the next several months, and by 21 months the child's behavior and perceptions of the world have changed dramatically. Vision is dominant and the child is both visually alert and visually tense. He approaches activities and people with caution. His spatial orientation to the environment, particularly in new areas, becomes much more tentative. There appears to be more thought given to situations where only a few months earlier he seemed to act with little thought about the consequences.

By 2 years the child may have a fascination for small objects. At this age he uses words such as "where" to gain information concerning spatial perception. The ability to decode language by hearing it spoken allows the child to reinforce perceptual experiences. Like all of the child's perceptual experiences, meaningful language is concrete and does not deal with abstractions of an object or a situation. At 2 years there is also increased eye-hand coordination. Although fine motor tremors are still observed, the child has adequate control over gross movements.

The 2½-year-old child is easily distracted. The slightest movement in his peripheral vision will capture his attention. The best method to hold this child's attention to a task is to keep him involved manually and visually. At this age he has difficulty planning ahead; he is still occupied by the here and now. The 2½-year-old demonstrates increasing ability to discern differences through vision and other senses. This is an important development because the child uses past experiences to examine relationships. If the relationships about an object or situation are not detectable as a difference, then the child will interpret them as the same, such as when a child cannot feel the difference between a rectangular shape and a square shape.

At the age of 3, unlike at 2½ years, the child will plan in advance and show greater organizing ability. Eye-hand coordination is more accurate, and the child is not so distracted. He is more central in his attention, as observed in his paper and pencil work. He can confine himself to boundaries while drawing, whereas six months earlier he scribbled all over the paper. The 3-year-old also shows a preoccupation with the wholeness of things, or perceptual closure. He tries to organize things in symmetrical relationships and will become upset when the organization is broken.

By 3½ years the child becomes uncertain of his abilities, anxious in new situations, and he tends to cling for protection. He appears to view things in a segmented manner, and the organized holistic qualities previously exhibited seem lost in the child's confusion about relationships and parts. He will indicate a fear of high places and will appear generally clumsy.

By the age of 4 years the child again perceives symmetry in relationships. He has become very assertive, and the introspective qualities of the 3½-year-old have disappeared. His perception of the whole continues, but he is now also able to see the parts of a whole and the whole as parts.

The 5-year-old seems more stable than the 4-year-old. He appears much more in charge of things and knows his limits. He prefers dealing with one thing at a time and enjoys the accomplishment of finishing a task. The child has enough control to make vertical and horizontal strokes but is still unable to draw an oblique line. These perceptual patterns are related to the maturation level of his oculomotor system. The 5-year-old also discriminates according to size, position and form. He can demonstrate perceptual constancy by matching or grouping by size and form, but prefers to position in a vertical line. He is able to see parts without separating them from the whole.

Within a few months' time the static and stable 5-year-old turns into a reactive, unstable 6-year-old. This eruptive period marks a transition to a more complete and controlled child. The child often suffers from physical ailments, allergies and frequent infections. His motor behavior may be very clumsy, and binocular coordination shows fluctuations and momentary monocular shifts. The child will attempt to master the oblique stroke and demonstrate a variety of body shifts and paper rotations.

By 7 years of age the child's eruptive behavior dissipates, and he becomes a more stable personality. The 7-year-old is withdrawn and pensive. Thought precludes actions, and he appears to be reorganizing his thought processes and experiences. The visual process actively engages thought, experiences, and interpretation of information while it guides motor responses. Through self-organization the child develops habits that may appear somewhat fanatical. He carries himself to the extremes of a task and lacks self limits. The frustrations observed are an indication of inner tension and conflict. With this characteristic self-control, the child will also begin to print smaller.

The 8-year-old is expansive, similar to the 6-year-old. The child moves out on all levels. He is increasingly social and demonstrates a strong need for peer companionship. The 8-year-old draws from the organizational skills he developed as a 7-year-old as he learns to commit himself by drawing conclusions. He is able to grasp the totality of situations and to work through tasks without making imposing short-term goals or limits necessary. There are increased gross and fine motor coordination skills exhibited. His writing becomes more balanced and uniform, and his drawing indicates an increasing awareness of perspective relationships. This appears to be related to improved time and space orientation. In grasping the totality of space and the relationship to time, the child shows increasing ease in shifting from near to far activities. This differs from the 7-year-old who could work in only one plane, near or far, at a time. At this level the child also develops the concept of directionality.

The 9-year-old shows a growing sense of self-awareness, motivation and responsibility. He seeks responsibility and follows through on tasks. Expansiveness is counterbalanced by self-awareness as he realizes that the frontiers to explore are not only in the external world. He focuses attention on one activity at a time, an important implication for the educator.

By the age of 10 the child becomes less focused in attention and is more able to deal with his new self-awareness and the external world simultaneously. The 10-year-old, like the 5-year-old, is realistic, seeks accomplishment, and is well-oriented in his world. In general, he is a more balanced individual.

Chapter 9

PERCEPTUAL DEVELOPMENT OF THE CHILD WITH A VISION IMPAIRMENT

William V. Padula

The effects of both partial and total vision loss on the development of the child are discussed in this chapter. Before examining adaptations the child must make to a vision loss, a review of the development of the child with no visual impairment will be described, as well as the importance of vision to normal development. The purpose of examining the effects of vision impairment on development is to further emphasize the profound relationship of vision throughout all phases and aspects of a person's life. The goal is to tie together the model of vision, discussed in Chapter 1, with function and performance.

The discussion and statements describing the developmental stages have largely been derived from research that includes observations of many children and are based upon population norms.[1] It must be understood that for every fact related to human maturation there is an exception. With that in mind, the reader should use the text to form a broad understanding of development for the visually impaired child and the profound relationship of vision to development.

To understand the importance of the various senses in the perceptual development of the child, think about your own development. What is the very first experience that you can remember? Does it involve a visual experience, a motor experience, a tactile experience, an auditory experience, or a combination of sensory and motor experiences? How do you think the partially sighted or totally blind individual would respond to this question? Now you can begin to understand the function of individual senses in developing perceptual experiences.

The sighted newborn infant has a nondiscriminatory, sensorimotor system. Observation of the newborn finds random motor activity that is uncoordinated and segmented. Just as arm and leg movements are uncoordinated, so are ocular movements. The child will glance momentarily at a moving object with monocular fixations. In a baby's development a rudimentary form of binocularity occurs at about 8 weeks when he first fixates monocularly and then converges both eyes for momentary fixations. The infant now begins to develop a binocular space world through a reinforcement of vision and motor (eye-hand) coordination.

The maturing infant develops coordination of his motor and sensory functions through a process of utilizing sensory information to guide motor activity. The newborn infant has undifferentiated motor and sensory systems that begin to respond to sensory and motor information through reflexes and matching of information between sensory and motor processes at appropriate stages of development. The child must learn that his senses supply information that will yield economy and efficiency to his motor functioning. The process will involve learning how to control and manipulate the senses, while at the same time using motor reinforcement to form relationships.

The infant soon learns that his visual system will supply him with information about the environment that no other sense can. However, the visual process develops from the activities of a motor system. As Gesell et al.[2] so aptly stated, *"Vision is an act mediated by eye and brain, which emanates from a growing action system."*

The coordination of the visual-motor system permits the infant to begin to explore his environment. Visual-perceptual experiences develop from reinforcing vision with other motor-sensory experiences. The infant will prop himself on hands and knees and begin to creep at 7 months. The creeping movements become a visual exploration of his environment. Eventually the ability to stand erect at 10 months leads to walking at 12 months.

At this stage, motor activity is led by vision. The ability to maintain balance on two feet at 10 months is reinforced by matching information from the visual, vestibular and kinesthetic systems. These systems inform the child about position when he is perpendicular to the floor. Vision becomes more dominant as a sensory system as the child begins to walk. The visual system dynamically relays information about balance and movement, interrelating the motor and other sensory systems. However, as in crawling and creeping, the initial purpose of walking is to explore the environment and this movement is stimulated and led by the visual sense.

The infant begins to trust his visual process as he develops visual perceptual experiences that are reinforced by the other senses: audition, touch and kinesthesia. Of the three million nerve impulses that travel to the brain each second, two-thirds are generated from the eye.[2] Approximately 70% of the sensory nerve fibers in the entire body originate from the eyes. From these statistics we can begin to understand the profound importance of vision as a process affecting development of the child and the learning process.

Your personal experience that provided an answer to the original question, "What is the first experience that you can remember?" is usually relevant to this discussion. For most people the first thing that is remembered is a visual scene with a secondary awareness that it involved a motor activity. It is important to note that the experience stemmed from a very early point in your development and, for most individuals, vision was the primary experience and motor activity often the secondary experience. This illustrates the important relationship between the visual sense during early perceptual development and its link to motor development.

The Child with Low Vision

If we were to ask a congenitally blind individual the same question about the very first experience that he can remember, do you think his response would differ from the sighted or partially sighted individual? Since he would probably not be able to recount the experience visually, he would relate an auditory experience or a feeling. Also, if asked when this experience occurred, he may have more difficulty estimating the time period because there is no visualization of age or other experience allowing him to make a relative judgment. The experience that he recalls may be later in development compared to that of the sighted individual, because the child formulates perceptual experiences from individual senses at different developmental stages. Since vision is the dominant process, a sighted child will most often use vision to develop his first experiences, relating the other senses to the visual experience.[2] A congenitally blind child must learn to attend more formally to information received from the other senses. Since it is more difficult to initially utilize information from other senses to develop perceptual experiences such as object constancy, distance relationships, localization and direction, the child must wait for certain maturational levels before he can interpret the information and form perceptual relationships.

An interesting experiment by Fraiberg, Siegel and Gibson[3] showed that the normally sighted infant develops visual object constancy for a bell during the second quarter of his first year. In their experiment the low vision infant was unable to develop auditory object constancy until the last quarter of the first year. However, the low vision child was able to develop auditory object constancy to his mother's voice at the same age as the normally sighted child. Several factors may be involved. Under the experimental conditions, there was no survival instinct related to the bell. An infant does, however, learn to rely on his mother for nutrition and protection. If it is assumed that the newborn attends to auditory information for survival, he may develop auditory object constancy to tones important for survival, but not for interest. A loud noise may indicate danger and initiate a crying response. The mother's voice signals warmth, nutrition, and protection and may initiate a smile. As a developmentally dominant sense, vision supplies information about survival and also allows the child to continually scan the environment for interest and stimulation. The sighted child may initially respond to a sound auditorily but will use his eyes to visually manipulate and reinforce information about the sound source. This ability to continually reinforce audition with vision, and vice versa, seems to help a normally sighted child develop the ability to maintain auditory object constancy at a younger age than the visually impaired child, who may have more difficulty reinforcing one sense with another.

Perceptual experiences are derived through matching sensory and motor information and are developmental in nature. Also, since vision is the dominant process, early perceptual experiences will develop mainly through reinforcement between the other senses, the motor systems and vision. Because vision allows the child to manipulate and scan the environment, it will be the leading force to draw the child to the environment.

The blind child will prop himself on hands and knees at the same age (10 months) as the sighted child. However, the blind child will not advance himself by creeping until 12 months. Instead, the blind child will begin to rock back and forth, thereby replacing the visual stimulation with kinesthetic and vestibular stimulation. Thus the lack of vision interferes with the development of the infant. The delay in perceptual growth causes developmental lags.

The blind child's chronological age, or age from birth, is of less importance than is his developmental age. The developmental age is based on the child's perceptual and physical abilities and should be emphasized. This concept applies not only to visually impaired children, but to all children.

Developmental lags are apparent and expected for the blind child.[2,4] However, for the child with a partial sight loss, developmental lags may or may not be present with either presence or absence possibly related as well to a variety of factors such as intelligence, environmental influences and physical abilities.

As is the case for all children, the visually impaired child may use his intellect to adapt to and compensate for his disability. The visually impaired child may also use a variety of sensorimotor abilities to compensate for and eventually adapt to his visual impairment. Therefore he may skip a developmental stage or master an advanced stage early. Thus there is no direct relationship between degree of impairment and degree of developmental lag for those with partial sight.

The percentage of sight loss does not equal the percentage of vision loss. As described in previous chapters, *sight* is physical and refers to the eye and optic nerve sending information to the cortex. *Vision* encompasses physical attributes and psychological disposition; it refers to the dynamic process of matching information between sight and other sensorimotor modalities. The matching process is not passive. It is an active manipulation and examination of the details of our environment. The relationship of these details understood through this matching process forms a perception of the environment that is unique to each individual. When a child is unable to compensate for and adapt to sight loss, the matching process is affected. A developmental lag occurs because *vision* has been interfered with. While the relationship between *sight* and development is an indirect one, *vision* is directly related to development.

A developmental lag may be determined through observation of behavior. However, to accurately test, diagnose and classify the problem requires an experienced clinician. Since it is not within the scope of this text to give detailed methods of testing and scoring, it is suggested that the reader refer to sources listed on the web sites of the American Foundation for the Blind and/or the American Printing House for the Blind.

Development of the Blind Child

The development of the blind or visually-impaired child will proceed in a manner similar to the sighted child, but the lack of visual influence will cause developmental lags to become evident earlier than in children with sight. As previously described, just as normally sighted children have varying developmental lags because of different genetic, environmental and psychological backgrounds, blind and partially sighted children will also exhibit developmental lags. The amount of developmental lag is not directly proportional to the amount of acuity or field loss.

Table 9-1 summarizes the development of the totally blind child between birth and 5 years of age. It has been adapted from work by Gesell et al.[2] and Barraga.[5]

The discussion of development for the blind child is limited to the age of five because the variations in the child's ability to adapt and compensate for the lack of vision increases with age. Therefore, the accuracy of any developmental schedule for the visually-impaired child becomes more difficult to predict with increasing age.

TABLE 9-1. DEVELOPMENT OF THE BLIND CHILD

Age	Visual Development
16 weeks	• Hands to midline • Facial expressions • Searching eye movements • Auditorily attentive to familiar sounds • Exaggerated limb movement
28 weeks	• Transfers objects from one hand to the other • Hand preference may be noted • Shows greater recognition to familiar sounds • Greater oral tendencies for blind child • Tendency for prolonged rubbing of eyes • Sitting up may be delayed due to lack of visual interest and support; this will develop in several weeks
40 weeks	• Uses tactual and auditory cues to explore objects • Demonstrates interest with feet • Expresses first words • Props on hands and knees but does not creep; rocks back and forth
12 months	• Accurate scissors grasp • Strong motor drive by creeping • Continues to show curiosity with feet • Rocks continuously in seated position • Localizes sounds by directing hand toward sound source • Stands only if prompted
15 months	• Walks with one hand held • Gait is widespread with short steps
18 months	• Walks for brief periods

- Easily disoriented
- Will drop to floor to regain orientation
- Unable to use sound for orientation
- Releases objects into cup and retrieves them
- Lacks understanding of three-dimensional space
- Begins to develop concept of distance through audition and tactual-motor reinforcement
- Developing object constancy

24 months
- Walks with greater control
- Walks toward familiar sounds and voices
- Able to use sounds for orientation
- Tactually inquisitive

30 months
- Able to identify shapes of familiar objects
- Uses sound to explore consistency of objects and to further develop concepts of time and distance

3 years
- Begins to match information between motor movements and audition to develop three dimensional concept of space
- Improved motor-coordination and balance seems to keep the child motorically bound and very much aware of peripheral sounds
- Able to construct vertical row of blocks with one hand

4 years
- Appears to regress in many areas
- Timing and coordination falter
- Anxious and cautious of new situations
- Seems unable to cope with more than one action at a time
- Peripheral sounds or activities can cause frustration with the activity at hand
- Segmented understanding of space
- Appears disorganized

5 years
- Has developed a concept of body symmetry and, when touching body parts of another person, will search for corresponding eye or arm, etc.
- Motor-coordination improves
- Seems more in control of situations and likes to be actively involved

The 16-week-old blind infant will meet most of the diagnostic developmental norms of the sighted infant (see Table 8-1). However, deviations in behavior will be noted as a result of his visual loss. The blind child will bring his hands to his midline and demonstrate active, spontaneous fingering of his hands. This is also seen in sighted infants. When the child expresses excitement he will breathe heavily and laugh spontaneously. The blind child will also demonstrate a searching or groping type of pursuit movement with his eyes when attempting to locate objects with his hands. The blind infant may appear to listen more than the sighted child.

Although all developmental norms in the blind child are met at this stage, various motor movements and postures may be observed that are different from those of the sighted child. Head rotations may appear restricted, and there may be exaggerated movements of the head and limbs. Both sighted and non-sighted children will cease all movement upon hearing a familiar sound or voice. It appears as if the child is attempting momentarily to suppress all other sensory stimuli, including vision for the sighted child, to direct his attention to sound. The primary difference will be that the sighted child will then attempt to direct his vision to the sound, thereby allowing him to transfer information between sensory modalities.

At 28 weeks the blind child continues to meet developmental norms. He will transfer objects from one hand to the other and on a tactile cue will reach out for an object with one hand. A hand preference may be noted at this time. His hands will be open more than during previous ages. He is able to roll to a prone position. At this age the child will also begin to show greater recognition and partiality to certain sounds that have become important to him.

The child will lift his head from the supine position and should be able to sit erect momentarily and support his weight when in a standing position. However, due to the lack of visual stimulation, motor development such as sitting and standing may not appear at this time. Since the child lacks vision, he may not be interested in sitting or standing. Within a short time this behavior should change.

At this age the blind infant will show greater oral tendencies than the sighted child. He may often touch his tongue with his fingers. Mouthing of objects allows the blind child to reinforce tactile experiences concerning form and substance. As his sense of touch becomes more developed, he will have less need to gain information by mouthing objects. Other deviant behaviors may include frequent and prolonged rubbing of his eyes.

By 40 weeks the blind child, with tactual and auditory cues, will explore a small object with his index finger and pick it up with a pincer grasp. He will also show an interest in his feet and will play with them often. At this age his expansion into the near environment also leads him to exploration of distant parts of his body. His first words (mama, dada) are usually spoken at this age, and he becomes more social. He will be aware of disapproval and will become upset when scolded.

The sighted child at this age will creep on hands and knees about his crib or the floor. The blind child will prop himself up on his hands and knees but will not begin to creep. Instead, he will rock back and forth. Since he lacks visual stimulation, he has no need to move forward, so he will seek kinesthetic stimulation by rocking. Any forward creeping movements will be a consequence of seeking kinesthetic stimulation. The age of 10 months usually marks the first sign of a lag in development, and it clearly relates to visual loss. The child will sit up straight but will not pull himself to a standing position unless helped. His postures and movements, particularly in the prone position, although better coordinated than at 28 weeks will still appear disjointed and impulsive. He will continue to mouth his hands and objects with more than normal frequency.

The 1-year-old blind infant will show an accurate scissors grasp and transfer an object from one hand to the other. He will not be satisfied by only listening but will demonstrate a stronger motor drive. He will creep without prompting and, in general, will show an exploring behavior. With prompting and support, the child will stand and take a step or two. In the supine position he will continue to show curiosity for his feet. In the seated position he will rock constantly. He will localize sounds and direct hand movement. This marks an important phase in the child's development of spatial perception.

By 15 months the child will walk with one hand held and begin to walk by himself. His gait will be widespread, and his steps will be short. To maintain maximum balance the child may shuffle along the floor.

The 18-month-old child will walk about the room for brief periods. If he does not come into contact with any objects, he will seek orientation by dropping to the floor. The three-dimensional space world through which he walks is boundless. The child should be encouraged to walk and investigate. Tactual stimulation, such as placing a large ball at the child's feet, will give him a sense of direction and orientation. As he shuffles his feet forward, he will come into constant contact with the ball as he dribbles it across the floor.

The child will also be able to drop objects into a cup and retrieve them. He will remain alert to auditory and tactile clues about his spatial environment. He will approach stairs and investigate them with caution. His comprehension of the steps in three-dimensional space is lacking; therefore, he will not attempt to climb them. The child will be able to discriminate various geometric forms tactually. A form box can be used to encourage the child to explore and retrieve different shapes from within the box. When the form is placed in the correct hole and falls in, the child experiences a tactile loss and hears the sound of the object as it falls into the box. The association of the tactual loss and sound will help develop object constancy for the child.

Since he does not have the visual abilities to manipulate and investigate his environment and develop various forms of perception, the child will, through sensory transfer, reinforce sensory information to construct his perceptual models. At this age the child will overturn a cup to find a hidden cube that was previously presented both tactually and auditorily. This is further evidence of the development of object constancy.

By the age of 24 months the child is able to stand and walk with greater facility, although his posture is rigid, stance wide and steps small. Sounds and familiar voices will stimulate the child to walk in that general direction. The child will take several steps and stop, attempting to reorganize information for orientation and direction. He may also squat intermittently to bring himself in contact with the floor to gain stability.

The child will begin to explore and may climb several stairs. This may be very disorienting to him since he has previously explored only flat planes such as the floor. The blind child lives in a flat, two-dimensional world. His visual deficit does not allow him to view the world from different perspectives; his only contact is through tactual and auditory means. When the child is picked up, he loses contact with his reference plane. He has no idea of the distance which he has traveled to his parent's shoulder because he has no relative reference plane.

By 24 months the child will build several wide blocks vertically. For that activity he should be encouraged to use one hand to gain information about the position and location of the tower of blocks. Blocks may be introduced by tapping them on the table to give him a sound cue. At this age he will be more tactually inquisitive and will show random motor movement.

The 30 month old blind child will identify the shapes of familiar objects such as a ball or box by manipulating them. After he has identified the object, he will shake it briefly with one hand and then release it. The sound of the object hitting another surface is then associated with the release of the object from the hand. In that way, the child begins to build a time and space relationship without active movement from one place to another. Previously in his development, time and space relationships were formulated by an active motor movement such as creeping or walking from one position to another. By approximately 30 months the child will begin to explore the environment, using himself as a reference point. His horizon will be extended from the limits of his reach to the limits of sounds which he can create by throwing an object.

By 3 years of age the child will begin to examine his relationship with the ground below him. He will take objects placed on a table in front of him and move them to the edge of the table where he will release them. From the sound of the objects coming into contact with the floor, the child further constructs his perception of the three-dimensional world. When the object is retrieved for the child, he will respond by duplicating the act, much to the dismay of his kind-hearted teacher. It may appear as if the child is purposely attempting to be aggravating; however, the simple retrieval of the object has fascinated him. From the retrieval, he has learned the permanence of things. There are limits to his world, and sounds created by objects coming into contact with another surface represent a limit on structure to his environment.

At 3 years the child will sit erect but will show exaggerated head movements. When manipulating an object, he will rotate his head into various positions while rolling his eyes in a random movement. His coordination has improved to the extent that he can pedal a tricycle and delight in the sensation.

The 4-year-old in many respects will appear to regress in development. His timing and coordination will falter. He may also become very cautious and show fear in activities that he accomplished with no difficulty six months previously. He will become frustrated and even rebellious at certain tasks.

The 4-year-old's conceptualization of space is segmented. At an earlier age (3 years old), he was able to construct a tower of blocks at his midline using one hand to locate the position and the other to place them. At 4 years old the child will attempt to build them with both hands. He loses the relationship of one block to another. His concept of the whole has been temporarily disorganized. This is a period of regrouping and reorganizing perceptual experiences and skills.

The rapid advancements in perceptual development during the first four years of the blind child's life closely parallel that of the normal child. Because of his visual deficit, developmental lags occur. Those lags will vary from month to month. The child may appear to be developmentally behind six months at one age and then show almost no lag when observed at another age. At one age the child may be unable to utilize other sensory information in place of his vision to create a particular perceptual experience, and a lag occurs in development. Within a few months the child is able to utilize the same information in a new way that becomes meaningful to him, such as utilizing another sense in place of his vision. This allows him to establish the perceptual experience. Upon establishing this experience and finding a new way to examine his environment, he may decrease his developmental lag in a relatively short period of time. From 5 to 9 years of age the development of the blind child will be more stable in advancement but will show fluctuations according to his particular developmental level. The developmental lag should also stabilize. It becomes apparent that the first four years are perhaps the most important of the blind child's life. It is during this time that he constructs the framework which he can build on later.

By understanding the major influence of vision on development, we can be more effective in designing therapeutic programs for children and rehabilitation programs for impaired individuals. It is important to examine the use of current terminology as it relates to any impairment to increase uniformity within the field for classification and treatment.

The most commonly used terminology describing vision difficulties includes: visually impaired, visually handicapped, low vision individuals, sight deprived, partially sighted, legally blind, blind and sight impaired. These are often very misleading and vary in popularity according to geography and from one agency to another. The federal government sometimes sets trends through the use of various descriptive terms in existing legislation and grants.

Because of misconceptions concerning what vision is, finding a single general term to describe the anomaly of impairment has not been a simple task. The most popular terms presently used are visually handicapped and visually impaired. However, the use of the word "visually" implies a condition well beyond the scope of present standardized testing, diagnosis and treatment.

The standards set by the Department of Health and Human Services for determining the proper classification of visually impaired, legally blind and blind stem from the measurements of the individual's visual acuity and visual field. The definition of *legally blind* states that a person must have a visual acuity of "20/200 or less in the best-corrected eye, or less than a 20-degree visual field." Typically, "20/70 or less in the best-corrected eye" is the standard for partially sighted, visually disabled or visually impaired. These definitions describe measurements that are taken during an eye examination and may not describe how the individual functions in his environment. The visual acuity and the visual field measurements indicate the impairment to the eyeball and to the individual's sight but do not necessarily indicate functional-perceptual abilities.

The static measurements of visual acuity and visual fields are measurements of eyesight. Vision, on the other hand, is a process by which visual input is related to motor movement, balance, thought processes, endocrine function, metabolism or any other action within the body. The relationship is not a one-way process but an interchange between motor, sense, thought, and physiology, which influences function and perception. Vision, therefore, is a dynamic process and should be analyzed as such.

An individual with impaired acuity or field has impairment to his sight but may not be impaired visually. The converse is also true; an individual may not be sight-impaired but may have other problems (e.g., visual midline shift syndrome) causing deficits in visual abilities. The impairment to sight may cause impairment to vision. However, the extent of visual impairment cannot be predicted or measured by assessment of only acuity and field.

The term low vision is presently used very broadly. It describes the concept or general classification under which other classifications and services are provided and should not be used to describe the individual. Measurements taken while testing to determine the low vision classification really determine only sight impairment.

The type of treatment most commonly available to those with sight impairment is the low vision examination. This includes testing of sight and the prescription of optical aids to improve sight. These aids are very important to the rehabilitation of the sight-impaired individual. But there are many individuals who receive various optical aids and are not successful in using them.

Providing that the aids have been accurately prescribed, one of the reasons for the lack of success is the inability of the individual to adapt his visual processes to accommodate the optical aid. For these visually-impaired individuals, neuro-optometric rehabilitation can often provide the understanding of their complex visual processing dysfunction that is interfering with success in using optical devices. It involves developing the use of the *process* of vision, not just eyesight.

Within the area of low vision utilization, some professionals have already begun investigation and treatment. Terms such as vision stimulation, visual efficiency and visual functioning have been used to describe the programs that have been developed to improve the visual process of visually-impaired individuals.[5-8] Training in how to use optical aids is also included in this category.[9,10]

Because of the importance vision has to the development and learning process, most of the work that has been developed in this area has been directed toward children.[11] Programs to improve visual abilities in adults have, in general, been overlooked by those working in the low vision field. Much more investigation into new techniques and methods of treatment is needed.

Chapter 10

EXAMINING THE CHILD WITH PHYSICAL DISABILITIES

William V. Padula

The child with motor impairments in addition to visual impairment has complex functional and habilitative needs. As described in the chapter about development and vision, the learning experience of a child with a motor impairment is limited, sometimes severely, because information cannot be matched accurately between motor and sensory input. The impairment often affects speech patterns, visual discrimination, movement, balance, posture and sensory discrimination. Having to deal with a motor impairment as well as sight impairment frequently causes medical and educational professionals to overlook the often serious visual difficulty.

Both sight impairment and/or vision impairment have been called "the hidden disabilities" because in most instances they cannot be seen. On the other hand, a motor impairment such as a deformed limb, abnormal posture, or increased or decreased postural tone is more obvious. While their intentions are good, professionals and lay persons usually treat the motor impairment as soon as possible with medical and therapeutic techniques. Progress in educational and habilitative therapy is often limited because the sight and/or vision impairments are not treated at the same time.

Unfortunately, most children with physical disabilities do not receive appropriate vision services until they are of school age and particular problems with visual discrimination are observed. The exception is where a child has strabismus and the eye turn is visible. In this case a referral will often be made for the consideration of surgery. While this at least enables the child to have an eye examination, this form of treatment often does not consider the relationship of visual function and performance to the overall neuromotor and functional abilities of the child.

Previous discussions have emphasized that the motor system provides a base for visual function. It is critical that the motor-impaired child is evaluated not only in terms of eye health, ocular motility and alignment, but also with regard to the functional relationship between the visual and neuromotor processes. The motor system, through the influences of the kinesthetic and proprioceptive systems, will affect how the child utilizes the visual process. This effect will take the form of variations in eye alignment, tracking ability, accommodative function, fixation abilities, and a variety of other functional behaviors.

Case Report

At the time of the evaluation, Andrea was 3 years old and diagnosed with cerebral palsy with increased postural tone. She demonstrated a right esotropia and an inability to track and fixate when she was placed in a sitting position. While in the seated position her head and neck were flexed and postural tone increased. When placed on her back on a mat with her pelvis lifted onto the examiner's knees, tracking patterns as well as alignment of the eyes improved.

The postural change affected Andrea's functional use of vision and demonstrates that the motor system does influence visual function. It particularly shows that stress in the neuromotor system will affect eye alignment and ocular motility. The sensory function of the visual system can be limited as well.

Developing a model of vision that incorporates the neuromotor system as the base for visual function enables us to understand how postural tone (hyper or hypo) develops. In turn, imbalances in the neuromotor system can affect the visual function and performance. It is therefore imperative that the multi-handicapped child be examined in a variety of positions to observe the effect of the neuromotor state on the visual system. When possible, the occupational and/or physical therapist should assist the optometrist or ophthalmologist in discussing the motor impairment and determining the appropriate positioning for the child. The following discussion will offer some guidelines for evaluating the multi-handicapped child with the understanding that there will always be individual exceptions.

Examination Procedure

When introduced to the child, the examiner should first observe the postural tone and whether a flexion or extension pattern exists. Flexion means that the child is leaning forward, typically with his head down and tucked to the chest. In the extension posture the child is positioned with head back and arms out. Hypotonic (low) muscle tone or hypertonic (spastic) muscle tone can occur in states of either flexion or extension. Secondly, the examiner should note if the child is leaning to one side, indicating a possible imbalance due to a weakness of the right or left side. Also, the examiner should review the type of chair, head supports or other prosthetics that may affect his posture and in turn affect vision. If the child is ambulatory, the examiner should observe the child standing and walking. When the child is able to stand on two feet, previously observed motor patterns may change. Bearing weight on the feet may cause a child who was in a flexion pattern while in a seated position to show extension postures or weight shifting to the right or left side while standing.

Head position is very important. The examiner should continually observe whether the head is rotated differently in standing or walking postures than in sitting postures. Also, is postural tone different in the standing or seated position?

If possible, a thorough history should be taken with the parent, therapist and educator accompanying the child. Information concerning the birth or any traumas incurred, as well as medical treatment and medications should be reviewed. If the child has had any seizures that information should be included with dates of occurrence. When the history reveals active seizures, the examiner should take caution not to flash lights directly into the eyes of the child since flashing lights, or even stimulation from a penlight turned on and off repeatedly, have been known to initiate seizures.

The examiner should then complete a thorough ocular health assessment, including external and internal evaluation of the eyes. If nystagmus (a constant and simultaneous jerk of both eyes caused by neurological problems) is present, a thorough evaluation should be made in the cardinal positions of gaze while the child fixates on an object. The nystagmus should also be evaluated when posture is varied, such as when the child is lying on his back or on his side. Changes in position that influence the vestibular and kinesthetic systems will sometimes change the amount of nystagmus. This is common in children with cerebral palsy. Often when the child lies on his back or side, nystagmus subsides and fixation abilities can improve.

A cover test in a variety of positions should be performed to evaluate eye alignment. Changes in kinesthetic and vestibular stimulation will often affect eye alignment. Not only should strabismus be evaluated, but the examiner should pay attention to states of phoria. The convergence ability of the child should be assessed. For a young or low functioning child, an interesting accommodative stimulus should be used. Not only should the quantity or extent to which the child is able to converge and maintain eye alignment be assessed, but the quality of his performance should be evaluated as well. That is, does the child work hard at converging his eyes, and does the examiner observe frequent fixation losses and an inability to sustain fixation on an object?

A thorough refraction using trial lenses and retinoscopy should be performed. Since the phoropter will affect the child's posture and position, it should not be used. Variations in posture will also affect the refraction. It is important that the child be placed in a position that is comfortable and supportive. A reclining position on a mat provides support and can enable the examiner to perform the refraction effectively. If the child is spastic, he needs to be supported with pillows or rolls so that his legs are not left suspended, and support to the back and neck is complete.

A near refraction should be performed after the distance refractive state has been analyzed. With the refractive corrections in place, the near refraction may be done while the child fixates on a small silver bell, a hand-held puppet, or another visually stimulating object. The near refraction should analyze whether accommodative (focusing) states are equal and balanced for the two eyes. In addition, the grasp and release of accommodation and how easily accommodation is sustained at the plane of regard must again be assessed. The near refraction should always be done in varying postures and fixations to different points of focus. When accommodation lags or varies, plus lenses should be introduced, and changes in fixation and accommodation evaluated.

When possible, touch-point (reaching and touching) activities can be used and accuracy measured. Touch-point activities should be performed with and without the distance prescription and again with plus lenses or those lenses found to be most effective in improving accommodative function.

Information about eye alignment, convergence ability, fixation and tracking should be analyzed in a manner that allows the examiner to functionally assess the patient's abilities, and to develop a means for visual rehabilitation. It is extremely important to provide information to parents, educators and therapists with regard to compensations that the child must make for visual inabilities. For example, the child with a right esotropia who attempts to establish binocularity may turn his head to the right. Materials presented to the left of the child's midline will be in a field of lesser demand, enabling the child to have better alignment of the head and neck. This will affect the child's balance and will further support the child in reaching and in eye-hand coordination. Unfortunately, the examiner often overlooks the opportunity to provide this information which, in addition to improving the child's functional ability, will also establish the credibility of the optometrist with the parents.

Retinoscopy with trial lenses and a trial frame should be included in the examination. As stated before, a phoropter is an inappropriate instrument to use to determine the appropriate lens prescription. Although trial lenses require more time and expertise, a more accurate prescription can be produced. In situations where the child responds negatively to trial lenses, radical retinoscopy can be used. In this procedure the optometrist varies his working distance and uses the reciprocal working distance when the neutral reflex is measured to determine the power of the refractive state. For the exact technique, the reader should review other sources mentioned in the reference sections of this book.[1]

Near retinoscopy should be performed before and after distance retinoscopic findings. Often children who have motor and neurological impairments will show imbalances in accommodative abilities. Unless this is treated, the ability of a child to function at a near range will be greatly compromised. The examiner should add plus lenses to distance retinoscopic findings until a balanced near finding is achieved. The examiner should do this despite the fact that one eye may accept +2.00 addition and the other eye +0.75 addition. The goal is to achieve balance in the visual system.

Balance in the visual system must be understood with respect to the motor and neurological imbalances that affect autonomic function. Imbalances in the motor and neurological function of the central nervous system can cause stress, affecting the autonomic nervous system, thus altering the accommodative response. Conversely, by utilizing lenses that reduce visual stress, it is not uncommon to observe postural changes. A confrontation visual field test may be effective in analyzing the scope of field. Children who have cortical visual impairment often also have a visual field loss. The visual field loss may interfere with the ability to relate the ambient process of vision to postural adjustments. For example, a child with a right homonymous hemianopsia (right field loss) will often neglect his right side. Since the child does not see in the right field of gaze, he places visual emphasis on motor functions of the left side. The neglect to the right side may interfere with handedness, posture, and balance while seated or walking.

Visual field testing may require two individuals. One, seated in front of the child, has a toy with which he is attempting to obtain fixation. The other individual, seated behind the child, introduces a penlight or other stimulating object in a peripheral arc from behind the child to the front midline. By patching one eye, the monocular visual field can be evaluated. The individual seated in front of the child must monitor the child's eye position. When the child first sees the penlight through peripheral awareness, he will often make a fixation change from the toy to the penlight. A rough approximation in degree or scope of field can be made by the person seated in front of the child.

Often visual field testing and visual acuity testing cannot be completed during the limited time of the in-office examination. It is important for therapists, parents and educators to follow through at home or in school in order to average information over a period of time. Parents, therapists and educators should be encouraged to perform these tests and bring findings to follow-up visits. The examiner will then be able to spend more time in other areas of testing and treatment to improve relationships among vision, motor and balance processes.

Upon completion of this assessment, the examiner should work with appropriate lenses and prisms in an attempt to establish greater balance of visual and motor functions. The examiner should seek information from the occupational and physical therapists regarding the child's motor abilities. Since the motor system provides the basis by which ocular alignment and visual skills are established, it is important to evaluate the child in a position that will offer the least stress to the central nervous system. If the clinician has a limited understanding of cerebral dysfunctions that cause cerebral palsy, muscular dystrophy, etc., he should consult with the physical and/or occupational therapist to learn about the neuromotor dysfunction. Generally, seating a child upright in a chair that does not support the child's pelvis or thoracic area may cause stress and increase motor spasticity. This can affect visual functions and cause ocular malalignment, accommodative imbalances and/or spasms. The spastic child needs an appropriate seat that offers support. The best position for a young child may be lying on his back on a mat with legs flexed up onto the examiner's thighs. In this way the pelvis is extended in the posterior portion with flexion in the abdominal area. Also, a small roll may be placed under the neck to support the head, as described previously.

Examination of the spastic child in this position often will show visual states that are completely different from those taken when the child is seated or standing. Another effective position in stabilizing the visual state is to roll the child onto his side while supporting the neck with a roll or pillow. The kinesthetic, vestibular, and tactual stimulation that he receives in this position may also reinforce visual functions. The clinician may find that fixation, tracking and convergence abilities improve considerably.

For the child with hypotonic (low) postural tone, posture should be supported so the head does not flex forward or to the side. Whatever support is necessary to reduce stress in the neuromotor system should be provided. This includes holding the child or supporting his head and neck with rolls or pillows so that stress is not induced. Another position that is effective in examining the hypotonic child is to have the child lie on his stomach over a large ball or a cylindrical roll that supports the child on the midline of the body. This kinesthetic and tactual stimulation on the midline will help the child organize central nervous system responses. This may affect visual functions, thus enabling the child to have improved fixations on the midline.

Emphasis must be placed on the support of the central nervous system and the reduction of stress throughout the neuromotor system for the examination of the multi-handicapped child. When this is achieved, the visual state may be analyzed with the least interference from either high or low motor tone conditions. This cannot be overstated: *the analysis must be continued utilizing lens and prism combinations to further affect vision and neuromotor function.*

The discussion of various neuromotor states will be dealt with in another chapter. However, it is important to emphasize here that the examiner must recognize that these conditions interfere with visual function, and very often visual states will reinforce and even cause conditions of flexion and extension patterns. The examination of the multi-handicapped child should not end at the point of correction of refractive states. The examiner must understand that the child's performance depends upon his ability to differentiate neuromotor functions as well as visual perception. When there is difficulty differentiating motor movements and organization within the central nervous system, the child will have difficulty in his ability to fixate and track. The converse is also true. When visual states interfere with ability to organize information, the child's ability to extend this organization to other sensorimotor processes will be affected. If visual stress can be reduced, it will have a positive effect on the differentiation of motor responses.

The examiner should observe postural shifts or adjustments that may be related to ocular alignment. If a child has an esotropia or an exotropia that is either congenital or surgically induced, appropriate compensation with yoked prisms may be considered. For example, as noted previously, if a child has a right esotropia and he is attempting to achieve binocularity, he may turn his head to the right. The head turn and the esotropia will often cause a midline shift due to the visual and oculomotor imbalance. This midline shift will affect his ability to posture himself properly, in turn affecting other motor functions such as reaching or walking.

After the refraction and evaluation have been completed, the clinician may decide to work with yoked prisms. In the case of right esotropia described above, yoked prisms with base-right orientation would be appropriate. Prisms of equal power would be added to each eye and placed with base-out for the right eye and base-in for the left eye. The prisms would essentially shift the visual field over to the child's left side. This is the area that offers the least demand on the child's vision. If the child has attempted to turn his head to the right, essentially he has tried to posture the visual world to his left. The base-right yoked prism will accomplish the same by shifting his visual world to the left. *However, more importantly, the spatial effect from the base-right yoked prisms shifts visual midline to the right and reestablishes sensorimotor and ambient visual relationships.* This may cause a change in postural adjustment. The child may align his head more directly on the midline because he does not have to compensate for oculomotor imbalances. Shifting the head to the midline will affect posture in the neck and shoulder areas. Often multi-handicapped children with this type of oculomotor compensation and postural shifts will have spastic or fixed tone in the neck or shoulder areas. This fixed tone is often due to the compensations for visual imbalances. The base-right yoked prisms, by shifting visual midline toward the right and shifting the image to the left, will reduce the state of muscle tension in the neck or shoulder area.

The child with a bilateral esotropia will often exhibit postural imbalances of a more severe nature. The young multi-handicapped child without the ability to align both eyes will attempt to posture the visual world in an area of least demand on his vision. For example, the child will often show extension of the head and neck. He will tip his head back, attempting to posture the visual world below his line of sight. For the multi-handicapped child this can cause a hypertonic situation in the head, neck and shoulder areas. In turn, an inability to accurately carry out upper-arm movements develops. Usually this fixed tone is dealt with through physical or occupational therapy. However, it must be recognized that this condition, too, is often the result of stress in the visual system. By placing base-up yoked prisms of equal power before each eye, the visual world will be shifted downward, or into an inferior position of gaze. The child will not have to extend his neck and head backward and, in turn, the visual field being shifted to an area of lesser visual demand will often produce a situation of decreased head extension and increased capital flexion. This is a more normal posture. In addition to posture, other behavioral symptoms of this condition are deep wrinkles and lines in the forehead. Because the child is unable to circumduct, or to elevate the two eyes together by manipulation of the superior rectus muscles, efforts by the child to elevate the eyes are referred to the frontalis muscle. As the frontalis muscle contracts, deep furrows are formed in the forehead.

A further indication that the hypertonic condition in the neck and shoulder areas can cause spasticity in the frontalis muscle can be understood by studying the anatomy of the head and neck. The frontalis muscle is connected to the galea aponeurotica, a thin tissue that extends from the frontalis muscle over the skull to the trapezius muscle in the neck. As the frontalis muscle contracts and pulls on the galea aponeurotica, tension will be created in the trapezius and neck muscles, causing high muscle tone in the neck and shoulder area.

Bilateral esotropia will also interfere with the child's ability to stand and walk because with the head in extension and the hypertonic condition in the neck and shoulder area, the midline is shifted to the posterior portion of the body. When the child attempts to bear weight on the feet, there may be overcompensation due to the shift of the midline posteriorly. This may in turn cause the child to lose balance, thereby interfering with the ability to stand or walk. Base-up yoked prisms may be effective in changing the visual-motor orientation, thereby affecting neuromotor functions.

By understanding the profound developmental relationship between the ambient visual process and the sensorimotor process, one can recognize that any neurological impairment causing a physical disability will affect the spatial aspects of the visual process. The important relationship to grasp at this point is: *What affects the neuromotor and sensorimotor systems affects vision. Also, what affects the balance of the focal and ambient visual process will impact the sensorimotor system, eventually affecting neuromotor function.*

Chapter 11

PHYSICAL CHARACTERISTICS THAT INFLUENCE VISUAL FUNCTION

Christine Nelson

In this chapter we will examine the special needs of individuals who have disorders of the central nervous system that affect their control of posture and movement and, in a large number of cases, their functional vision. This is a population that generally has no clear injury to the eyes per se, and yet may have great difficulty organizing the visual system to utilize information received from the environment. A "functional disorder" may have been noted early on without being identified as a specific problem that could respond to intervention. Neuro-optometric rehabilitation is a process that considers the person's physical characteristics/problems, and their relationship to visual function. Through this approach the functional inabilities of the individual are more completely understood and there is greater potential for remediation. The ultimate goal of neuro-optometric rehabilitation is to reduce vision-related deficits thereby improving function, mobility, and quality of life through the therapeutic use of prisms, and lenses in association with remedial techniques.

In the general population there are children as well as adults who have physical problems that are unrelated to the functioning of their visual systems. They may have a coincidental problem with vision along with conditions that affect the muscular system, such as polio or dystrophy, or physical injuries. Another group, including children, has well-defined neurological conditions such as hemiplegia due to stroke, in which there is a strong likelihood that the responses of the eyes will mirror the responses of the body. There are also many who do not demonstrate visual complications with such neurological conditions. On the other hand, homonymous hemianopsia, a type of visual field loss, may be a complication of a brain hemorrhage or infection without any clear physical manifestations that affect that individual's posture and movement.

Neurological disorders that exist from birth or occur as the result of accident or illness are seldom as clearly defined as an adult hemiplegia, as they are often not due to a limited area of the brain being affected but rather to developmental dysfunction. Children who have had problems since birth or an early age have never known the clear automatic feedback of normal postural control against gravity. In those cases, the central nervous system fails to perform its function of coordinating control of the body and thus alters the functional base of all sensory systems. The fundamental movement patterns of the eyes have no base from which to mature, and there is a lack of synchrony between eyes and body.

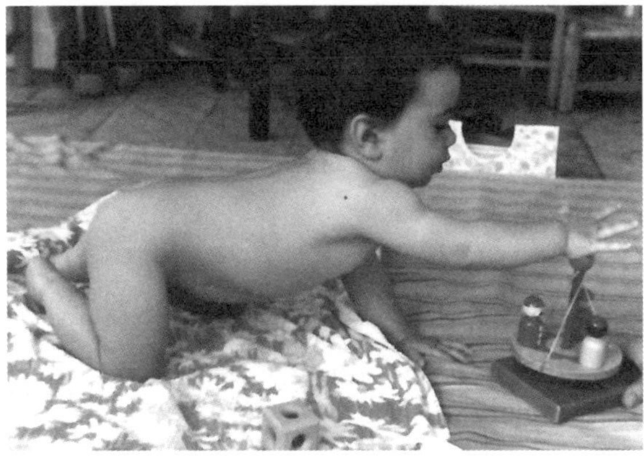

Figure 11.1. Normal posture. Normal posture control balances stability with mobility.

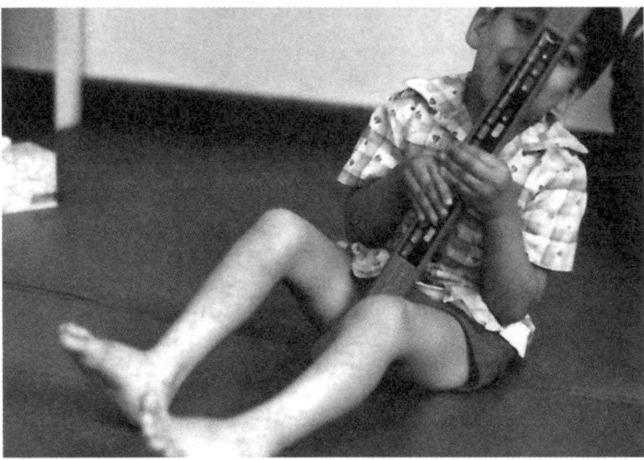

Figure 11.2. Abnormal posture. Excessive flexor tonus moves the center of gravity back and prevents comfortable floor sitting.

Conscientious evaluation is not easy. These children may have had more than the average number of disagreeable experiences with professionals merely because of their need for greater than average amounts of medical care. As infants and young children, they overhear comments that they don't understand, and are often handled in ways that are more efficient than sensitive. The similarity of any examination to these previous experiences may be disadvantageous to the optometrist. The ability to relate to the child beyond the disability will be a great strength. The fact that the small child can remain with his mother while responding to the optometrist also aids in establishing rapport. Brain-injured adults may also arrive in a very frustrated and depressed state, as many services offer diagnosis and general supervision rather than interventions that change their functional state.

A complete examination of any functional system requires that we take into account the lack of developmental experience available to that system. When we are considering the interaction of postural control, movement and vision, a child's seemingly simple play activity becomes complex. Dysfunction in any one of these systems, or limitations in their intercommunications, results in poor organization of environmental impressions. Children with cerebral palsy may have such inadequate postural reactions that they are dependent on another person or special equipment to position them against gravity. Movement may be disjointed and appear inappropriate to the task, even when the child understands clearly what needs to be done. When the message of the central nervous system is expressed in the form of inadequate postural and movement responses, all other systems must compensate to organize function. The visual system, due to its strength of relating directly to the environment, is one of the strongest sources of compensation. That means that the system learns to react in a way that maximizes the security of the person and delivers the best information about the environment.

As with substitute movement patterns, the compensatory efforts of the visual system reach their maximum effectiveness and then begin to interfere with further maturation. Adaptations that should be relegated to the preconscious level remain in a state of consciousness and interfere with new learning. Children with high postural tone, or spasticity, typically rely on total patterns of movement and may use eye movement upward to initiate extension. Relaxation of the eyes, then, reduces the high tonus and lets the head fall forward into gravity. The child who lacks postural control may have random, inappropriate movement of the eyes that mirrors the lack of postural control in his body.

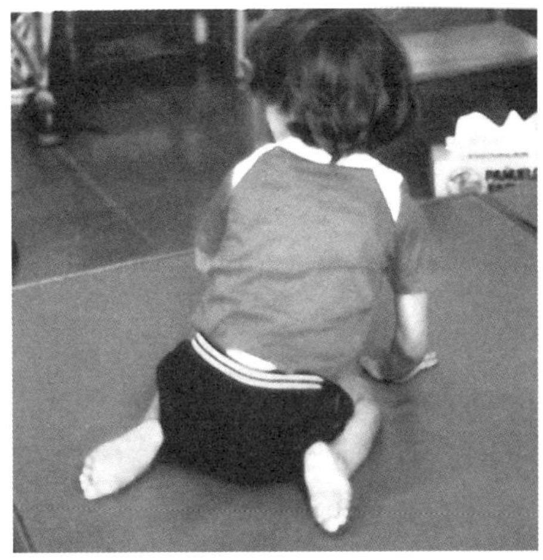

Figure 11.3. Sitting between legs. Sitting between the legs is to be avoided because it blocks active trunk adjustments for balance.

A functional orientation to the visual examination is essential for any person who has a neurological disability. Aside from the fact that it requires ingenuity and creativity to analyze the relationship between the visual system and behavior, these individuals will require even more specialized observations. In some instances the child is able to move his eyes without an ability to direct vision intentionally. This is comparable to extraneous movement sometimes seen in the physical body. When there is very low postural tone, or a basic inability to move the body, the child may capitalize on his control of eye movement. This type of child will use his eyes as a major form of communication, focusing repeatedly on what he wants or in the direction in which he wishes to be moved. Speech pathologists can take advantage of such reliable control of vision to fashion visual communication systems for the child who is unable to speak.

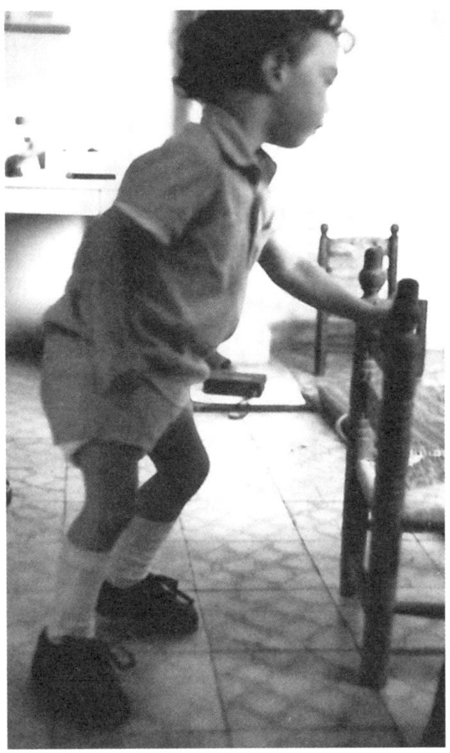

Figure 11.4. Poor control and high tone. High tonus limits normal sensory feedback and distorts the child's learning of movement.

To evaluate the functional state of the visual system, it is most important to know whether head movement is possible in all directions and to the fullest potential range of movement. Without free excursion of the head, there may be a limited visual field used. In some cases the eyes are able to compensate by use of extreme movements. In those cases there may be problems of focusing, poor conjugate vision, or visual stress due to the effort of compensation.

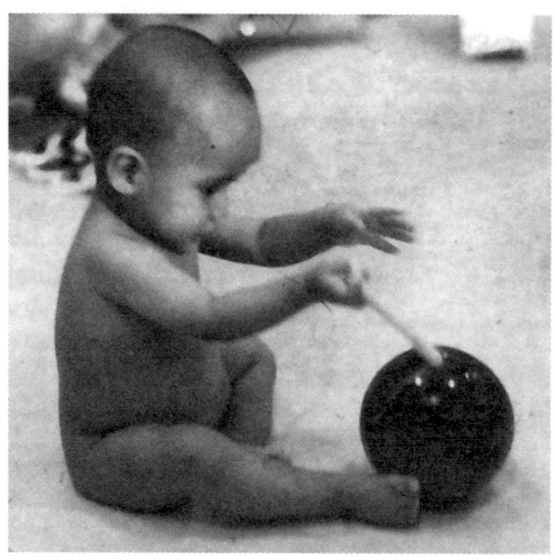

Figure 11.5. Normal fixing to focus. For the normal baby, visual focus is a skill closely integrated with movement.

Parents can offer essential information to help us understand their children. In cases of acquired brain injury the family can offer much information about the personality prior to the accident or illness, although that information is better acquired after the professional has demonstrated some ability to make a functional difference for the client. Parents will know or can observe whether the direction of the child's gaze correlates with the direction of the window from his crib. They can describe changes in head position when the child attempts a visual task or under which circumstances he loses interest in visual activity. When responding to a visual stimulus, the child may notably increase his postural tone. It is helpful perhaps to think of this as an abnormal exaggeration of the postural fixation observed in the young infant when he needs to sustain visual focus for examination of some intriguing aspect of the environment.

The nature of abnormal tonus is such that the individual associates it more closely with functional activity until the functional response does not occur without the tonus change and the abnormal tonus interferes with function. In the case of young children there is little or no normal sensory information to balance the abnormal, and consequently the child becomes more limited over time. We might think of the behavioral manifestations of the original disorder as increasing, although the brain dysfunction, per se, is a stable condition.

When assessing the outcome potential of a central nervous system disorder, we are trying to anticipate the compensatory skill of that total system to use alternate pathways and synaptic connections to substitute for the ones that have been injured or rendered dysfunctional. The compensatory ability of the central nervous system has been well documented with adults.

Bach-y-Rita,[1] a research neurologist, relates the story of his own father who suffered a severe stroke and made a complete physical, mental, and emotional recovery to full function. Years later, when he died of an unrelated cause, an autopsy revealed that one entire brain hemisphere had completely atrophied as a result of the hemorrhage and had remained that way for ten years, even though full function had returned. Young adults have remained in a coma for six months to a year, and two years later have attended classes in a community college. These possibilities are mentioned for the benefit of clinicians who may be uncertain as to whether they should follow their intuition to offer visual support for the traumatized child or adult who struggles to make a comeback.

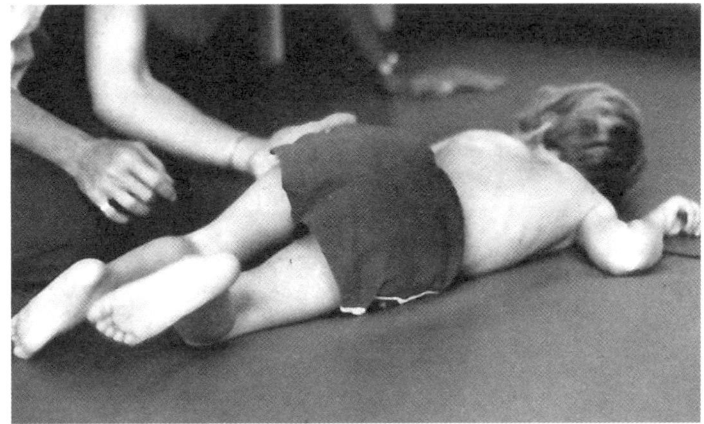

Figure 11.6. High tone movement. This boy has high intelligence but is unable to move his body in the way he knows it should move.

Abnormal Postural Behavior

In the presence of abnormal postural behavior, a lack of movement of the body away from the surface is an overriding influence. The proprioceptive system is not able to coordinate these responses, and therefore effort on the part of the child to readapt the posture of the body results in total extensor responses or reflexive patterns that do not support body function. Attempts to use the sensory systems to gather information about the environment are thwarted by the energy lost in efforts to control posture.

1. If a healthy adult is unable to move the child's body into a given position, the child will be unable to assume that position independently. This seems a simple premise until one observes that we frequently ask a child to reach for an object or keep his head in a given position without ever trying to move the body part into that position ourselves. A willingness to touch the affected individual and gently move a body part will reveal much about the amount of effort used by that person to make the simplest response. It may be impossible for the individual to control movement of the limbs in a predictable way. Eye blinks are often the most basic communication initiated by the individual and may be used to answer yes/no questions.

2. If we introduce or superimpose movement of a body part that consequently threatens balance or causes a total reaction of another part of the body, the person with brain dysfunction will intuitively avoid the first movement. This does not mean that he is unable to coordinate the movement, only that he cannot handle the consequences. As movement potential becomes chronically limited in range and diversity, the child loses the ability to perform the avoided movement and substitutes abnormal reactions in order to function. This is somewhat analogous to the physical atrophy that occurs in situations of limited use of a body part over time.

3. If the head cannot be stabilized with normal control, the eyes will not be able to function in a normal, automatic and effortless way. There will be some attempt

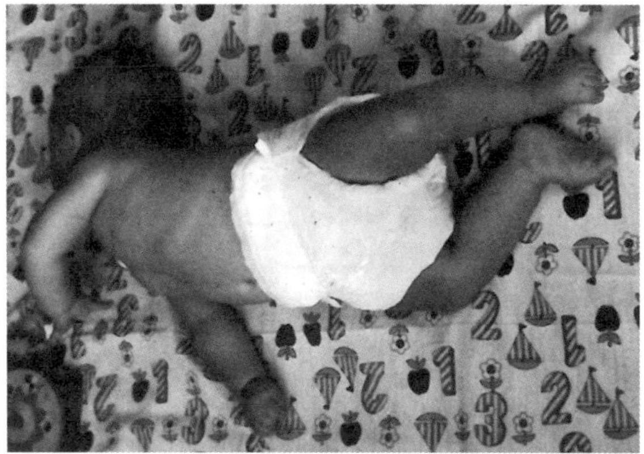

Figure 11.7. Abnormal posture with visual focus. Vision will lead postural adaptation even when the responses are abnormal.

to compensate as the child begins to use existing vision; the head may be fixed to one side or tipped back in a slightly extended posture, causing an apparent shortening of the neck. It will be helpful here to attempt to bring the head forward to feel the resistance and in some cases to ask the child to close his eyes while his head is brought forward. When the head can be brought forward with gentle assistance, there is less likely to be a significant structural limitation, and the child is a good candidate for effective use of prism lenses. While informed use of prism lenses can make dramatic alterations in postural adjustment by changing the environmental information that affects balance, the structure must be free to respond to these new messages. In this regard it is vital that the optometrist and the therapist work closely together. Prism lenses, especially when positioned base-up, have resulted in dramatic changes of the strong tonus in the flexor surface of the body that pulls a child into gravity. In other sections of this book the interested reader can learn more about the criteria for determining individual recommendations. Behavioral change and postural adaptation are the best monitors of successful change.

4. If there is no point of stable alignment, normal or abnormal, for the neck and head, there is no physiological base from which the eye muscles can organize their movement. This lack of stable alignment will result in a lack of postural control for the neck and, therefore, the eyes. There will be a tendency to scan with the eyes without the ability to control fixation or, consequently, to develop essential eye-hand coordination. Assisting the child by stabilizing the neck externally will aid the organization of physical movement for the eyes. This may be done simply with a towel rolled lengthwise and placed firmly in a position like that of a fur collar. It may be helpful to think of this as a temporary facilitation of eye movements, which have not previously been used, in order to stimulate use of the visual system. This is particularly important for the multi-handicapped child who has few resources, and for whom we need to demonstrate some sign of constructive intellectual activity. As better eye movement permits the visual system to mature in its function, such external supports may be reduced.

5. High extensor tonus of the neck tends to be associated with upward movements of the eyes. The backward movement of the head that results from this upward rolling of the eyes may be initiated either by an attempt to use the eyes or by an increase in extensor tonus in the back and the neck itself. Tonus distribution in extension is increased when the child rests on a firm support in a supine, or face

up, position. When the same child learns to sit or is propped in a sitting position by artificial supports, there are likely to be secondary compensations in the form of increased tonus over the flexor surface of the body. Being threatened with the constant possibility of falling backward, the child may use whatever force he has to pull himself forward into flexion. This forward flexion may sometimes be mistaken as representing a benign collapse, when actually there is considerable force in the forward movement, and the examiner will no doubt find it difficult to bring the child to an upright position. After several years of the abnormal adaptation, the vestibular system no longer differentiates the correct signals, and the body fails to support itself.

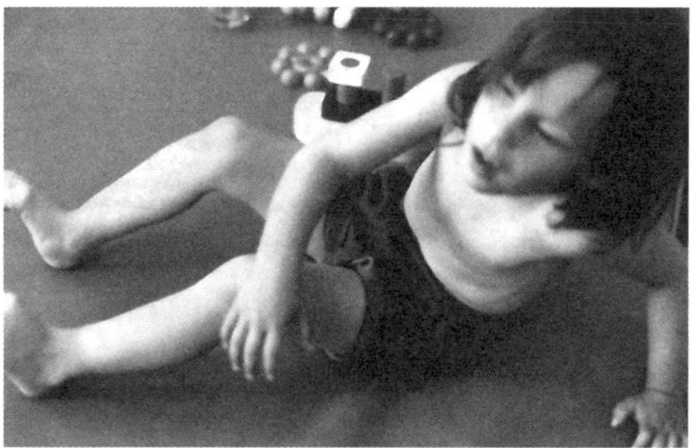

Figure 11.8. Sitting with asymmetry. Lack of rotation in the trunk increases the effort needed for postural change.

6. Avoidance of extension in the neck tends to be associated with keeping the eyes in a downward gaze. In this situation the eyes will assist the control of the body and avoid the takeover of extensor tonus, as described above. Bright children learn to do this early and may even appear to have a field loss or lack of awareness of visual stimuli above the horizontal midline. Movement of the eyes upward may result in a sudden loss of postural control, a frightening experience.

7. Lack of sensory awareness of one side of the body tends to be associated with less eye movement toward that side and/or less movement of the eye on that side. There may be less use of the eye on the more involved side to the point that acuity is actually affected. This is also influenced strongly by the body posture of the individual and takes into account the postural adaptations. The more affected side tends to be retracted, which creates a natural tendency to tilt the head toward the paper on the "better side" and to use that eye more. In reality, there is no "better" or "worse" side, as the seemingly less-affected side of the body soon attempts to compensate and may actually become almost hyperkinetic in its attempt to take over functions of the less able parts. In therapeutic physical handling it is essential to inhibit constantly the overactive responses as the less active postural responses are encouraged. The reactions of the total body must be given consideration, and the child must be helped to gain an experience of dynamic symmetry through careful handling combined with the proprioceptive firm pressure experience of weight-bearing. The adult must also be assisted to regain this sensation of postural symmetry, although the therapist will often work with the client in a seated posture in order to move in and out of a vertical midline orientation.

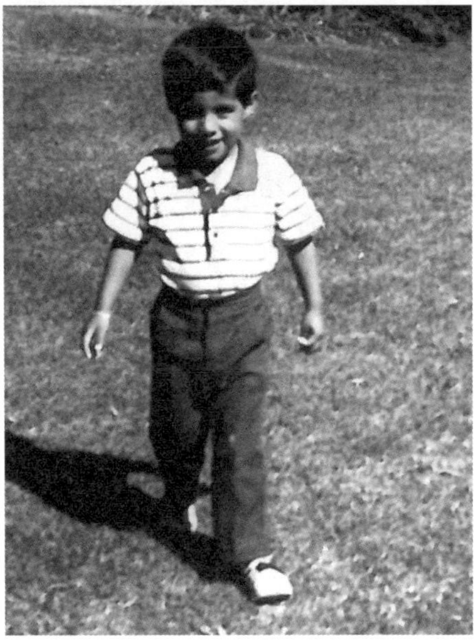

Figure 11.9. Skilled movement. To achieve control in an upright alignment requires preparation of many postural components.

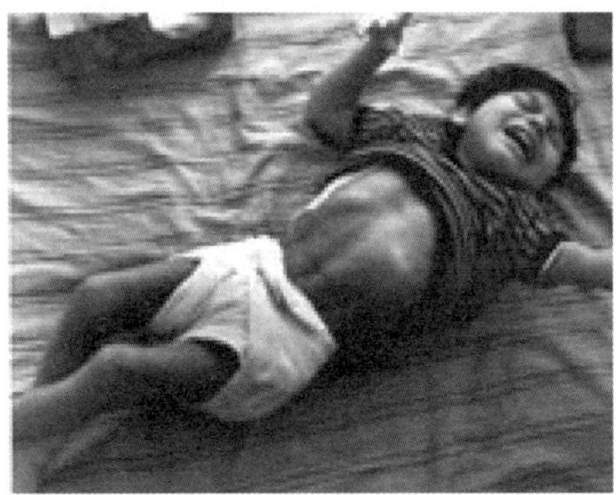

Figure 11.10. Severely involved child--multihandicapped. Significant neuromotor disability without treatment becomes more severe due to lack of movement experience.

Physical Manifestations of Lack of Postural Control

Developmentally, it is useful to think of normal extension of the body against gravity as starting at the neck and moving to the head and then down the length of the spine. Early righting reactions are further integrated by the equilibrium reactions to form a subconscious network of control against the force of gravity. Normally, we give no conscious thought to these reactions and are consequently free to put our attention on communication, creative thoughts, or concentrated intellectual pursuit. Our subconscious network of righting and equilibrium reactions should be available, as needed, to protect us and to stimulate movement against gravity. It is a fundamental concept that when a body part or functional system, such as vision, is involved in maintaining a body position, that same part or system is not available to perform its own specific function.

Chronic maladaptive posturing of the head may be due to malalignment of the cervical spine or lack of balance and muscle action, as well as a lack of balance in the use of the eyes. It is often apparent in casual observation of the child in the waiting area or in general visual tasks designed to put the child at ease. In the case of children who spend much of their school day strapped into special chairs, it is important to know whether the child usually has the option of moving his head for visual adjustment. Such a child may be dependent on positioning by the teacher, classroom aide or one of his physically mobile peers.

A lack of trunk control is often characterized by seemingly erratic tilting to one side and then to the other. This will include movements of the head that attempt to stabilize the trunk. Use of vision will be adversely affected by poorly designed straps or supports that compromise free movement of the diaphragm or the proper alignment of the spine. Poor correlation between trunk and head positions becomes chronic and limits the functioning of vision, vestibular reactions, and hearing, as well as the expression of fine coordination skill. The first line of intervention should

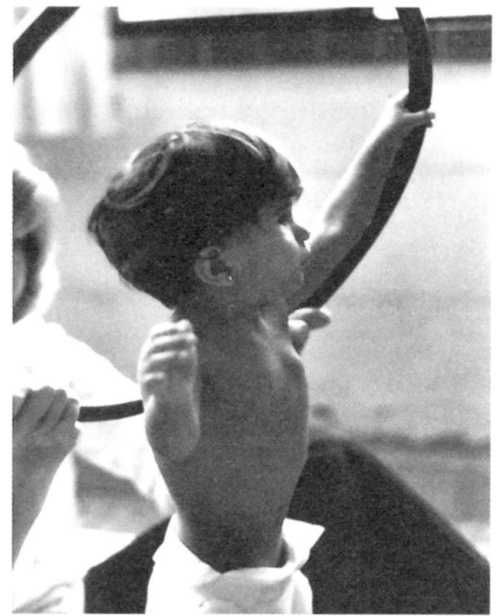

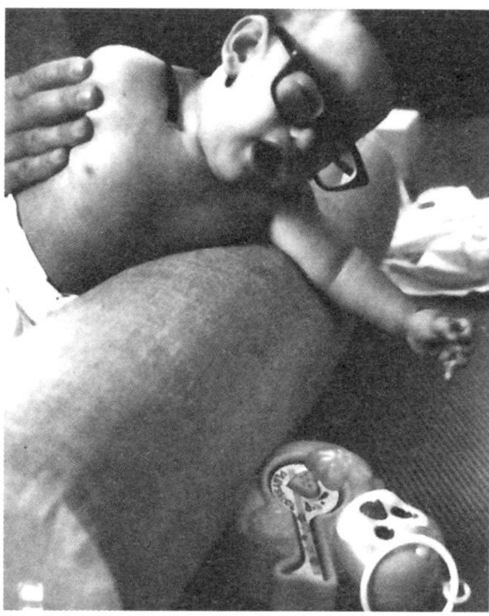

Figure 11.11. Active treatment. An active response on the part of the child is useful after adequate preparation in treatment.

be restoration of the structural alignment to stimulate optimal development. This suggests professional coordination between the therapist, optometrist, classroom teacher and the parents.

Poor control of limb movement may be general or concentrated in the upper or lower extremities or on one side of the body. A general problem may be reflected in inadequate trunk control, while disturbed coordination of the arms and hands may originate in a lack of stability or excessive tension of the shoulders. The latter may start with alignment problems of the spinal column or lack of developmental activation of the shoulders in infancy. There tends to be an inverse relationship between trunk tone and postural tone in the limbs, so offering more adequate support to the trunk often eases the struggle against gravity and normalizes the postural tone. In the case of chronic reactions in older children, it will be necessary to offer direct treatment experiences during which the child can experience a more normal dynamic alignment and the possibility of movement without such excessive effort. Quality movement responses proceed from well-aligned postures that are ready to change according to our needs.

Incoordination of righting and equilibrium reactions is generally accompanied by problems of postural tonus. Since the vestibular system is so closely aligned in its structure and its function with the visual system, there will usually be an attempt by the visual system to support posture against gravity. This fatigues the visual system over time and interferes with the delicate balance between focal and ambient processes of vision. Since righting reactions represent a fundamental coping with the influence of gravity, their lack of expression results in lack of movement. Equilibrium responses can be excessive in their expression when there is an imbalance within the proprioceptive system, with the vestibular input being stronger than that of the deep-pressure receptors. Persons with this condition tend to flail their

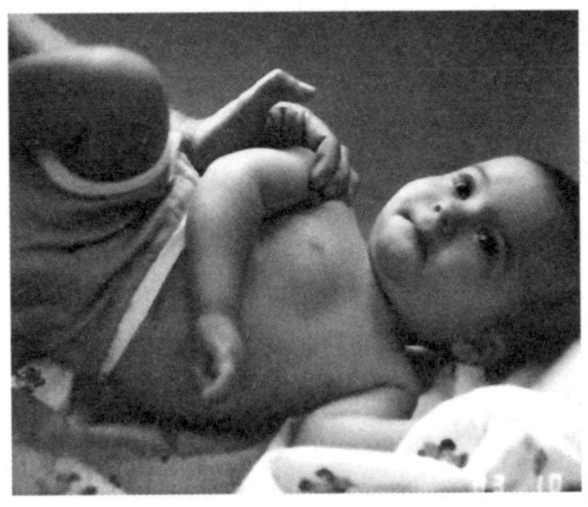

Figure 11.12. Therapy. The therapist gives the child the sensation of normal movement patterns that he has not achieved independently.

limbs and use excessive movement in tasks that require precision. Offering some compression to the trunk with simple hand pressure over the shoulders will assist the organization of movement. This clinical situation is frequently referred to as "athetoid-like" in movement quality, and the personality of this person tends to be rather labile with strong fluctuations in response.

Normal postural tonus should fluctuate within a range adequate to support us against gravity and low enough to permit effortless movement. There is a readiness factor in normal tonus that supports us in our intention to move at any time, even with significant changes in speed, such as dashing to answer a telephone. High tonus limits the initiation of movement; there is a fear of postural change and a lack of balance reactions. The person tends to orient the body to a symmetrical position and seldom moves from that alignment. In such a situation the stimulation of lateral movement of the eyes could be an important contribution to change.

The contrasting situation, that of excessively low tonus, reduces the amount of movement as the body weight is pulled into gravity. The limbs may move to touch an object or to interact with an adult, but the proximal body associated with that limb remains fixed. Kicking of the legs, for example, is limited in excursion and, more importantly, is not accompanied by the lifting of the pelvis, which also activates the diaphragm. Consequently, the child with low tonus tends to have limited volume to his voice. Ironically, the child who demonstrates excessive high tone or spasticity initially may demonstrate low tone once the spasticity is reduced with therapeutic techniques. This is sometimes referred to as spasticity with a low tone base. It is a difficult problem for the therapist since the low tone must be stimulated to a normal level without exciting unwanted spasticity.

A fluctuation of tone is referred to as athetosis, from a Greek origin meaning "a lack of posture." The child tends to fix proximal parts of his own body in position in order to control his movement responses, although this consequently limits his range of movement and the development of graded control. These uncontrolled movement responses are also seen in some cases of multiple sclerosis and degenerative conditions of the central nervous system. While most experienced clinicians agree that there is a significant reduction in the number of pure athetoid individuals from birth as compared to 20 years ago, there are still persons struggling with movement patterns that fit the general description, so the term is useful to know.

Positioning the Client for Examination

When confronted with either an adult or a child who has sustained a brain injury, it is a good idea to note the postural characteristics. Is there an ability to sit inde-

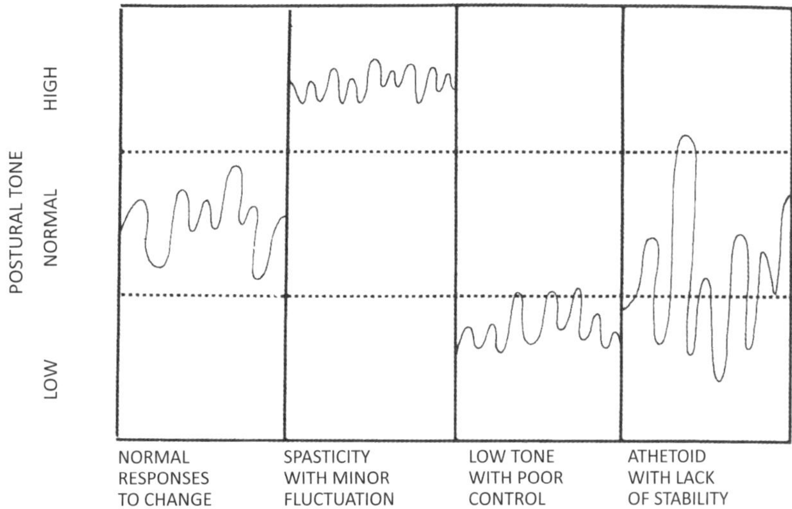

Figure 11.13. Normal and Abnormal Tonus.

pendently, or is the person relying on another person or a protective chair? Does movement tend to be free or restricted? Is there some symmetry to the position of the body? Does the person initiate movement or rely on care givers?

Don't be fooled by the overly solicitous family member who takes charge. Try to establish some rapport directly with the client. Most commonly in the case of central nervous system disorders the person understands more than he can easily express. Often there is a delay in the mental processing of a request so that the person may answer several minutes later with an appropriate response. Be alert to this phenomenon, especially in the case of traumatic injuries.

After noting the initial posture, attempt to make a simple change to determine the resistance to movement or even to your touch. In the case of a child who is obviously more secure in his mother's arms, you might wish to check some responses of the visual system first and then attempt the movement. A friendly lifting of the arm or leg in play will tell you much about the relative tone of the limb and the changes in the body position as a result of the change in balance.

If the person accepts your touch, you will have no difficulty placing the palm of your hand behind his neck. At first, this may give you very little information, but soon your experience will suggest whether the tension that you feel is sufficient to prevent lifting the head forward or to limit lateral excursion of the head and the eyes. A finger placed lightly on the chest or the shoulder while the eyes move to follow your stimulus will be enough to sense the stiffening, or increased tonus that tends to accompany visual activation. Knowing that this tension exists may suggest specific interventions at the visual level that might contribute to the lessening of the stress.

If the person is unable to turn his head to one side, it is a good idea to assist the movement. It is possible to feel whether there is a slow resistance throughout the

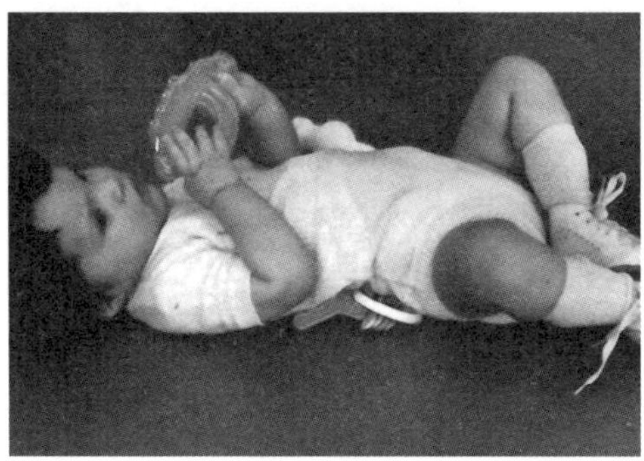

Figure 11.14. Baby with low tonus. Low postural tonus limits trunk movement, which is essential for good anti-gravity control, and visual experiences.

range that suggests a neuromotor involvement with an increase in postural tone as opposed to an abrupt stop in the movement that can represent a structural limitation. Tracking tasks may be assisted by having the person turn his head to one side. Individuals who have postural problems that originated in infancy, with the evolution of rotation of the body around the longitudinal axis, will successfully track an object from one side to the other with the head to one side after being unable to perform the same task with the head/eyes forward. By turning the face to the side, we introduce a rotation component in the posture that frees the vision and allows the eyes to move in a more differentiated way.

When presenting a visual task to a person with poor control of his physical body, it is best to offer additional postural stability. This might be in the form of cushions, a different chair, or the physical assistance of the parent or family member. The objective is to observe whether the quality of the response improves with the additional support. This information may alter recommendations for lenses as well as suggestions for classroom placement and educational management. Trunk stability can usually be improved by aligning the shoulders directly over the hips. This will offer a better possibility for the arms to move and the head to align with the trunk.

Performance on two or three tasks can be compared with and without supplementary postural support in order to understand the interaction between postural control and visual system function for the individual. Priorities in treatment and education as well as direct visual intervention will become clearer as this information is gathered.

Alternative positions may be close to the original posture but take advantage of a different type of support, a new relationship to gravity or a change in the surface texture. In cases of sensitivity to touch it is useful to realize that the central nervous system is calmed by firm pressure, smooth surfaces, and slow, predictable rhythms. Light touch, rapid staccato contact, and irregular surfaces are excitatory and even noxious to some systems. The support of one's own weight tends to be organizing and may assist the child in making a visual response. The small child may like to be in a prone, tummy-lying position with a small roll of towel under his chest. An older individual might be brought forward to take weight on his elbows in order to change the postural alignment of the trunk. Providing a support for the back of the head in a seated position removes the stress from the back of the neck and may also change the movement potential of the eyes.

While many therapists have had no experience working with the visual system, most will be interested in the contributions that visual change can make in the physical functioning of their clients. Distractibility is often reduced and increased awareness of the environment may motivate physical exploration. Specific reorientation of visual focus may even change the potential of an individual for independent ambulation. Changes in postural tone give the therapist greater possibilities for physical handling.

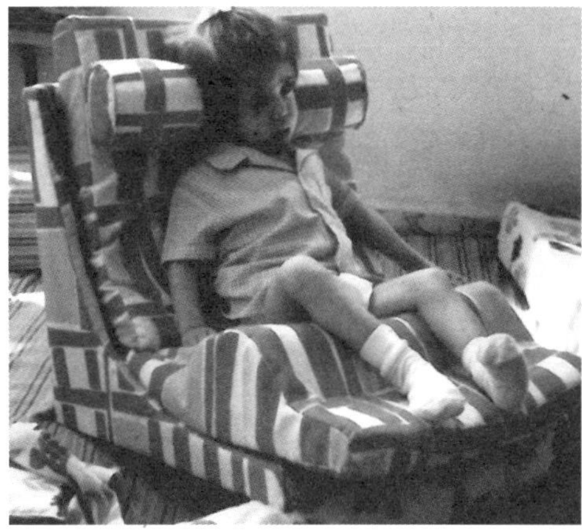

Figure 11.15. Positioning in sitting. Seating supports should maintain the child's position without reliance on the straps used for safety.

In exchange, the therapist who is trained in a neuro-developmental approach, or a similar holistic view of the many aspects of neurological dysfunctions, can offer fellow professionals specific guidance and assistance to supplement the suggestions made here. Eye movements are a fine level of differentiated movements that evolve with developmental control of the body. Direct therapeutic handling permits the system to experience more normal feedback with the assistance of the therapist. This direct experience is the essential cue for the central nervous system to initiate action that will provide feedback within the system itself. As normal responses begin to outnumber the abnormal ones, a shift in functional balance occurs, and the person changes posture, movement, visual function and behavior. Vision as a primary process influences both attention and concentration, and permits the function of higher cognitive ability through the focal process. The maintenance of support positions and dynamic postural control rely heavily on the ambient process.

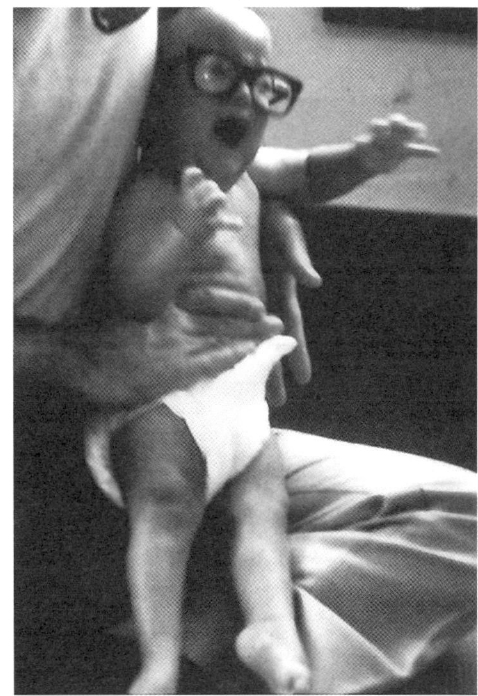

Figure 11.16. Positioning. Crying increases tonus and makes it difficult to adapt the child's body to a new position.

The combination of these visual processes, together with the righting and equilibrium of the kinesthetic postural system, is essential to facilitate optimal change in the physically disabled individual. By taking advantage of these dynamic, interactive patterns of the human being, neuro-optometric rehabilitation encourages problem solving by utilizing the special skills of multiple professionals to obtain functional change.

Chapter 12

AUTISM: A VISUAL PARADOX

William V. Padula

Introduction

Autism is defined by the Autism Society of America (ASA) as: "a complex developmental disability that typically appears during the first two years of life and is the result of a neurological disorder that affects the functioning of the brain, impacting development in the areas of social interaction and communication skills. Both children and adults on the autism spectrum typically show difficulties in verbal and nonverbal communication, social interactions, and leisure or play activities." Autism is estimated to affect an average of 1 in 110 children in the United States, and is four to five times more prevalent in males than in females (CDC 2009). While it is now understood that there are genetic aspects to autism spectrum disorders (ASD), there is also great interest in the interaction of genetic and environmental factors.

Any attempt to completely understand or even describe the visual world of persons with autism fails by the very nature of the condition. Autism has defied any accurate definition, including the one noted above, because it is such a diverse phenomenon. Physically, differences such as posture or toe walking can be noted in some persons, but not others. Behaviorally, some demonstrate perseveration, rocking and finger flicking, while others do not. Physiologically, mineral, enzyme and metabolic imbalances are found in some persons, but not in others. If there is any description that seems to fit autism spectrum disorders it is that autism presents a paradox and that what seems to be accepted by so-called normal or "*neurotypical*" society as logical and structured is in many ways nonexistent for those with autism. Autism is perplexing, and so is the visual world of persons with autism.

Sensory Differences

Varying degrees of abnormal responses to sensory input have long been described as common in those on the autism spectrum, and include responses to vision, hearing, touch, smell, and taste, with many persons having multi-modal sensory problems.[1,2] These may involve both hyper and hypo sensitivities, as well as unusual reactions to sensory inputs such as certain sights or sounds, while ignoring some that are meaningful such as when the child's name is called. Some of the more commonly described *visual* behaviors are lack of eye contact, eye pressing, finger flicking, staring at lights or fans, fixation on objects for extended time periods, difficulty with visual attention, appearing to look through rather than at objects, and increased use of peripheral vision including lateral glances, especially toward moving stimuli.

Persons with autism spectrum disorders have also been depicted as more likely to use visuospatial imagery in their thought processes.[3] In her book *Thinking in Pictures*,[4] Temple Grandin describes this, and how her visual thinking skills help her to "build" equipment in her mind.

> *"I think in pictures. Words are a second language to me. I translate both spoken and written words into full-color movies, complete with sound, which run like a VCR tape in my head. When somebody speaks to me, his words are instantly translated into pictures. Language-based thinkers often find this phenomenon difficult to understand, but in my job as an equipment designer for the livestock industry, visual thinking is a tremendous advantage.*

Developmental Aspects Involving Vision

There is a continuing effort to diagnose autism spectrum disorders as early as possible so that intervention can begin at as young an age as possible. Atypical behaviors are seen early in many babies on the spectrum, and among the possible early symptoms commonly cited as suggestive of autism are several involving vision including: the baby does not track objects visually, does not smile when someone smiles at him, does not make eye contact, looks out of the "corner of his eyes" (lateral gaze), and does not imitate other people or their gestures such as waving goodbye or pointing.

As the autistic child develops, various atypical visual exploratory behaviors for inanimate objects (AVEBIOs) have been described. (See Mottron et al.[5] for a review.) These include the some of the behaviors noted previously that are considered strong symptoms of autism such as repeated movements of the fingers in front of the eyes, spinning objects, prolonged staring at objects, etc. In the study by Mottron et al.[5] the frequency of lateral glance occurrences was clearly more common among the autistic children (9-48 months of age) than other atypical visual exploratory behaviors that were observed as part of the study. The lateral glances were "frequently associated with the presence of a moving object," (e.g. the child's fingers or an object the child was moving) and were "dramatically more frequent in autistic than in comparison children." A study by Ozonoff et al.[6] looked at atypical object use in 12 month old children who were at risk for autism because of family history. While there were "significantly more atypical uses of objects in the infants later diagnosed with autism/ASD, high rates particularly of one specific behavior—unusual visual exploration of objects" was also seen in these young children.

Visual Problems

The visual world of the child as well as the adult with autism can be very challenging. Along with vision related behaviors, vision itself may be atypical in many autistic children. While these children are often found to have 20/20 acuity, significant eye and visual perceptual problems appear to exist more commonly in those on the autism spectrum. There are reports of an increased incidence of strabismus,[7,8] astigmatism,[7] binocular vision problems,[7,9] convergence insufficiency,[10] decreased voluntary pursuit movements,[8] atypical optokinetic nystagmus,[11,12] impaired motion perception,[10,13] abnormal electroretinograms and evoked visual potentials,[12] decreased sensitivity to complex motion stimuli,[14] and deficient oculomotor responses.[15]

If we recall the chapters in this book on vision development and the importance of vision to the associated development of mobility, balance, fine motor control, etc., it is easy to understand how visual problems experienced by a child on the autism spectrum can significantly affect many other aspects of his development and behavior. For example, Brenner et al.[15] have described problems in ASD children involving oculomotor functions such as eye movement and visual search. These are considered possibly critical elements of attention, imitation, object identification, etc., and are thought to be crucial "ingredient functions" for language development.

On the other hand, hypervision,[14] and superior processing of fine detail and other types of perceptual tasks have also been reported.[11,13-18] Studies of enhanced performance have shown that this occurs in areas of detail processing such as visual search tasks, e.g., detection of static figures embedded in complex distracters, block design re-creation tasks, etc.,[11] or of identifying simple grating orientation.[13] Most of these studies show that superior performance in the autistic population has typically been found on low-level visual perceptual tasks.[13,14] Nevertheless, as Mottron et al.[13] have noted: "perception plays a different and superior role in autistic cognition."

Facial Recognition

In recent years there has been increased interest in the facial processing abilities of autistic persons including face recognition.[19] Impaired ability in this area has been and continues to be the focus of much research since it is one of the most frequently described aspects of the social awareness problems noted in this population. Faces reflect information about a person's identity, gender, emotional state, etc. Thus, as Jemel et al.[20] noted: "faces constitute one of the most complex classes of stimuli encountered by the visual system." In addition, the information provided by these facial stimuli is important for establishing appropriate social interactions. Babies learn to recognize their mother's face at an early age, and much as been published about the systems by which this is thought to be accomplished, how these face processing systems change as the child grows,[20] and the localization of areas in the brain that are involved in this process. For example, Uddin et al.,[19] using fMRI, found that children on the autism spectrum did not activate shared regions of the brain for self and other-face processing as would a normally developing child, and noted that this difference may be a "neural signature of reduced social engagement and understanding in these individuals."

There have also been many studies concerning the possible relationship between the manner in which facial recognition is accomplished and its influence on problems with social interaction for those with ASD.(See Behrmann et al.[21] for a review.) Research has shown individuals with ASD tend to use atypical strategies to process faces, to spend less time fixating on the eyes than do normal controls[22,23] and that they appear to use a part-based facial process.[13,20] Deruelle et al.,[24] using simultaneous matching tasks, reported that autistic children used different strategies in facial recognition, and that their performance was better when using high spatial frequency information, whereas the typically developing children had fewer errors when using low spatial frequency information. Electrophysiological studies have also supported a different manner of processing rather than a profound deficit,[20] with Sugiura et al.[25] finding support and "evidence of multiple brain networks for visual self-recognition." In recent years studies using MRI, fMRI and PET scans have been published suggesting that *underconnectivity,* that is, the "underfunctioning of integrative circuitry,"[26] is an important neurological factor in understanding characteristics of cognition, and perception in ASD, and that it appears to occur especially in the frontal and fusiform face areas.[26,27] However, Jemel et al.,[20] in a recent comprehensive review of face processing studies concluded that "the versatility and abilities of face processing in persons with autism have been underestimated.

The Vision Examination and Beyond

As a means to structure a discussion about neuro-optometric aspects of vision we will begin with the examination of the eyes since the traditional medical approach, delivered through optometry and ophthalmology, concerns itself with analysis of eye health, sight (seeing clearly), and function (coordinating the two eyes).

Examination of a person with autism is often a challenge for the practitioner using only traditional approaches, since many persons with autism have difficulty controlling fixation upon request. Also, most doctors rely upon the subjective portion of the examination when determining the proper prescription of lenses by asking the patient to discern the difference between lenses and state a preference, for example: "Which lens is better, number one or number two?" A person with autism is frequently unable to communicate in the expected manner, or cannot accomplish the task in the limited time frame provided in a busy managed health care office environment.

Persons with autism will often have difficulty fixating (looking directly) at the eye chart or fixating target; most of the time they will direct their eyes to a point away from the target. When asked to track an object they will often track it only briefly, if at all, demonstrating frequent fixation losses. An inability to focus or sustain focus due to neurological problems may be noted when examining their skills, and may be interpreted by the traditional approach of eye doctors as weak eye muscle control. Commonly noted self-stimulating behaviors can also be a problem during an eye exam.

Thus examination of the eyes often adds little to our understanding of the visual world of a person on the autism spectrum. To go beyond this we must also understand something about the way in which vision is processed in order to get a glimpse of what the altered state of vision is like in autism. In addition to looking at the results of studies of visual perception, we need to listen to how individuals with autism have been describing their visual worlds.

In her book about living with autism, Temple Grandin[4] describes her vision as "fragmented". This is an interesting description and is difficult for most so-called "normally" sighted persons to understand. However, many persons with autism describe "fragmentation" or other similar characteristics when discussing their vision: a world of pieces and parts that sometimes briefly form a glimpse of wholeness.

One young man explained that as he attempted to look directly at something, the object appeared to break apart into lines, colors, shadows, etc. At times, each of these forms became a figure emerging from the background obscuring its relationship to the original object. This figure lasted only a moment and then would be blended and overtaken by yet another as part of detail; the lines of a person's face would be overtaken by a mosaic of color and so on. This first occurred when he was three years old. He remembered that he used to "play" with the visual changes by staring for a time and then shifting his gaze away. He found that by viewing with his side or peripheral vision, he could blend the pieces and parts back into a sort of wholeness that he could deal with functionally. As he became older, it became more and more difficult for him to use his peripheral vision to reestablish wholeness to his visual world. The broken world became more intense. He found that if he moved or if something or someone else moved, his visual environment became a chaos of details. As difficult as it was to live with this way of seeing, the detail and constant changing of the environment became stimulating to him. There were times that he would spend hours reaching out and hitting an object like a leaf or branch to watch how the movement caused it to break apart into a vibration of colors, lines, and contours.

Penelope McMullen[28] writing about her vision noted: "I have a hard time finding something when I don't already have an idea of where it is because there are too many other things around from which to distinguish it. I don't like to shop for that reason, and I hate it when I go to buy something I'm familiar with and the packaging is changed so I don't recognize it.... I consciously try and often succeed to give eye contact, but if I have to work hard to get my words out, then I have to look away (at space – at nothing, really) in order to concentrate on speaking. If I look at the face, then visual overload interrupts the words."

The above noted descriptions of visual perception defy all logic regarding the visual world that many of us experience as reality. We tend to take for granted the balance of our bimodal vision and the stability it provides in the visual-spatial environment. However, for those with ASD, compromise of this balance in visual processing causes instability with ambient (spatial) processing which can be projected into the visual environment.

What Can We Learn from Post Trauma Vision Syndrome

Attempting to understand what causes vision to be so unstable and what can be done to help the autistic person reduce the symptoms, those of us practicing neuro-optometric rehabilitation recognized that many of the characteristics and symptoms of persons with autism are not unlike those presented by persons with TBI, such as: 1) a predilection to see the visual world as detail; 2) seeing double (diplopia) intermittently; 3) difficulty attending and concentrating; 4) difficulty focusing; 5) glare sensitivity (photophobia) and difficulty adapting to changes in lighting and the environment. Research with traumatic brain injured (TBI) persons,[29] which is described in Chapter Five, *Post Trauma Vision Syndrome,* proved that many of these characteristics and symptoms were not from the eyes but from an imbalance in the visual process.

The symptoms described in the above paragraph are related to problems of visual processing. When discussing visual processing in autism, one must refer back to the description of the bimodal processing system[30] and the importance that the ambient portion of that system has to spatial organization (see Chapter One). You will recall that twenty percent of the visual information from the eyes, i.e. the ambient aspect, is delivered to an area of the midbrain where it matches up with information that has been received from the sensorimotor system (kinesthetic, proprioceptive, and vestibular systems). The sensorimotor system matches up with information from this peripheral visual process, and the integrated information organizes concepts of space. An example of this is the awareness of our body position in relationship to the ground for the purpose of balance, coordination, and anticipated movement. This spatial information is then sent through a feedforward mechanism to major portions of the cerebral cortex, including the occipital cortex. In a sense, the ambient visual process is attempting to preprogram how we look at and organize the images that we see. The ambient process occurs before we become conscious of what we see; it is preconscious.

You will also recall that the occipital cortex is a focal processing system that looks at detail and that it is the ambient visual process that provides spatial organization to the focal system. This enables us to take the spatial details and put them together so that we can recognize wholeness in our visual world. If we did not have this ambient visual process, our visual world would be detail bound. This means that when looking at a person's face all you would see would be lines and shadows, perhaps an eye, nose, lip, or ear, but you would not be able to organize the details to recognize the person you are looking at. It is the ambient spatial visual process that organizes and relates the details so we can recognize a person's face and see wholeness in objects.

From the very earliest moments of life, we learn to balance the way in which we organize information from both the ambient and the focal visual processes. You will recall from previous chapters that it is the ambient visual process that grounds the focal process. The ambient visual process allows us to anticipate change. In a sense, the focal process isolates us onto detail and the ambient visual process facilitates the release from the fixation to the new point of visual reference. It allows us to shift our gaze from point to point in our environment. Without the ambient process we would become locked in on detail and have a very difficult time releasing from it. While it is the focal process that has been described as being preferred by autistic children,[31] it is noted that autistic children are also portrayed as often using peripheral vision for activities for which one would usually employ focal vision.[32,33]

When a person becomes focally bound, they not only see everything broken apart or fragmented in detail, but every time they move their eyes the objects in the environment will appear to jump, shift, and even break apart or *fragment.* A page of words becomes isolated letters and when such persons attempt to move their eyes, they experience the letters jumping and moving about. The same thing can happen in a busy crowded environment. The movement of people walking in a shopping mall or supermarket is usually organized spatially first by the ambient visual process. There is a stability that the ambient system provides. When the ambient visual process is compromised, the person begins to see all the objects and people as detail. Any movement of persons walking in the peripheral vision becomes isolated detail but appears chaotic and random. It is a very confusing and disordered visual world that can cause increased anxiety and emotion due to the visual stress that the person experiences. As described in Chapter Five, these symptoms have been called *Post Trauma Vision Syndrome* because they were initially observed in patients having suffered some type of trauma to the brain. However, if we look at the symptoms of visual processing difficulties described by those who have autism, the similarities are very obvious. A person who has autism frequently has compromised balance between the ambient and focal visual process and, as noted, many show a tendency to be focally bound. This can result in a confusing and chaotic visual state such as was described above, can thus cause increased stress under varying conditions, and can interfere with learning and daily living skills.

Balance in the visual system is the goal in treating many visual perceptual problems, and must be understood with respect to the motor and neurological imbalances that affect autonomic function.[32] The use of binasal occlusion can often reduce visual stress by providing spatial structure to the field of vision and limiting the portion of the visual fields in the area where they overlap. It also has an effect on binocular integration.[29,34] Thus in working with autistic persons the ambient process can often be positively affected by using binasal occlusion, sometimes in conjunction with mild base-in prisms for peripheral visual field expansion.[29,31]

In addition, dysfunction of the ambient visual processes can directly interfere with posture and balance. It can also produce a distortion of visual space that will cause the concept of the visual midline, which is learned very early in life, to be shifted. (See Chapter Seven.) The ambient visual process is responsible for balancing the peripheral visual space and giving the person the opportunity to remain erect and upright or perpendicular to the ground. The vestibular, proprioceptive and kinesthetic systems are also involved in providing information with regard to any variation in posture relative to the ground and gravity. When the ambient visual process becomes compromised, the person may shift the concept of visual midline laterally, as well as anteriorly or posteriorly (forward or backward). Recall that when the visual midline shifts, it will cause the person to lean towards the direction of the shift. In the case of autism, a lateral shift of midline can occur. However, with over-focalization, the midline is frequently shifted anteriorly or forward, and experience suggests that this is the more common VMSS seen in autistic persons. This causes the (preconscious) ambient visual process to distort the spatial world and to interpret the plane of the floor as tilting downward. Some autistic persons will consciously see and interpret this, describing it as if they are constantly walking down a hill.

In most cases, individuals will not be able to describe this phenomenon because, as noted, it is preconscious. Instead, they attempt to realign their bodies to be perpendicular to their perception of space, which is a floor tilted downward. In their attempt to do this, they will lean forward. It is impossible to lean forward while still maintaining your weight on your heels. The reader can try this and will quickly discover that as you lean forward, you must brace yourself with your toes or you will fall forward onto your face. Clinical observation has found that persons who have autism and a visual midline shift anteriorly will soon learn to balance themselves while walking on their toes, and this toe walking may be constant or intermittent.

It has been found clinically that by utilizing yoked prisms to shift the midline to a more centered position, in many cases individuals will begin to extend their stride forward in a heel-to-toe gait pattern and will stop walking on their toes. Sometimes, this treatment can produce immediate results, while at other times it requires extended use of prisms in conjunction with neuro-optometric rehabilitation and/or physical/occupational therapy. Yoked prisms have also been reported to be used with autistic patients to try to change aspects of motor and sensory organization regarding spatial awareness, posture, visual coordination and orientation.[34, 35]

A combination of yoked prisms and low plus lenses can be an effective means to help stabilize the visual process.

Experience in working with autistic persons using the above interventions has often shown that they are better able to organize their vision and report less fragmentation. They may also show better eye contact and less of a tendency to look down at the floor while walking. As the visual process becomes more organized, improvement in behavior and emotional stability may also be seen.

Case Study

Thomas was diagnosed with autism at age two. According to his parents, Thomas was full term and had a normal birth. During the first year his parents thought that growth and development appeared to be normal and they described him as "a gentle and loving child." He had no significant health issues with the exception of a high fever which he spiked after the last inoculation at twelve months of age. However, they reported that at about 14 months of age they began to note changes in their son's behavior; he became more withdrawn, started to spend time rocking back and forth, and they began to notice a change in babbling. Motor ability also regressed and instead of walking Thomas would drop to the floor and begin the rocking behavior. Over the next few months he began to repeatedly follow the horizontal lines of counter tops, table tops and any horizontal surface with his eyes and head motion in the direction of scan. This behavior would continue for 30 minutes or more. There were also periods of time when he would begin finger flicking to the side of his eyes while he rocked. During these intervals he would tilt his head to the side. The parents also reported that Thomas became very upset with loud noises or when in busy crowded environments. Fluorescent lights seemed to cause increased rocking behavior.

At seven years of age he was brought by his parents for a neuro-optometric rehabilitation examination. They reported that they had enrolled him in their public school where he was in the regular classroom for half of the day and in a special education program for the other half, with a full time aide. While still showing similar rocking and occasional finger flicking behaviors, he no longer would drop to the ground. He was now walking but had developed a *toe-walking* behavior and would often rock repeatedly forward onto the toes of one foot and then back to the toes of the other foot. When walking he brought his hands and arms close to his chest.

His mother said that Thomas was not interactive in the classroom and that he was receiving occupational therapy and speech therapy in school. He occasionally seemed to participate briefly with the speech therapist by mimicking speech sounds.

The examination was performed through observation and objective methods. Thomas was fearful of the examining instruments and would frequently jump up from the chair and toe-walk about the room while flicking his right hand and fingers to the right of his eyes. A head tilt and turn to the left was noted. He would hold a fixation for only one second and would then appear to be looking elsewhere. His parents were working with his teachers and therapists to try to develop increased fixations and eye contact, but he was not responding.

No strabismus or deviation of an eye was found. When attempting to elicit a convergence movement, Thomas would look away yet seemed to be very much aware of the position of the target as it came closer to his face. When the target was within 6 inches, he moved his head around the target and stood up.

The refraction found a low amount of hyperopia (farsightedness) in both eyes of +0.50. Dynamic accommodation tests found no accommodative response due to a lack or avoidance of fixation. Low plus lenses were introduced before both eyes by holding a handheld rack of lenses; however, he moved his head away from the lenses. When the lenses were changed to +2.00 before each eye and the same puppet held at 14 inches, he initially pulled his head away from the lenses and began to rock, but then brought his face back to the lenses for a moment. The examiner continued to hold the lenses in the same position, and Thomas repeated this behavior of moving toward the lenses and looking through them and then pulling his head away. At one time, he looked through the lenses for a period of 10 seconds and showed intermittent fixations on the puppet for the first time.

Thomas would not let the examiner touch his face or his eyes. When the external examination of the eyes was performed at a distance of approximately 15-20 inches, no abnormalities were found. Biomicroscopy could not be performed. Thomas would not permit an attempt to dilate his eyes, and direct ophthalmoscopy could not be accomplished. Instead, the examiner attempted monocular indirect ophthalmoscopy using an ophthalmoscope with a plano lens and a hand held +10.00 lens briefly held up in front of the eye being examined. The examiner decided not to risk having Thomas react to the indirect ophthalmoscope. He had become somewhat use to the handheld ophthalmoscope since it was the same size as the retinoscope and fixation light. Using the technique described, the examiner found a moderate reflex with normal color and the media clear. The vessels as well as the optic nerve of both eyes were observed briefly. No abnormalities were seen.

Observations were then made while Thomas was moving. He walked on his toes with head and eyes directed toward the ceiling. When gaze was directed upward, capital extension was produced, and it was observed that he was leaning anteriorly and to his right. Yoked prisms were place before his eyes; however, he immediately reached up and pulled the prisms off. This was attempted several times with the same behavior.

The examiner asked the parents to stand on either side of Thomas and for each to hold one hand to help him maintain use of the prisms. The examiner spoke directly to Thomas as he had done throughout the exam. Thomas appeared to listen and if the examiner told Thomas what he was going to do before it was done, Thomas seemed to have more of an ability to accept the procedure or activity. Twelve-prism diopters base down and left at axis 280 degrees were introduced before each eye while each parent held one of his hands. Thomas initially tried to break their grasp but within a few moments he began to look around the room and quieted his body. It was interesting to observe that up until this time he did not show differentiation between eye and head movement and he maintained capital extension. He now reduced the capital extension and showed differentiation of saccadic fixations without head movement. His parents were asked to gently try to encourage movement forward. With his first few steps the capital extension returned as he also attempted toe-walking. However, after three steps he extended to heel-to-toe and developed alternation of heel strike and no capital extension. Eye gaze then became directed around the room and to the floor with appropriate capital flexion of the head and neck.

The examiner discussed the findings with emphasis on dysfunction of the spatial or ambient visual process affecting spatial orientation, posture and balance. It was explained that Thomas seemed to be strongly oriented to focalization with the peripheral part of his eyes. Further, when his parents and teachers thought he was not paying attention, Thomas most likely was very aware visually but was looking at them with peripheral or eccentric viewing. The examiner explained that for some persons with visual spatial dysfunction (e.g. Post Trauma Vision Syndrome), the spatial collapse leaves the focal process without the spatial support or construct to function properly. In turn, the focal process isolates on detail to the extent that the visual environment becomes a mass of detail. Since the focal process utilizes primarily the macula of the eye for central fixation and focalization, often the person will develop a way of looking at objects and people with side (peripheral or eccentric) viewing, because the peripheral vision helps them begin to establish more complete spatial relationships instead of just detail.

Recommendations were made for two pair of yoked prism glasses, one pair with stronger yoked prisms (12 prism diopters base down and left at axis 280 degrees) for both eyes. These glasses were to be worn for up to two hours per day in conjunction with any physical, speech, or occupational therapies. The remainder of the time Thomas was to wear a less strong pair of yoked prisms (5 prism diopters base down and left at axis 280 degrees for both eyes). The glasses were prescribed and Thomas was seen for a follow-up visit four weeks later.

Thomas' parents reported the he wasn't able to wear either pair for the full amount of time but that he was beginning to wear the stronger glasses for up to an hour and the lesser power glasses intermittently for several hours. During the time with the stronger prisms the parents reported that Thomas spent most of his time walking in heel to toe gait. With the lower power prisms Thomas seemed to be less agitated and exhibited fewer visual stimulation behaviors. The occupational therapist also sent a report confirming these behaviors as well as stating that Thomas was demonstrating an improvement in eye contact for brief periods.

Thomas was next seen six weeks later at which time he was tolerating the weaker yoked prism glasses for most of the day. He still would only use the stronger yoked prism glasses for about an hour per day. He was now walking with heel to toe gait even with the lesser power prism glasses unless he became upset. There was also less visual stimulation behavior and less agitation reported.

Use of the two pair of prism glasses has been maintained and improvement in eye contact has continued. Over the course of a year facilitated communication was developed through speech therapy, and Thomas began to develop rudimentary communication skills. The speech therapist reported significant improvements with this work when Thomas was wearing the stronger yoked prism glasses.

Conclusion

While an increased incidence of neurological differences, eye problems and visual perceptual differences has been recognized in persons on the autism spectrum, often ignored is the visual imbalance that can also produce dysfunction. The conditions of Post Trauma Vision Syndrome (PTVS) and Visual Midline Shift Syndrome (VMSS) are prevalent in persons with autism. These syndromes are often overlooked and/or misdiagnosed as dysfunctions caused by other conditions. Treatment for both Post Trauma Vision Syndrome and Visual Midline Shift Syndrome can be accomplished through the use of prisms and binasal occlusion. Balance between the visual processing systems can be developed through this approach but requires intervention through neuro-optometric rehabilitation.

Autism is a phenomenon that continues to perplex researchers and clinicians. However, the development and increasing use of neuro-imaging and electrophysiological techniques provide the potential for revealing areas of the brain and neuro-integrative mechanisms that are associated with the different and complex behaviors of those who have autism spectrum disorders.[36,37] As these studies lead to a better understanding of the underlying disordered sensory systems and their inter-relationships, improved interventions and management can hopefully be developed.[38]

The visual paradox of autism is a hidden phenomenon. It is one that cannot be seen by looking at the person unless we first try to understand the issues that may be producing the symptoms which we observe. By considering these behaviors not as causes but as symptoms, we may be able to discern and better understand the chaotic and often disturbing visual world of a person who is experiencing that which we call autism.

Chapter 13

A THEORY OF VISUALLY BASED STEREOTYPICAL BEHAVIORS ASSOCIATED WITH AUTISM

David F. Delacato, Antonio Parisi

Introduction

Do autistic individuals have visual awareness of the world around them similar to ours? Why is it that an autistic child can wander about in a room with a seeming lack of conscious attention, yet be completely aware of activities, conversations, etc.? If we were able to find where consciousness is located in the brain, measure it and develop a precise definition of it, perhaps we could answer these questions. If we were able to find the neural seat of autism and its biological markers, and were able to measure them, we could get closer to understanding autism spectrum disorders without basing our diagnoses on subjective measurements. Through understanding vision we are beginning to have a better perspective.

In fact, consciousness is a sensation, something deeply intimate, that even though it is born of a physical system—the brain—it cannot be transmitted "directly" to another brain. Usually we attempt to circumscribe it by using the terms of other experiences. Thus if we attempt to explain the private sensation of seeing the color blue we refer to things perceived as blue, such as the sea or sky. Personal experiences such as the smell of roses or the interpretation of the color of sunset are what philosophers call "qualia" and physiologists call perceptions. Thus what we transfer are not the perceptions but the actions (words, behaviors) related to our sensations. Therefore, even though we are not sure what others perceive, we can reasonably assume that they, too, perceive similar experiences because they behave and speak as we do about their experiences involving vision and other senses.

It is obvious that the already limited scientific study of consciousness also has a methodological limit when we want to demonstrate the level of consciousness of autistic people who often do not have speech and behave in a different way. A scientific theory that wants to consider autism has to take into account all the data regarding the evolution of the nervous system, the ontogenetic development of the human brain, neuroanatomy, and neuropathophysiology involving the study of perception through the primary process of vision and other senses.

Since vision is the primary process among the senses, vision influences the development of perception. Perception is a process that is very difficult to understand. Even when the brain is healthy and works perfectly, it does not just provide us with a photocopy of the world through our perceptions. To use a vision example, each person's unique visual perception of the world is the result of the *visual process* influencing how the brain sees through the eyes. Sensory organs send electrochemical impulses to the brain. However, the interaction of brain processes through feedback and feedforward influences how each person sees or otherwise perceives their world. The brain utilizes this information and makes *deductions* about the environment. However, the brain does not passively organize information coming from the world but creates active images and associations of the environment based on accurate and on inaccurate matching of information through the senses. For example, each time we "look" at the environment our brain predicts tridimensional space starting from a visual picture that impacted our retina as light energy with only two dimensions. Using this limited information our perception corresponds to an anticipation based upon the sensations which were sent to our brain. This anticipation is a function of the action system.[1]

Autism is the consequence of brain dysfunction that destroys its ability to organize and select the important elements from within the host of information that impacts our senses and populates our memory.

Visually Related Stereotypical Behaviors Associated with Autism

The first attempt to describe autism systematically was carried out in the 1940s,[2] at which time the primary symptoms were seen as atypical speech/language development including lack of speech, problems with non-verbal communication, and impaired social interaction including eye or body contact. Another characteristic pathological sign was described as repetitive meaningless gestures or movements, which were then called *stereotypies.*

At that time and even later, it was assumed that autistic behavioral disorders stemmed from unconscious maternal rejection of the autistic child so that normal parent-child relationships were not developed. The child's behavior was considered a strategy in response to his mother's rejection which enabled him to avoid his mother, but also isolated him from the world around him.

However, this psycho-dynamic interpretation of autism had two major faults: autistic children's mothers did not exhibit any conscious or unconscious rejection towards their children, and the classic symptoms of autism could not be explained on the basis of psycho-dynamic conjecture.

The repetitive behaviors of autistic children, though they might differ in frequency and intensity, were often of a similar nature. Hands flapping in front of the eyes, toe walking, spinning objects, etc., were observed in the majority of autistic children. Yet these children who developed similar stereotypies lived in different environments thus making the psycho-dynamic theory implausible.

A more logical explanation was that autistic children showed similar stereotypical behaviors because their nervous systems, the one thing they had in common, must have suffered functional damage. Thus organic theories of autism, based on observation and unprejudiced by psycho-dynamic theories, began to develop. However, the stereotypies were still difficult to explain.

From direct observation and mothers' reports it appeared that the first signs of autism presented quite early in life, but were difficult to understand in isolation. While the child's development was grossly normal during the first months, seemingly insignificant differences were noticed. For example, sensitivity to sound, intolerance of prolonged body contact, problems making eye contact with the mother, and toe walking were described. A crucial factor that worried parents more frequently was poor speech development, or cessation of speech development at about age two and a half.

These children also did not engage in play as a way to relate to other children, and frequently seemed to be self-absorbed in repetitive behaviors instead. The most recurrent behaviors they exhibited as specific stereotypies of autism were: hand flapping, spinning objects, head rotation, arranging objects in a row, tearing paper, opening and closing doors and drawers, tapping objects, playing with saliva, rocking, running to and fro aimlessly, paging rapidly through books or magazines, watching TV very closely, and biting objects. When the autistic children were engaged in one of these repetitive behaviors they appeared totally isolated from the world around them. The common link between these stereotypies seemed to be vision since the majority of the stereotypical behaviors exhibited by these children appeared to involve stimulation of the visual system.

Dr. Carl H. Delacato attempted to interpret these stereotypies.[3] He believed that these children were unable to select sensory inputs properly as a consequence of a mild, diffuse brain injury. He also believed a hypo- or hyperalteration of the incoming sensory signal occurred so that the perception of this information was modified. Facing difficulty in transforming the sensation into perception, the child tried to reproduce or avoid the stimulus in his attempt to restore an appropriate perceptive process and this caused the repetitive stereotypical behaviors. It was Dr. Delacato's opinion that the perception of any of the five senses—taste, vision, hearing, smell and touch—could be affected, and some or all could be altered to result in a hypo- or hypersensitivity, with stereotypical behaviors being set off by these dysperceptions.

Thus Delacato thought that a child who covered his ears could be experiencing a hyper- or hypo- alteration of the sounds he was hearing, and with this behavior tried to avoid the bothersome stimulus. A child with poor tactile sensitivity (hypotactility) would try to repeatedly bite himself or other objects. However, in order to interpret the stereotypical behaviors appropriately, Delacato felt it was not enough to connect them to a specific sense, but rather that the child's behavior had to be examined globally, especially when visual stereotypies were considered.

Vision related stereotypical behaviors have always been the most frequent and difficult to understand. The visual system is so complex that is not easy to say when the stereotypies are triggered by the system itself and when instead they are the result of the visual system trying to make an adjustment.

One behavior that many autistic children have in common is rocking sideways. One interpretation of this behavior is that it could be related to the child's need to modify his visual system through movement. Yet it is not rare that these children have a very high pain threshold and have difficulty feeling their own bodies. If this is the case, the rocking could be the means to ground or re-establish the motor component of vision. From studying blind or partially sighted individuals, we know that without visual information tactile and auditory inputs provide important information that can be relied upon. Many persons who are totally blind from an early age have an above average ability to perceive certain aspects of sound. Similarly totally deaf persons, especially those who use sign language from an early age, have better visual skills in some areas. Delacato believed the same process occurs in autistic children. If tactile perception is not reliable they try to use visual-vestibular information by rocking, and if their auditory system is not trustworthy in analyzing sounds, once again they will try to organize their perception of the world through vision.[1]

Thus in order to understand a stereotypy involving the visual system, all sensory channels must be evaluated to learn the manner in which they are altered. We can then ascertain whether a certain repetitive behavior comes from a dysfunction of the primary visual areas or is an attempt to compensate for distorted sensory information. Thus sensory screening is the most suitable tool for defining vision related stereotypical behaviors.

Once the stereotypies have been isolated, it is necessary to consider the physiology of the visual system and the visual means to process information in order to interpret them correctly. Knowledge of how that sensory system has been modified during human evolution can be very helpful. While it is possible to perceive a sound or an odor without knowing its source, and to do so in daylight or darkness despite certain obstacles, the eyes can only perceive sensory input if it is in front of them and there is adequate light. If there is an obstacle in the way it will block vision, yet even if central vision is blocked there is still ambient vision to support posture, balance, and movement. Therefore, from an evolutionary point of view the eyes have become the most sophisticated tool we have.

Why do we rely on such a substantially limited system? By comparing vision with other senses we will find that only vision can perceive the movement of the objects around us in the moment it happens. The hypothesis then is that during our evolution perception of movement proved important for survival and thus much space was given to the system that best enabled us to perceive it. If we now look at the anatomic and functional evolution of the eyes we will see that everything advanced in the direction of being able to see movement.

By analyzing primitive eyes we discover, for example, that a frog can catch a fly only when it is moving, or that the rabbit's eyes are sensitive to the slightest movement so that it can skillfully escape predators. In other situations they live in a kind of constant haziness.

More evolved types of eyes belong to animals with more complex lives. Marmoset monkeys that live in the forest need to be able not only to perceive movement, but also to detect food on the ground. This is why they have developed the ability to see colors. However, this occurs in a very limited way because female monkeys have three-color based vision, and males have two-color based vision. But this is a very interesting aspect: the less they are able to see colors, the more sensitive they are to the perception of shine and reflection.[4]

In the forest, the light filters through the thick vegetation and color variations are minimal. It is easier for an animal that cannot see colors to visually perceive something based on its brightness. Marmoset monkey males can detect the food camouflaging itself with the ground because of their color vision, albeit limited, and their ability to evaluate variations of brightness in conjunction with movement and parallax.

The visual information associated with either movement or brightness is related to motor ability, i.e. to catch prey, escape predators, or gather food. Such an immediate motor reaction to visual perception of movement and/or shine is possible only in the presence of an associative cerebral area where visual and motor neurons release information at the same time.

The first associative cerebral areas of vision-mobility are already present in phylogenically very old neural structures such as in the pons and midbrain; others are diffuse in the medial temporal cortical area (MT), medial superior temporal area (MST), and fundus of the superior temporal area (FST) which is connected with Brodmann's area 7 of the posterior parietal lobe. The older brain areas of the pons and midbrain match visual and motor information in a way that we could define as pre-established: a certain motor action corresponds to a certain visual stimulus. However, the cortical area combines visual and motor information in a much more complex manner. This is due to the fact that medial temporal, parietal, and frontal pathways are connected; as a consequence the motor processes are based on much more information.

In the subcortical areas of pons and midbrain visual information can determine rotation of the neck and trunk followed by a ballistic arm movement forwards without the person who makes these movements being aware of them. In the parietal-occipital area a visual stimulus can make the arm stretch toward a target preparing the hand to grasp an object. In this case, too, there is no awareness of the movement, but motivation in addition to the visual stimulus is needed in order to elicit the arm movement.

Pons, midbrain and posterior parietal areas receive stimuli from the retina's receptors: the cones and rods. The rods work in low light conditions and are commonly considered receptors for movement, but it is more accurate to say that these receptors are able to see details of moving objects. From the periphery of the retina information goes to the occipital striate cortex (V1), and to the subcortical and cortical areas MT, MST and the posterior parietal area, to begin the reactions described above.

The infant's visual development goes from peripheral to central retina (see Chapter 1); in fact, rod cells start to activate earlier than cone cells. In this way the infant becomes ready to recognize light variations and perceive movement, and his reactions will initially be just head rotation to follow the movement of an object, and arm extension to grab it. Later, around seven months of age, the focal process, through the cones, starts to develop functional maturity which enables the infant to see outlines of objects better. Motor reactions are still limited to head, trunk and arm movements, but little by little control of the upper limbs will improve so that the infant will learn to grasp without ballistic movements. The young infant's color detection is very similar to that of the marmoset monkey. Babies initially learn to distinguish an object in a group based not on color but on brightness.

By knowing the evolution of the visual system and some aspects of its physiology, we can now begin to develop an understanding of visual stereotypies in autistic individuals.

Based on Dr. Delacato's diagnostic hypothesis, autistic children could have dysfunction of primary visual area V1 subsequent to mild and diffuse cortical damage. In this area all of the information from the retina is gathered and we know that during the first months of life the eye is ready to respond to variations of brightness and details of moving objects. Later, when the cones reach functional maturity, information regarding the outlines of shapes will also arrive at V1. At this time, inhibitory pathways will be activated in the first layer of the visual area. These are aimed at limiting the analysis of the visual stimuli coming from the peripheral retina in favor of the ones coming from its center. Functional alteration of V1 could hinder proper inhibition of information concerning brightness and movement, and limit significantly the perception of stimuli regarding shapes. Should this happen, V1 would continue to analyze inputs coming from the periphery of the retina unloading this excess of information into areas V5 (MT), V5a (MST) and the posterior parietal area, as well as into subcortical areas, resulting in hyperconnection.

Since the subcortical areas and posterior parietal area activate motor pathways, the ultimate effect of this process would be to start up a series of aimless motor reactions: stereotypies.

Without inhibitory control an excessive number of stimuli will be delivered to the posterior parietal area, and in turn they will initiate an exaggerated movement of arms and hands resulting in a constant arm flexion-extension or hand flapping or finger twisting. Motivation is lacking because the whole process was caused by too much information coming from V1. Thus frontal areas do not exert any control on the action and the movement is not relevant to a real context.

From V1 information also goes towards subcortical areas that arouse a repertoire of stereotyped behaviors when they are excessively stimulated. In this case the child will react to any light source in an indiscriminate way and tend to bend his head sideways to favor peripheral vision causing an imbalance of ocular-motor function.

We can assume that color detection, too, is limited since V1 has difficulty in inhibiting information about movement and brightness, resulting in these children responding to a lack of inhibition to brightness. This could explain why autistic children are often seen manipulating objects so that light hits any angle.

If perception continues to be linked primarily to movement, autistic individuals will tend to devise strategies to comprehend objects. One of them is to grasp an object with their fingertips, and wave it in front of the most peripheral part of the eye. As described above, excessive peripheral vision will cause imbalance in the motor function of eyes. It could happen that by using central vision very little, the moments of fixation are very few. Fixation is, of course, a visual perceptual act of focalization, but it is also a function of a motor action of the eyes that allows the ambient process to spatially orient to the location of the target, then in turn permitting focalization on the target. The movements that back up the fixation are the saccadic ones. Therefore the eyes will move spatially through ambient domain until they focus the fovea on the target. Once fixation has occurred, the piece of image that has been selected is transmitted to the brain. However, the ambient process must release the focalization to enable another saccadic movement so that eyes can select another piece of the image. When sufficient focal and ambient spatial information has been obtained, the brain will establish relationships to perceive the image as a whole.

We started with the hypothesis that in area V1 there is an inadequate number of inhibitory mechanisms for information coming from the peripheral retina, and that this results in problems with perception of information collected by the central retina. When visual pathways charged with the analysis of shapes do not get the information they need, they will have great difficulty in activating all the neural pathways involved in saccadic movements. These movements will occur anyway, but not in a functional way to allow integration of further details of the image. The consequence of this would be the perception of only details of a scene or an object, resulting in potentially devastating effects on behavior.

An individual perceiving the world in this way has a difficult time defining the edges of what he sees and evaluating spatial information. It is possible then that he will develop some unique mannerisms to compensate for his disorder and that he will eventually demonstrate true visually induced stereotypical behaviors such as: opening and closing doors and drawers to control their real size through movement; pouring water to check the capacity of the container; putting objects in a row along the edge of a table to understand its outline; or placing objects in the same position to facilitate spatial recognition.

Once one has a greater knowledge of the neurological substrate of those with autism, especially the connections between the motor and visual systems, the stereotypical behaviors of autistic persons can be better understood. As David F. Delacato described in his foreword to the book *Children Who Do Not Look You in the Eye: The Secrets of Autistic Behavior*[5]:

"You will need an open heart to fully understand the world these children are trapped in. I must constantly remind people that the behaviors of autistic children are the result not of psychological issues but of an altered perception of the world; they act appropriately for their perceptions. If we could create in you the same perceptions these children suffer from, you too would act in this manner."

Chapter 14

THE AUDITORY SYSTEM AND ITS INTERACTIONS WITH THE VISUAL SYSTEM

Jennifer McCullagh, Stephanie C. Nagle, Diantha Morse, Frank E. Musiek

Introduction

The auditory system and how we hear has influenced what is known about the visual system. Hearing and seeing together provide immense amounts of information about our environment. In this chapter the focus will be on the auditory system, but some brief yet relevant side journeys into visual phenomena will also be included.

Both the auditory and visual systems have well-defined peripheral and central segments, with each being responsible for specific functions that complement each other. The auditory system is sensitive to sound waves, which are simply the expansion and contraction of air molecules secondary to the vibrations of objects in our environment. Loud sounds have bigger vibrations and high pitch sounds have faster vibrations compared to soft sounds and low pitch sounds, respectively. These sound waves are funneled into the ear through the ear canal and strike the eardrum, which causes it to vibrate and places the middle ear bones in vibratory motion. The most medial middle ear bone, the stapes, imparts vibratory energy into the inner ear, or cochlea. The cochlea transduces vibratory energy into electrical impulses so the auditory nerve and the brain can utilize this energy. As this chapter will discuss, the cochlea also codes loudness and pitch and passes this code on to the auditory nerve which carries it to the brain. The auditory nerve is part of the VIII cranial nerve and connects the cochlea with the brain. The external ear through the auditory nerve is considered the peripheral auditory system. Once the electrical impulse enters the brainstem, it travels through the central auditory system which processes these impulses into meaningful signals – the most important signal being speech. This chapter will describe the key anatomy of the central auditory system and discuss some relevant functions.

The chapter will also mention what happens when the peripheral or central auditory system doesn't work properly – hearing loss. Hearing loss can take many forms and is tightly linked to auditory anatomy. Each major structure, either in the peripheral or central system, if damaged, leaves a particular mark that often can be interpreted in a manner that leads to a diagnosis. Electrophysiologic measures elicited from nerve arrays in the auditory system are termed evoked potentials, and can indicate appropriate function or dysfunction of the system.

How and why do visual and auditory signals interact? What happens to the central auditory system in blindness or the visual cortex in deafness? These questions will be addressed in this chapter and will lead the reader to realize these systems, although different in many ways, share certain similarities as well. At the end of the day, these systems do summate to provide vast amounts of critical information to our minds.

PERIPHERAL AUDITORY SYSTEM

The peripheral auditory system is comprised of the outer ear, the middle ear, the inner ear, and the auditory nerve. The middle and inner ears, auditory nerve and portions of the outer ear are encased in the temporal bone of the skull. As sound enters the outer ear and travels through the middle and inner ear, it is transformed from acoustic energy (the vibration of air molecules) to mechanical, hydromechanical, and then neural energy, which then travels through the neurons of the central auditory system.

Outer Ear

The outer ear has two major components: the external auditory meatus (EAM) or ear canal, and the pinna or auricle (see Figure 14-1). The pinna is the portion of the auditory system visible to the naked eye. The function of the pinna is to capture and funnel sound into the ear canal, and also to aid in its localization.

The EAM or ear canal is a bony tunnel which begins at the concha and ends at the tympanic membrane. The ear canal amplifies certain frequencies of incoming sound, typically around 2700 and 5000 Hz.[1]

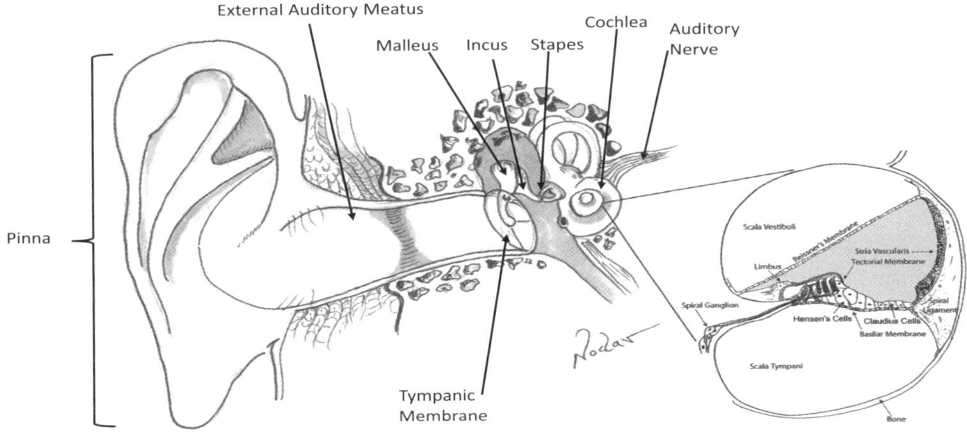

Figure 14-1. The main structures of the peripheral auditory system and a cross section of the cochlea.

Sound travels through the air as acoustic energy, compressing and rarefacting air molecules. This energy is captured by the pinna and funneled into the ear canal, where it travels down the length of the ear canal and hits the eardrum.

Middle Ear

The middle ear is an air-filled cavity bounded by the tympanic membrane (TM), or eardrum, on one side and by the bony cochlea on the other (see Figure 14-1). The middle ear space contains the ossicles, or bones of the middle ear, and 2 small muscles. The tympanic membrane is a thin, taut membrane that is made of epithelial tissue making it an efficient vibrating surface.

The ossicles are the three smallest bones in the body. From lateral to medial, they are the malleus, incus, and stapes. The manubrium or long process of the malleus is connected to the medial side of the tympanic membrane. The malleus connects to the incus, which in turn connects to the stapes. The stapes is shaped like a stirrup and has a flat plate at the bottom part of the bone called the footplate. The footplate of the stapes sits inside the oval window of the bony cochlea. The two small muscles of the inner ear, the stapedius and tensor tympani, attach to the stapes and malleus, respectively, and have a reflexive function to protect the ear from loud noises.

After sound energy is captured by the pinna and funneled into the ear canal, it hits the tympanic membrane and sets it into vibration. This, in turn, sets the ossicular chain into vibration. The motion of the stapes results in a piston-like movement of the stapes footplate in and out of the oval window of the cochlea.

In addition to conducting sound energy from the outer ear to the cochlea of the inner ear, the middle ear also acts as a transformer. As the sound energy moves from the air-filled middle ear to the fluid filled cochlea, a mismatch in impedance takes place. Impedance is the amount of resistance to flow of energy that exists in a medium, and is affected by mass, density, and stiffness of a medium. The air of the middle ear has lower impedance than the fluid of the inner ear, which means that it is more difficult for energy to move through the inner ear, and that more force is needed to do so. As a result, the amount of sound energy being introduced to the middle ear must be amplified before it reaches the fluid-filled inner ear, in order to compensate for the difference in impedance between the middle and inner ears. If no compensation took place, there would be a net loss of sound energy of approximately 30 dB in the middle ear. Altogether, the middle ear functions as an efficient energy transformer, amplifying enough sound energy to make up 26 dB of the 30 dB that would be lost due to impedance mismatch.[1]

Inner Ear Anatomy

The inner ear lies deep within the temporal bone of the skull, and can be divided functionally as well as structurally. Functionally, the inner ear contains both vestibular structures, which are part of the balance system, and auditory structures. Discussion of the vestibular structures is beyond the scope of this chapter. Structurally, the inner ear contains 2 labyrinths: a bony labyrinth and within that a labyrinth of membranes and fluid. The bony labyrinth provides the outer bony shell of the snail-like cochlea, as well as the vestibule where the round and oval windows are located. The cochlea contains a bony core, the modiolus, as well as a bony shelf, the osseous spiral lamina, which spirals up and around the modiolus from the bottom, or base, of the cochlea to the top or apex.

The membranous labyrinth of the cochlea contains three channels or ducts: the scala vestibuli (upper), scala media (middle) and scala tympani (lower) (see Figure 14-1). Each duct is filled with fluid. The scala vestibuli and scala tympani are filled with perilymph, a neutral liquid similar in composition to cerebrospinal fluid (CSF); the scala media is filled with endolymph, a fluid high in potassium, with a charge of +80 mV. The scala vestibuli and scala tympani are separate channels at the base of the cochlea, and spiral up and around the modiolus to the apex of the cochlea, where they meet at the helicotrema. Reissner's membrane forms the boundary between the scala vestibuli and scala media. The basilar membrane separates the scala media from the scala tympani.

Within the scala media, the stria vascularis lines the lateral wall of the cochlea, and a structure called the Organ of Corti sits on top of the basilar membrane. The stria vascularis provides the blood supply and nutrients to the cochlea. The Organ of Corti contains several important structures, including the inner and outer hair cells which are the specialized sensory cells that are largely responsible for the transduction of sound. There are approximately 13,500 outer hair cells arranged in 3-5 rows, and 3,500 inner hair cells arranged in one row.[2] The hair cells have stereocilia, or small hairs, on their superior surface. For the outer hair cells, the tips of the stereocilia are embedded in the underside of the tectorial membrane, a gelatinous membrane that lies on top of the Organ of Corti. The stereocilia of the inner hair cells, however, do not make physical contact with the tectorial membrane, but are closely apposed to the underside of it. The inferior aspect of both inner and outer hair cells is the site of attachment for the auditory nerve fibers (mainly afferent).

Inner Ear Physiology

The piston-like movement of the stapes footplate in the oval window results in a specific pattern of fluid movement in the cochlea. The speed of the stapes footplate movement corresponds to the frequency of the sound in cycles per second. The in and out movement of the stapes footplate creates a traveling wave of fluid and basilar membrane movement. This traveling wave starts near the stapes footplate at the basal end of the cochlea, and travels through the cochlea until it reaches a point along the basilar membrane at which it resonates. The resonance of the basilar membrane varies throughout its length, based on the changing physical characteristics of the basilar membrane. At the basal end of the cochlea, the basilar membrane is stiff, thin, and narrow; at the apical end, it is floppy, thick, and wide. The physical gradients of stiffness, thickness, and width of the basilar membrane lead to a continuum of resonant frequencies along the length of the basilar membrane, ranging from 20,000 Hz at the basal end to 20 Hz at the apical end. This physical arrangement of frequencies along the basilar membrane is the first example of tonotopicity in the auditory system. The principle of tonotopicity refers to a physical map or arrangement of frequencies, and recurs in each auditory structure from the cochlea through the auditory cortex.[2]

The vibration of the basilar membrane increases when the traveling wave reaches the point on the basilar membrane that has a resonant frequency matching that of the original sound. This is called maximum displacement. Frequency is encoded by the cochlea via the *location* of the maximum displacement of the traveling wave on the basilar membrane; intensity is encoded by the *magnitude* of the displacement, as waves that are larger in amplitude activate more hair cells around the maximum displacement area.

When the basilar membrane moves up, the stereocilia of the hair cells are bent toward the lateral wall of the cochlea by the movement of the fluid and tectorial membrane. This causes ion channels in the stereocilia to open, allowing ions from the positively charged endolymph into the negatively charged hair cells. This, in turn, causes depolarization of the hair cell, the release of a neurotransmitter from the hair cell to the afferent auditory nerve ending attached to the inferior end of the hair cell, and subsequent depolarization of the auditory nerve fiber.

Auditory Nerve Anatomy

The auditory nerve is also known as the eighth cranial nerve (CN VIII), and is approximately 22-26 mm long, connecting the cochlea of the inner ear to the cochlear nucleus of the brainstem. The dendrites of the auditory nerve fibers attach to the bottom of the inner and outer hair cells, and the fibers then travel through an opening in the osseous spiral lamina. The nuclei of the auditory nerve fibers, or spiral ganglia, are located in a bony tunnel called Rosenthal's canal. From there, nerve fibers travel into the modiolus, the bony core of the cochlea. The individual nerve fibers join together as a bundle in the modiolus, with the fibers connected to the apical end of the cochlea forming the core of the bundle, and the fibers from the basal end forming the outermost part of the bundle. The auditory nerve exits the modiolus area, and then courses through another bony canal, the internal auditory meatus, across the cerebellopontine angle (CPA) to the brain stem. It terminates at the cochlear nucleus, located at the ponto-medullary junction of the brainstem.

The auditory nerve is composed of two types of auditory fibers. Type I fibers comprise approximately 90-95% of auditory nerve fibers, and connect to inner hair cells, with multiple type I fibers connected to each individual inner hair cell. Type I fibers are partially myelinated. In contrast, type II fibers make up the remaining auditory nerve fibers, and connect to outer hair cells, with each type II fiber connecting to multiple outer hair cells. Type II fibers are not myelinated.[2] Most of what is known about the physiology of the auditory nerve is derived from the study of type I fibers.

Auditory Nerve Physiology

The tonotopicity of the cochlea is preserved in the auditory nerve, since the excitation of auditory nerve fibers is dependent on excitation of the hair cells they are connected to in the cochlea. Following depolarization or hyperpolarization of the hair cells of the cochlea, ions travel across the synapse between the hair cell and auditory nerve fiber dendrite to cause excitation or inhibition of the auditory nerve. Auditory nerve fibers that form the core of the auditory nerve are responsive to low frequency sounds, since they are connected to the apical (low frequency) end of the cochlea. Conversely, auditory fibers on the outside of the auditory nerve respond to high frequency sounds, as they are connected to the basal (high frequency) end of the cochlea. Additionally, the auditory nerve also encodes frequency temporally. Auditory nerve fibers have the capacity to lock onto a sound and fire regularly in correlation to the compression and rarefaction cycle of the sound; this is called phase-locking.[2]

Different auditory nerve fibers have different capacities for encoding intensity, and no one fiber has the capacity to encode the entire range of intensity for human hearing. Some fibers encode low intensity sounds, some encode moderate intensity sounds, and some encode high intensity sounds. Auditory nerve fibers work in concert with one another to encode the entire range of sound intensity.

CENTRAL AUDITORY SYSTEM

Brainstem Auditory Nuclei

The brainstem auditory nuclei consist of the cochlear nucleus (CN), superior olivary complex (SOC), lateral lemniscus (LL), inferior colliculus (IC), and medial geniculate body (MGB). Each of these successive structures is responsible for coding the frequency, intensity, and temporal characteristics of the incoming signal.

The VIII cranial nerve fibers project from the auditory periphery, synapsing with neurons in the first structure of the central auditory nervous system (CANS), called the cochlear nucleus (CN). Each CN receives input from the fibers of the ipsilateral auditory nerve. The CN is located in the brainstem at the level of the pontomedullary junction. Many different cell types have been found in the CN, each of which has a different physiologic response to the incoming acoustic signal.[3] The neural outputs from the CN take three primary paths to synapse, both ipsilaterally and contralaterally, with CANS nuclei higher in the system. These three pathways include the ventral, intermediate, and dorsal acoustic striae.[4]

The superior olivary complex (SOC) is the next major group of nuclei in the ascending auditory pathway. The SOC nuclei are relatively small and diffuse within the caudal pons. The SOC receives primarily contralateral inputs from the CN, making it the first group of nuclei along the ascending auditory pathway to receive inputs from both ears (see Musiek and Baran[5]). Outputs from the SOC synapse with neurons in the lateral lemniscus (LL) and inferior colliculus (IC).

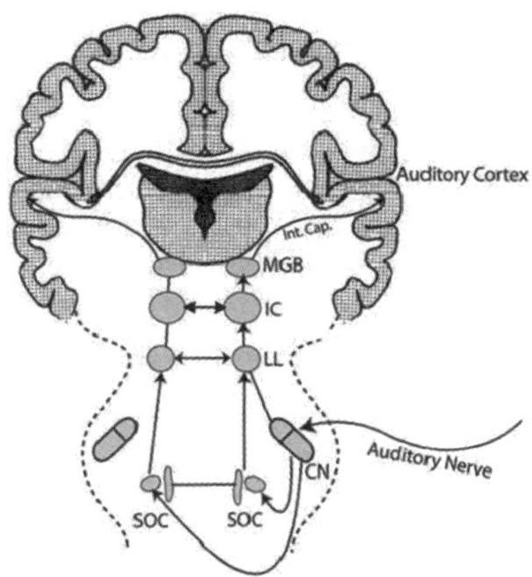

Figure 14-2. A schematic view of the central auditory nervous system. CN= cochlear nucleus; SOC= superior olivary complex; LL= lateral lemniscus; IC= inferior colliculus; MGB= medial geniculate body; Int. Cap.=internal capsule.

The LL consists of a major auditory pathway in the brainstem, as well as two nuclei groups. The LL pathway is formed by fibers exiting the CN, as well as the SOC. This fiber tract courses superiorly in the brainstem along the lateral aspect of the pons and terminates at the IC in the midbrain. The nuclei of the LL on the left and right are connected by the commissure of Probst.[5]

The IC is located in the dorsal midbrain along with the superior colliculus. Inputs to the IC come from the CN (contralateral), SOC (ipsilateral and contralateral), and the LL (ipsilateral and contralateral) (see Ehret[6] for review). Outputs from the IC primarily course ipsilaterally through the brachium of the IC to the medial geniculate body (MGB). In addition, outputs from the IC course contralaterally through the commissure of the IC to the MGB as well as the thalamus.[5]

The MGB is located on the underside of the posterior thalamus. The MGB, along with other auditory responsive structures in the thalamus receive ascending inputs from the IC. Neural outputs from the MGB course through the basal ganglia to the caudate and putamen. In addition, outputs from the MGB course through the internal capsule, laterally to the primary auditory cortex (Heschl's gyrus). This pathway consists of primarily auditory fibers.[7] Other outputs from the MGB course through the inferior internal capsule to the external capsule where they connect to the insula. This pathway not only includes auditory fibers, but also somatosensory and possibly visual fibers.[8,9] Fibers from the MGB also course to the amygdala linking the auditory system to emotion.[10]

Each of these brainstem structures, CN, SOC, IC, and MGB, are responsible for coding the frequency, intensity, and temporal aspects of the acoustic signal. Similar to the auditory nerve, frequency coding in each of these CANS structures can be attributed to tonotopic organization. Intensity is coded in the CANS by nerve fibers which have different dynamic ranges, or intensity ranges at which the neurons respond. Therefore, some neurons respond to high intensity sounds, while others respond to middle or low intensity sounds. Like the auditory nerve, temporal coding in the CANS is related to the ability of neurons to phase-lock onto periodic stimuli.

Since the SOC is the first structure along the CANS pathway to receive binaural inputs, it is responsible for localization of acoustic information. The convergence of inputs from two ears allows the SOC to analyze differences in the neural impulses that relate to intensity and timing of the auditory signal as it arrives at each of the ears. Binaural processing of the acoustic signal continues in each of the subsequent auditory nuclei in the brainstem.

Auditory Cortex

The primary auditory area in the cortex is located in the temporal lobes along the Sylvian, or lateral, fissure. The primary auditory area, Heschl's gyrus, courses posterior-medially along the superior temporal gyrus. Evidence suggests that Heschl's gyrus is larger in the left hemisphere than the right.[11] Heschl's gyrus has extensive intrahemispheric connections. Some neural connections from the primary auditory areas course posteriorly to Wernicke's area (responsible for understanding speech) then the signal is sent through the arcuate fasciculus to the frontal lobe. Heschl's gyrus also has connections with the planum temporale which is located directly posterior to it. Similar to Heschl's gyrus, the left planum temporale has been shown to be larger in the left hemisphere than the right.[12] Since the left hemisphere is typically the dominant hemisphere for speech, the planum temporale may be responsible for receptive language function in humans.

In addition to the structures of the superior temporal plane (Heschl's gyrus and planum temporale), other cortical areas have been shown to have auditory responsive areas including: the supramarginal gyrus, angular gyrus, inferior aspect of the postcentral gyrus, and inferior aspect of the precentral gyrus.[13]

The primary subcortical structure that responds to the auditory stimuli is the insula. The insula lies medial to the Sylvian fissure and is covered by parts of the temporal, frontal, and parietal lobes. Similar to Heschl's gyrus and planum temporale, the insula has been shown to be larger in the left than the right hemisphere.[14] In addition to auditory functions, the insula is responsible for processing visceral, motor, vestibular, and somatosensory information.[15,16]

Physiologically, the auditory cortical structures are responsible for coding frequency, intensity, and time. Like the brainstem auditory nuclei, Heschl's gyrus is tonotopically organized. Intensity is coded in Heschl's gyrus by neurons that respond to high, middle, and low intensity sounds. The auditory cortex is highly sensitive to the temporal, or timing, characteristics of the acoustic stimuli such that it is capable of segregating responses to brief stimuli only 1 to 2 msec apart. This degree of temporal precision is especially essential for the accurate coding of speech (see Musiek & Baran[5]).

Interhemispheric connections between the two auditory cortices are the result of the corpus callosum. The corpus callosum is a heavily myelinated pathway that connects the two hemispheres by transferring information from one hemisphere to the other. The region of the corpus callosum responsible for transferring auditory information is called the sulcus. Located posteriorly to the sulcus is the splenium which transfers visual information from one occipital lobe to the other. The corpus callosum is not only responsible for dichotic listening (processing auditory information from both ears), but also for pattern perception with a verbal response.[5]

Dysfunction in the Peripheral and Central Auditory Systems

Hearing loss can occur in the auditory periphery (including the outer, middle, and inner ears and the auditory nerve) or the central auditory nervous system. Hearing loss related to pathology beyond the cochlea is often referred to as retrocochlear. This term is often utilized when discussing VIII nerve pathology.

Peripheral hearing loss can be separated into two primary categories: conductive and sensorineural. Conductive hearing losses occur when the acoustic signal cannot pass through the outer or middle ear. Congenital malformations of the pinna and external auditory meatus can lead to conductive hearing losses. In addition, otitis externa, occluding cerumen, perforation of the tympanic membrane, ossicular discontinuity, and otosclerosis can lead to conductive hearing losses in the affected ear. In children, the most common pathology that results in conductive hearing loss, although transient, is otitis media with effusion. Often times, but not always, conductive hearing losses can be repaired.[17]

Sensorineural hearing losses are the result of damage to the cochlear structures, most often the hair cells and subsequent degeneration of the auditory nerve fibers. A common type of sensorineural hearing loss related to aging is presbycusis, which is the deterioration of the outer hair cells, followed by the inner hair cells. It is characterized by a progressive bilateral symmetric sensorineural hearing loss. Due to the tonotopic organization of the cochlea (high frequencies at the basal end; low frequencies at the apical end), high frequencies are affected first, and the loss progresses toward the lower frequencies. Over time, soft speech sounds become difficult to hear, and these individuals will complain of difficulty *understanding* speech. Noise-induced hearing loss (NIHL) is another common type of sensorineural hearing loss. NIHL is the result of the exposure to high intensity sounds, particularly over long periods of time. NIHL may be unilateral or bilateral depending on the location of the noise source relative to the individual. NIHL can either be temporary (temporary threshold shift) or permanent (permanent threshold shift). Temporary threshold shifts occur following exposure to high intensity sounds at, for example, a concert, but will recover within a day or two. Permanent threshold shifts can occur if noise exposure is repeated over time. The repeated exposure to high intensity noise is transmitted through the outer and middle ears to the cochlea where the hair cells become over-stimulated and over time degenerate.[17] Permanent threshold shift can also occur following only one exposure if the intensity of the sound is high enough.

Retrocochlear pathology is defined as pathology beyond the cochlea, including but not limited to the auditory nerve. Vestibular schwannomas are a common VIII nerve pathology. A vestibular schwannoma is a benign tumor of the vestibular branch of the VIII nerve. Depending on the location and size of the tumor, the VII and V cranial nerves may also be affected. These tumors are often slow-growing and for this reason, might be present for years without the individual experiencing symptoms. Symptoms typically include both auditory (unilateral hearing impairment, tinnitus, and aural fullness) and vestibular (off balance, vertigo, nausea, vomiting) complaints.[18]

Difficulty hearing does not have to be related to dysfunction in the peripheral auditory system, but may be the result of pathology and/or dysfunction in the CANS. Inaccurate and/or distorted perception of sounds, in spite of normal peripheral hearing sensitivity, is often the result of disordered central auditory processing abilities. Central auditory processing disorders are characterized by having difficulties in one or more of the following areas: sound localization/lateralization, temporal processing, auditory discrimination, and auditory pattern recognition. Individuals might also have poor auditory performance with degraded or competing acoustic signals.[19] Large numbers of neurons need to respond accurately and synchronously to incoming acoustic stimulation in order to accurately perceive the auditory message. If neurons fail to do so along the ascending auditory pathway, a breakdown in auditory processing occurs and the individual will "lose" some of the message. The degree to which the message is mis-coded, or not coded, is related to the number of neurons affected by the CANS pathology (see Chermak & Musiek[20]).

VISUAL EVOKED POTENTIALS AS PART OF VISUAL-AUDITORY RELATIONSHIP

Evoked potentials (EPs) can be recorded from humans in both the auditory and visual modalities. These EPs can be used in research in regard to physiology of the auditory and visual systems and/or in clinical diagnosis of underlying problems. Both auditory and visual EPs can be used for the determination of deafness or blindness in those that cannot respond behaviorally. More specifically, degrees of hearing loss and visual impairment can be approximated by using these EPs. Therefore, these potentials have the capability of revealing much about these sensory systems from the periphery to the cortex.

Both auditory and visual EPs are best recorded when the stimuli are robust and abrupt. In the auditory system, clicks are the abrupt stimuli often used to evoke auditory potentials. Tones can also be used, but they must be relatively abrupt (short rise - fall times). The visual EPs are usually obtained using two kinds of stimuli which are classified as luminance and pattern forms.[21] A bright flash stimulus and the background on which the flash is presented must meet standards of use for

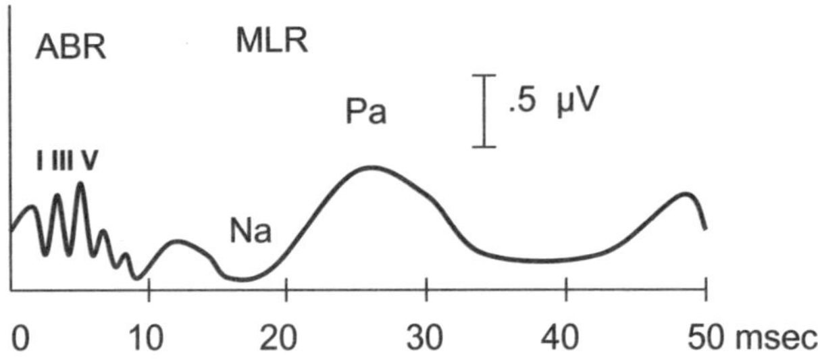

Figure 14-3. An example waveform of an auditory brainstem (ABR) and middle latency (MLR) response.

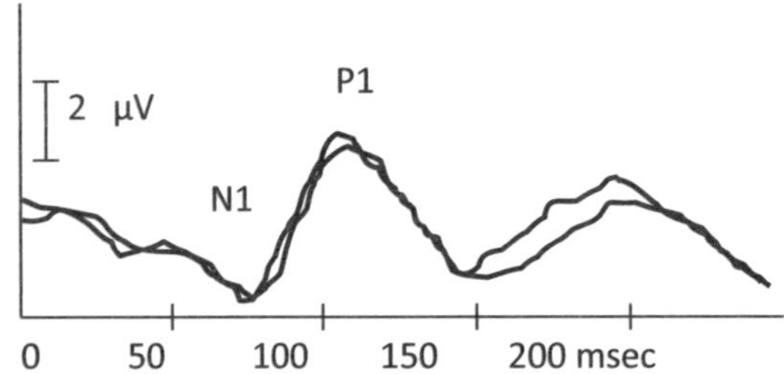

Figure 14-4. An example of a visual evoked potential waveform.

these kinds of stimuli.[22] Pattern stimuli are usually black and white checks and can be presented in an on – off or reversal fashion to trigger a response, again with standards set forth.[22] The auditory and visual EPs are extracted by the signal-averaging of neural activity emitted from the scalp, which is then filtered and amplified. Electrodes are commonly placed at the vertex and referenced to the ear for auditory EPs, and are placed on the occipital area and referenced to the frontal area for visual EPs.

Several types of auditory EPs exist, but three common types are the auditory brainstem response (ABR), the middle latency response (MLR) and the late potentials including the P300 (see Figure 14-3). The ABR occurs in the first 5-10 msec after stimulus onset and is characterized by three main waves I (from the auditory nerve), III (from the low pons), and V (from the mid to upper pons). Abnormalities in the function of the peripheral system, auditory nerve, or brainstem result in the delay or absence of these waves. Strategies using ABR have been developed to separate peripheral from central auditory involvement (see Musiek, Bornstein, Hall, & Schwaber[23]). The middle latency response (MLR) occurs between 15 – 70 msec post-stimulus onset and reflects thalamo-cortical activity and integrity. The important waves in this response are referred to as the Na and Pa responses and are larger (about 1 microvolt) than the ABR (0.5 - 0.7 microvolts). The late potentials are composed of the N1 and P2 responses which occur at about 100 and 200 msec, respectively, post-stimulus onset. The P300, which is also considered a late potential, will be discussed later. The N1 and P2 are large responses, usually greater than 3 microvolts, and are primarily generated by the auditory cortex. The MLR and the N1 and P2 are sensitive to dysfunction of the higher auditory areas (cortex) and are often reduced in amplitude or delayed in latency in central auditory system disorders.[24]

A major difference between auditory and visual EPs is that the visual system does not have an EP comparable to the ABR. There are early visual EPs (25 – 30 msec) called P1 that occur during similar time domains as the MLR, but these are not highly reliable and not well investigated. The visual system does have an EP similar to the N1, P2 with an N response at 75 msec, a P2 response at 100 msec and another negative (N) response at around 140 msec (see Figure 14-4). These later visual responses are sensitive to dysfunction along the visual tract leading to, and including the visual cortex. For example, people with multiple sclerosis may have delayed P2 and N responses if the visual tracts are involved.[21,25] Furthermore, researchers have also used visual EPs to document dysfunction in the visual system in individuals with Post Trauma Vision Syndrome (PTVS).[26]

The P300 EP can be obtained for both the visual and auditory system. Although the responses appear similar, differences between the two do exist.[27] The P300 is obtained using an oddball paradigm which is characterized by the inclusion of frequent and rare stimuli. A series of frequent tones, or flashes, during which occasionally one stimulus differs from others in the train (rare stimuli) are presented. The individual is asked to note the different stimulus. This mental recognition and decision result in a large EP (10 – 20 microvolts) called the P300. This involves the sensory and cognitive systems and is sensitive to aging as well as higher auditory or visual cognitive dysfunction. This EP can be compared across modalities to determine specific versus more general cortical involvement. Though direct comparisons between auditory and visual P300 cannot always be made, this approach can yield valuable information about these systems.

Deafness and Blindness & Brain Interactions

Evoked potential and more recently, imaging studies, have indicated significant plasticity in the central nervous system (CNS) in individuals who have congenital blindness, or congenital deafness. Neural plasticity is defined as the changes in the physiological and/or anatomical properties of neurons related to environmental demands.[28] Individuals who are congenitally blind rely on other sensory modalities, such as audition, to interact with the visual world. Likewise, individuals who are congenitally deaf rely on other sensory modalities, such as vision, to interact in the hearing world. The reliance on other sensory modalities to function and interact with the visual and auditory worlds results in use-dependent plasticity. Use-dependent plasticity is related to the changes in cortical response properties as a function of behaviorally relevant stimuli.[29]

Researchers have shown in both animals and humans that early auditory or visual deprivation can lead to altered neural pathways in the brainstem and cortex (for a review, see Bavelier & Neville[30]; Bavelier, Dye, & Hauser[31]). In animals, researchers have shown that ablation of the superior colliculus and the ascending auditory pathways results in the development of permanent projections from the retina to typically auditory-responsive neurons in the medial geniculate body.[32] Not only do these projections form, but they are functional and retinotopically organized.[33] At the cortical level, neurons in the auditory cortex of these animals have receptive field properties similar to those of the visual cortex.[34] Animal research has also indicated plastic changes in the activation of the visual cortex following visual deprivation such that neurons in the visual cortex become responsive to auditory stimulation.[35,36] Furthermore, increased neural density in the auditory cortex has been shown to occur following early visual deprivation indicating greater demands on the auditory system when the visual system is impaired (for review, see Bavelier & Neville[30]). These studies indicate that cross-modal plasticity occurs in animals following early deprivation of either auditory or visual input.

In addition to animal studies, evidence exists suggesting that anatomical and physiological alterations occur in humans following auditory or visual deprivation.[30,31,37] Research indicates reorganization of the auditory cortex in individuals who are deaf.[30] Results of functional Magnetic Resonance Imaging (fMRI) studies indicate auditory cortical neurons are recruited to process visual stimuli in individuals who are deaf.[30,38] Additional research suggests visual activation in the auditory cortex during visual language processing tasks in individuals who are deaf.[39] These studies demonstrate that visual stimuli are processed in typically auditory-responsive areas in the cortex in individuals who do not receive auditory input due to profound hearing impairment.

Similar to the changes in the cortical response patterns in deaf individuals, research also suggests that auditory stimulation evokes activation of neurons in the visual cortices in early blind individuals (for review, see Burton[37]). Imaging studies have shown visual cortex activation in sound localization tasks[40] as well as in spoken word tasks.[41, 42] Furthermore, investigators have used magnoencephalography (MEG) to show the expansion of tonotopic areas around the primary auditory cortex using low and high frequency tone bursts.[43] Expanded tonotopicity in the auditory cortex indicates more neural substrate responding to frequency-specific stimuli in individuals who are blind. Anatomical and physiological alterations in the visual and auditory cortices as a result of blindness do occur in humans, but the extent to which related functional changes happen is still unknown.

The plastic changes seen in the auditory and visual cortices of deaf or blind humans have not been directly linked to functional changes. To date, absolute sensitivity thresholds in either the visual or auditory modalities have not been shown to be affected by the plasticity that takes place in those individuals who are deaf or blind (reviewed by Bavelier & Neville[30]; Bavelier et al.[31]). Although these changes haven't been shown to affect threshold sensitivity, it is likely that functional changes do occur for more complex tasks. Individuals who are deaf have been shown to have enhanced visual attention, such that they process events in the peripheral visual field more accurately than hearing individuals.[44] Similarly, early blind individuals can process sounds faster and localize sounds more accurately than sighted individuals.[43,45,46,47] Given these findings, future research is needed to investigate the extent to which these functional changes are directly linked to neural plasticity in the auditory and visual cortices.

Associations between Auditory and Visual Processing

One of the possible interesting clinical relationships between the visual and auditory systems is the ambient visual process and the more rostral aspect of the efferent auditory system. In the visual system the ambient process is critical to the appropriate function of binocular vision. In the auditory system, the rostral afferent/efferent system is not as well understood or defined. However, it is thought that it feeds back to the cortex and may in some manner modulate input to the auditory cortex. In some animals this area is well integrated in terms of combining auditory and visual functions. The anatomy and physiology of the ambient process and the rostral efferent, and possibly the afferent system do show some similar aspects. As Padula et al.[26] relate, the ambient process is preconscious and appears to orient to anticipatory temporal/spatial information. The ambient process targets the midbrain, specifically the superior colliculus, and is involved in a neural feedback loop to the cortex.

In the auditory system, from an anatomical perspective, the midbrain is also involved in an efferent feedback system, but it is the inferior not the superior colliculus that is involved (see Musiek and Baran[5]). The inferior colliculus is part of a feedback loop that involves the auditory cortex, medial geniculate body and inferior colliculus. The function of this feedback loop may be controlling the afferent system at this level, but this is not well substantiated.[48] Although these interactions are not well substantiated in the human, animal models might serve as a model for these interactions. The barn owl's tectum is a structure that might correspond to the human midbrain that uses both auditory and visual functions to integrate spatial relationships so they can fly and locate prey accurately.[48] Thus the barn owl may serve as a model of how visual and auditory areas of the midbrain work together to analyze spatial relationships and forward these cues on to the cortex.

Like the barn owl, a human's perception of his world is largely the result of hearing and vision, often working together to localize and identify information about the environment. Although our ears are head-fixed, our auditory environment has the advantage of extending in all directions and providing information despite darkness or obstacles that may be present. The environment of the visual horizontal field of view for a forward facing human is about 190-degrees.[49] Much of this involves peripheral vision, but the eyes can move without head movement, providing an illusion of a greater range. Usually, a response to an auditory stimulus involves turning one's head in the direction of the stimulus producing occasion so that vision, often more accurate, can then both refine the spatial information and provide further information about the occurrence. Thus "each sensory system can provide 'missing pieces.'"[50]

As related in Chapter One, the visual system has images mapped directly onto the retina with topographic representation to higher levels of the cortex, a system that provides great accuracy for spatial awareness. However, as described below, sound localization has to be computed by the brain from cue differences between the ears. In order to obtain a coherent mental impression of spatial cues, the cortex must integrate the sensory information from both vision and audition.

The ability to integrate spatial information for localization from visual and auditory cues is often chosen as an example of sensory integration (see Bulkin and Groh[50] for a review). Auditory localization is important both from the standpoint of focusing attention on a person or incident, and for avoiding dangerous situations. Having binaural auditory spatial information is also important when listening in noise.[51] As has already been described in this chapter, auditory localization is largely based on interaural differences involving timing and intensity of the stimuli arriving at each ear. Interaural latency differences (ILD) are especially important for signals below about 1500Hz and provide horizontal spatial information. Interaural intensity differences (IID) also provide horizontal spatial information, especially above 1500Hz and are largely based on the effects of head shadow. Spectral peaks and notches in the acoustic signal, which are related to the anatomy and acoustic properties of the pinnae and external auditory meatus, also provide spatial information, especially for front/back and elevation cues.[52] The auditory cues used for spatial localization change during growth and development of the head and external ears, and thus recalibration is ongoing. Both auditory experiences and visual integration are considered to be an important aspect in this recalibration.[53-56] However, integration of visual and auditory space is ever changing since the position of the eyes, and the position of the head move, altering the localization cues.[57-60]

In situations where there is a discrepancy in the multisensory integration of auditory and visual cues, vision usually dominates (see Welch and Warren[61] for a review). Vision can affect and dominate the spatial localization of the auditory stimulus likely because of the high spatial resolution of the visual system.[62] Behaviorally, the use of visual illusion by ventriloquists is frequently cited as an example of visual dominance. The ventriloquist is able to produce an illusion by separating the auditory from the visual stimuli. The audience will tend to focus on the visual stimuli which is usually more reliable.[63] Misaligned cues, when repeatedly presented, cause the perception of auditory space to be shifted. This "visual capture" of sound occurs regularly in the movies and on television where sound appears to be coming from the actors, but in reality is coming from speakers situated in various locations.

A number of studies have experimentally demonstrated vision's superiority over audition in sensory conflict situations. For example, the use of prisms in barn owls to shift visual spatial information also resulted in a shift of the auditory neural representation of space.[53,64] Zwiers et al., using human subjects and special lenses to compress visual space, showed that the "spatially scaled vision induces systematic and adaptive changes in sound localization that restores the spatial calibration between the two modalities."[65]

Vision can also have a marked influence on auditory speech perception, and in difficult listening situations "lipreading" cues can be critical to speech intelligibility. Increasingly neuroimaging is being used to explore how visual speech provides linguistic cues.[66] The McGurk effect also provides evidence of the multimodal information involved in speech perception and what happens when the stimuli are conflicting.[67] For example, if one sees the lips form the phoneme /ga/, but the auditory input is /ba/, it will often be perceived as the phoneme /da/. Previously in this chapter there was a discussion of cross modal brain plasticity in which early deafness or blindness results in physiological changes to the visual or auditory cortices. It is thus of interest that recent research has shown that most children who receive a cochlear implant before the age of two and a half will exhibit the McGurk effect, but later recipients of an implant will usually not.[68] Such findings underscore the importance of early identification of hearing and vision problems.

Hearing can also dominate vision, especially when temporal information is involved[69] (see Shimojo & Shams[70] for a review). For example, Recanzone[62] found that normal subjects were better at discriminating auditory than visual temporal rates, and that an "auditory distractor" could significantly change the perceived rate of visual temporal stimuli, though the visual stimuli did not affect the auditory rate percept. In a study of temporal representations both visually and auditorily, Guttman et al.[71] concluded that "visual temporal structure is automatically and effortlessly transformed from its inherently visual form into an accurate auditory representation."

Auditory stimuli can also produce a visual illusion as when multiple auditory stimuli accompanying a single light flash causes the flash to be perceived as two or more flashes.[72,73] There is evidence suggesting that by adding an auditory stimulus there can be "multisensory enhancement," as when the number of omissions of visual stimuli decreased during a series of these stimuli when accompanied by sound;[74] when perception of the intensity of a visual stimulus was increased by sound;[75] or when detectability of a visual stimulus improved when accompanied by an abrupt tone presented synchronously.[76]

In trying to determine the neurophysiological basis of multimodal integration and conflict, much of the work has been done using primates, owls, ferrets, and other animals. In non-human primate studies the superior colliculus has been shown to contain multisensory cells (see Driver and Noesselt[78] for a review). While an understanding of the process of sensory integration in humans is still limited, recent advances in the investigative methods of neuroscience in both humans and animals have shown multisensory integration in areas of the brain that were previously thought to be unimodal, including areas of early sensory processing[77,78] (see Ghazanfar & Schroeder[79] for a review).

Every day we rely on our brain to integrate environmental information from all of our senses in order to increase the accuracy and reliability of our perceptions. Visual and auditory inputs are critical parts of this largely unconscious activity. A better understanding of vision and hearing and how they work together can be helpful to practitioners involved in many aspects of patient care.

Summary

The auditory system is responsible for coding the frequency, intensity, and time characteristics of the incoming sound signal. Any dysfunction related to conductive or sensorineural hearing losses, or central processing disorders in the auditory system results in inadequate coding of these acoustic characteristics. Poor coding will result in poor perception of acoustic signals, particularly those which are most complex, like speech. Electrophysiologic measures have been utilized for years to evaluate the function of the auditory nerve as well as the central auditory nervous system. Auditory and visual evoked potentials, as well as imaging studies, have shown cross-modal plasticity occurs in either the central visual or auditory systems as a result of visual or auditory deprivation. These two systems have been shown to change anatomically and physiologically as a result of congenital blindness or deafness. Functional changes have also been shown in individuals who are congenitally blind or deaf, although these changes have yet to be linked directly to anatomical or physiological changes in the central visual or auditory systems.

For those with normal hearing and vision, their daily experiences most often include concurrent stimulation by several senses. The psychophysical literature suggests considerable integration and interactions among the various modalities, including hearing and vision. The visual system can influence auditory perception and is often dominant, especially in areas of spatial information, while the auditory system can influence visual perception, especially regarding temporal aspects. When these complimentary systems are both working well, the integration of information from each can provide our minds with a unified perception that improves detection, localization and specificity of our environmental surroundings.

Chapter 15

NEUROPSYCHOLOGY AND NEUROPHYSIOLOGY OF VISUAL PROCESSING

Marc A. Zola

This chapter will examine the neuropsychology of visual processing and visual impairments in relation to brain-generated automatic processes, developed abilities, and learned skills involved in the daily lives of human beings. Both bottom-up and top-down influences of visual processing, in addition to visual impairments, on cognitive, social, behavioral, and emotional adaptive behaviors are discussed.

Neuropsychology: A Primer

All of our perceptions, thoughts and actions are the result of our brain's ability to integrate and process multisensory input. The brain's information-processing functions and related structures underlie our intellectual, emotional, and social lives, which are central to our mental health, our physical well-being, and our ability to function competently and independently in ordinary activities. Variations in processing strengths and weaknesses are normal and may vary greatly among individuals.

These normal variations, however, become disorders when they interfere with a person's ability to function at home, at school, at work, or in relationships with other people. The causes of disorders may be inherited, related to prenatal, perinatal, or postnatal problems, or acquired during childhood development—or later in life—by way of illness, accident, injury, toxicity, tumor, surgery, trauma, or chronic stressors. Each person's unique pattern of strengths and weaknesses is the result of inherited predispositions in confluence with the what, when, how, and for how long any given incident may have produced a neurological insult to the brain, thereby negatively affecting its structures and functions. In children, such affronts to the brain can have negative consequences for the still-developing, higher-order abilities; in adults, these incidents can result in a loss of specific brain functions.

The field of neuropsychology is concerned with the relationship between brain dysfunction and its behavioral manifestations. In general, neuropsychology focuses on the brain structures responsible for cognitive abilities, social skills, emotional regulation, and behavioral functioning that affect a person's quality of life at home, at school, at work, and in relationships with other people. Pediatric neuropsychology, one of several subspecialties, concentrates on learning and behavior in relationship to the developing brain of the child.

The Neuropsychology of Visual Processing

In recent decades neuropsychological models of visual processing have been influenced by the *two streams* theory. This theory of visual processing proposes that two separate, yet interdependent, pathways emanate from the primary visual cortex (V1): an occipitotemporal network, the *ventral stream*, projecting to inferotemporal cortices, and an occipitoparietal network, the *dorsal stream*, projecting to posterior parietal cortices. The ventral stream and the dorsal stream were first described as *object vision* and *spatial vision,* respectively,[1] or the *what* and the *where* streams. They were later challenged and retheorized as the *vision-for-perception* and the *vision-for-action* streams,[2,3] to emphasize the role of "real-time control of action, transforming moment-to-moment information about the location and disposition of objects into the coordinate frames of the effectors being used to perform the action." Thus, the ventral stream is understood to be responsible for recognition of objects and their attributes, whereas the dorsal stream is responsible for location in space and for motion.

Models of the functional visual system related to attentional control are significantly more complex.[4] Top-down attentional control of endogenous, goal-directed behavior, such as that involved in selective spatial attention, is believed to be regulated by a dorsal parietofrontal network[5] consisting of the dorsal occipitoparietal stream of visual processing, particularly the superior parietal lobule, intraparietal sulcus and precuneus, in addition to the dorsolateral prefrontal cortex, precentral gyrus, frontal eye fields, supplementary eye fields, and anterior cingulate cortex. Bottom-up processing of exogenous, sensory-driven, reflexive attention, such as the detection of movement in the periphery or responsivity to high stimulus salience, is believed to be controlled by the ventral temporofrontal network involving the ventral occipitotemporal stream, including V2, V3, V4, superior colliculus, inferotemporal cortex, plus the middle frontal gyrus, inferior frontal gyrus, anterior cingulate, anterior insula, pulvinar and cerebellum.

In general, the respective neural networks involved in endogenous, versus exogenous, attention are typically non-overlapping, with the former employing more dorsal anatomy and the latter more ventral anatomy of the frontal, temporal, and parietal regions. The anterior cingulate, which has been shown to be the only brain region sensitive to both emotional and attentional focus,[6] is critical in mediating control and resolving conflict between competing top-down endogenous, goal-oriented demands for attention and bottom-up exogenous, sensory, and arousal-driven demands.

The temporofrontal network has been demonstrated to subserve the regulation of reflexive, amygdala-generated arousal to fearful or threatening stimuli,[7,8,9] albeit the anterior cingulate response in anxiety-vulnerable individuals is altered.[10] People prone to anxiety have anterior cingulate response biased towards bottom-up processing. Anxiety-prone individuals, who display increased activation in the amygdala, the ventral prefrontal cortex, and the anterior cingulate cortex, also demonstrate abnormalities for visual processing,[11] such as abnormal flicker fusion threshold,[12] fixation of focal spatial attention,[13] plus altered visual perception, attention, and memory of complex visual scenes.[14] Damasio[15] described the anterior cingulate cortex as "a particular region in the human brain where the systems concerned with emotion, attention, and working memory interact so intimately that they constitute the source for the energy of both external action (movement) and internal action (thought, animation, reasoning)."

This increased activation in the anatomy responsible for mitigating both affective arousal and attentional allocation, as described above, provides a compelling mechanism for understanding the high incidence of visual processing deficits in clinical populations who present with primary or comorbid anxiety disorders. For example, consider children diagnosed with an autistic spectrum disorder. These children—both low and high functioning—with either autistic or Asperger's features, share in varying degrees several debilitating impairments that diminish the quality of their daily experiences. The common features of the autistic spectrum disorders constitute impairments in communication and social interactions, and repetitive patterns of behavior, interests, and activities. Underlying intractable and debilitating anxiety holds sway over the cognitive, emotional, social, and behavioral faculties, which produce the dysfunctions that autistic children suffer throughout their lifetimes.

The symptoms associated with autism vary from child to child. Communication impairments may be delayed or disordered and characterized by mutism, gibberish, jargon, or echolalia; or they may be intact yet display impairments in social use of and in understanding of language, such as the ability to discern literal versus non-literal meaning, double entendre, sarcasm, humor, exaggeration, understatement, eye gaze, facial expressions, and gestures.

Restrictive and stereotypic behaviors in lower functioning children may involve playing with toys in an unusual manner. For example, some lower functioning children may repetitively turn and stare at the wheels of a toy car. In contrast, restrictive and stereotypic behaviors in higher functioning children may present as a preoccupation, or expertise, with one specific area of interest, such as Spider-Man™ or trains, to such an extent that they frequently inappropriately intrude their fixation into otherwise unrelated activities and conversations.

Social interaction difficulties span the gamut from isolation and parallel play to social awkwardness. Other behaviors may be present such as the following: poor tolerance for a change in routine or expectations, temper tantrums, self-stimulatory behaviors, physical aggression, self-injurious behaviors, short attention span, impulsivity, hyperactivity, and unusual sensory processing (e.g., high pain threshold, oversensitivity to touch).

Children on the autistic spectrum with epigenetic cognitive difficulties invariably fail or are delayed in the development of adaptive, higher order social, emotional, and behavioral skills. Poor frustration tolerance and affect dysregulation develop in association with constant social and cognitive demands that exceed limited capacities. Emergent destabilizing anxiety often motivates stereotypic behaviors in efforts to self-soothe, for example, lining up objects by those at the lower end of the spectrum, and overly narrow areas of preoccupations or expertise at the higher end of the spectrum. Maladaptive psychological behaviors develop in an effort to avoid or escape unpleasant cognitive, academic, and social circumstances; taking the form of disruption, aggression, oppositionality, and defiance.

Deficits in visual processing play a critical role in the developmental cascade of impaired cognitive, social, emotional, and behavioral abilities that present as the varying signs and symptoms of autism. The two most compelling theories on autistic development involve abnormalities in *mirror cells* in the brain and impaired facial recognition. Mirror cells are specific neurons that facilitate the ability to perceive emotions and pain in others. These play a role in empathy; in how we understand what other people might be experiencing or feeling, a marked area of difficulty for children with autism. Research has suggested that mirror neurons enable language development, which critically depends on an infant's visually mediated, socio-emotional connection with the mother to learn cooing and babbling and ultimately social and communication skills. Infants with deficits in facial recognition are able to recognize their toys but not their mother's faces, and consequently they fail to develop the social-emotional connection to their mother or their caregiver necessary for language development. Visual processing defects, which are dysfunctional to the development of early cognitive, emotional, social, and behavioral maturation, continue to distort real-time experiences and shape the developmental landscape throughout the lifetime of the child with autism.

Neuropsychological Assessment

Measuring the brain's neuropsychological abilities allows us to determine an individual's unique strengths and weaknesses, not only the complexities that may underlie a problem, but also—and more importantly—the neuropsychological processes, abilities, and skills that they perform most efficiently. In this way, we can more precisely understand an individual's difficulties, rather than just assign a diagnostic label, thereby developing effective interventions that promote or restore healthy cognitive, social, emotional, and behavioral functioning.

Neuropsychological assessment is a comprehensive process conducted over multiple sessions, involving directly measuring processes, abilities and skills related to cognitive and academic abilities and social, emotional and behavioral functioning. (*Neuropsychological Assessment* by Lezak et al.[16] provides an excellent review of the subject matter.) What follows is an introduction to the neuropsychological investigation of higher cortical functions, as it pertains to the examination of visual processing and related integrated functions. References to specific instruments are included as examples.

The main components of the neuropsychological examination include a thorough patient history, interview, observations, and assessment; pertinent and accessible patient records undergo review. History-taking involves reviewing the presenting complaints in addition to identifying and chronicling current, previous, or long-standing problems related to a range of functional domains, such as sensorimotor functioning, executive and attentional abilities, learning and memory, language abilities, nonverbal skills, academic or work-related performance, and behavior. Routinely, detailed data collection is conducted; this includes an interview about the mother's pregnancy, the child's delivery, birth, developmental milestones, medical history, and family history, social history—including educational and work history. A battery of parent, teacher, and patient self-report questionnaires and instruments yield critical clinical information regarding emotional, behavioral, social, and adaptive functioning (e.g., see Behavior Assessment System for Children, Second Edition [BASC-2][17]; Vineland Adaptive Behavior Scales, Second Edition [Vineland-II]).[18]

Objective assessment procedures consist of one-on-one and face-to-face valid, reliable, normative-referenced, standardized test protocols administered in several formats including paper-and-pencil and hands-on activities, verbal/auditory responses and performances, and computer-administered assessments. Domain areas measured include sensory and motor functioning; attention and response control in both auditory and visual modalities; executive functions; motor speech and articulation; receptive and expressive language abilities; visual perception and visual-motor abilities; learning, memory, and retrieval for both verbal/auditory information and visual/nonverbal material; intelligence and fluid reasoning; in addition to academic abilities and crystallized knowledge.

From a practical point of view, the comprehensive and detailed neuropsychological investigation of visual processing involves an evaluation of basic vision and visual processes related to the peripheral sensorium and subcortical pathways, those related to higher-cortical visual object and spatial perception, and those related to integrated and mediated processes, abilities and skills including sensorimotor functioning, visual attention and response control, executive skills, visual/nonverbal learning and memory, reasoning and intelligence, and academic skills.

A thorough history may reveal evidence of longstanding problems in visual development or other acquired difficulties, indicated by delayed milestones, poor motor coordination, emotional difficulties, behavioral problems, or inadequate development of visually mediated academic skills for reading, writing, spelling, and math. Diligent observation of an individual's gaze, posture, gait, ambulation, balance, and the quality of test performance—especially dialoging, object handling and using paper and pencil may reveal signs of strabismus, nystagmus, defective accommodation and convergence, field-cuts, displaced visual attention, midline shift, or other abnormal visual processing behaviors that warrant further evaluation by a neuro-optometrist.

The sensorimotor examination of visual processes with the Dean-Woodcock Neuropsychological Assessment System Battery (DWNAS)[19] includes an evaluation of near-point vision with Snellen notation to assess visual acuity; visual confrontation of upper and lower, nasal and temporal visual quadrants to identify inattention, hemianopsia, quadranopsia, or other field defects; plus naming pictures of objects to detect dysgnosia for drawings. However, in individuals with spatial dysfunction and associated impaired imago visual representation, the sensorimotor examination may also reveal deficits in tactile perception, such as astereognosia (the inability to perceive form by touch) and dysgnosia (a cognitive problem, especially related to disease or mental illness) on tactile object identification; asomatognosia (lack of awareness of one's body parts) and tactile projection on tactile finger recognition; and asomatognosia, tactile projection, and right-left confusion on tactile simultaneous localization. Coordination on visually mediated tests may be impaired, for example, on finger-to-nose and hand-to-eye examination; on free walking, heel-to-toe, hopping, and on station examination. Individuals with visual processing difficulties may also evidence confusion for left-right movements, and ideomotor dyspraxia for mime movements.

The formal assessment of visual processing, per se, involves the utilization of valid, reliable, and normative-referenced tests for evaluating visual fields, motor-free visual perception, and visual-motor integration. In addition to confrontation of the visual fields, cancellation tests detect hemianopsia or quadranopsia related to pathology of the subcortical visual pathways, plus visual inattention, visual neglect, or visual extinction related to posterior parietal lesions. Cancellation tasks are among the most frequently utilized neuropsychological measures of visual processing. These are commonly administered in paper and pencil format and consist of an array of rarely occurring target stimuli displayed among frequent foil stimuli. The cancellation paradigm requires the patient to find and mark the target stimuli. Performances are analyzed for omissions, commissions, and quadrant differentials. Timed cancellation tests yield additional information about visual scanning, sustained and selective attention, visuomotor activation, inhibition, speed, and coordination.

Color perception is assessed for evidence of achromatopsia (hereditary lack of cones for color vision) and color imperceptions, agnosia (versus anomia) and amnesia. Basic visual recognition and evidence of agnosia is evaluated by using tests that measure the ability to match or discriminate between two similar visual figures (e.g., visual discrimination) and the ability to accurately recognize and identify objects (e.g., object recognition). More complex recognition, involving visual analysis and synthesis, is measured by tests that assess the ability to recognize objects from unusual views and angles (e.g., position in space), the ability to recognize stimulus figures that are incomplete or have missing parts (e.g., visual closure), and the ability to recognize stimulus figures from their disarranged parts (e.g., visual integration).

Tests involving discernment and recognition of objects when they are obscured in complex backgrounds (e.g., figure-ground, embedded figures, or hidden figures) measure complex object recognition in the presence of visual interference. Recognition of familiar faces and evidence of prosopagnosia (face blindness) are typically assessed with tests requiring the identification of famous persons. Recognition of unfamiliar faces is measured via paradigms to match faces after a brief delay and paradigms to match faces presented from different angles. Visuospatial abilities and defects are measured via tests of localization in space, judgment of direction, judgment of distance, spatial thought, and topographical orientation. These tests include the ability to discriminate right from left, directionality, and angulations. Tests of visuomotor integration typically measure the ability to draw guided by visual boundaries (e.g., eye-hand coordination), speed of marking or matching of target stimuli (e.g., visuomotor speed), speed and accuracy of connecting visual stimuli in sequence or in alternating sequencing (e.g., trail making), accurately copying drawings (e.g., design copy), and rapid, accurate assemblage of three-dimensional constructions from a model (e.g., block design).

The computerized evaluation of complex variables of attentional regulation and response inhibition has become a standard for attentional assessment during the past decade. Weaknesses in attention are predictive of emotional, behavioral, and social outcomes. Early attentional dysfunction has been associated with an increased likelihood of substance abuse, legal problems, and job-related difficulties later in life. The Integrated Visual & Auditory Continuous Performance Test (IVA+Plus)[20] analyzes responses to intermixed auditory and visual stimuli presented under high (i.e., frequent) and low (i.e., infrequent) demand conditions. It yields standard scores for composite attention and response control as well as respective component variables.

Deficits in executive functions are common in many disabilities and disorders of childhood and adulthood. Visual and spatial processing are foundational to executive functioning in the ecology of everyday human activity. Correspondingly, developmental and acquired visual processing weaknesses contribute greatly to the delay or dysfunction, respectively, of executive abilities.

For school-aged children, executive difficulties are frequently associated with ADHD; autism and Asperger's; and with learning disabilities in reading, writing, and mathematics. In adolescents and adults, executive difficulties are commonly associated with the same, in addition to traumatic brain injury and other acquired assaults to the brain. Executive difficulties have also been associated with medical diseases, metabolic disorders, and mental illnesses in children and adults. Executive difficulties may be present in individuals with or without learning disabilities, both challenged and bright alike. Persons with executive difficulties tend to be unproductive in school and inefficient at work as adults. Specifically, these individuals may have difficulty starting and completing assignments, remembering to do their assignments (e.g., homework), managing emotions, being timely, and carrying out long-term projects.

There is general agreement that executive abilities represent a complex set of cognitive and emotional skills for self-regulating goal-oriented behavior, which is primarily mediated by the frontal lobes. Executive skills have been compared to the conductor of an orchestra: organizing and coordinating the brain's processes, abilities, and skills with the intention and effort to accomplish short-term and long-term goals enabling us to supersede our immediate automatic behaviors in favor of organizing self-guided efforts over time to maximize our future benefit.

Executive functions "draw upon the individual's more fundamental or primary cognitive skills, such as attention, language, and perceptions, to generate higher levels of creative and abstract thought" (Delis–Kaplan Executive Function System™).[21] These include the following: the ability to design a strategy to reach a goal (i.e., planning), the ability to arrange required materials according to a system (i.e., organization), the ability to begin a task in a timely manner without procrastination (i.e., initiation), the ability to follow through purposefully and efficiently in the completion of a goal (i.e., persistence), the ability to observe and evaluate one's own performance (i.e., self-monitoring), the ability to hold important information in mind while maintaining another train of thought for problem solving (i.e., working memory), the ability to anticipate the consequences of your actions before you act (i.e., response inhibition), the ability to suspend expression of emotions in order to achieve a goal (i.e., affect self-regulation), and the ability to revise plans and adapt to changing conditions (i.e., flexibility).

Executive functions are measured subjectively both via self-report questionnaires and by parent, teacher, and significant-other questionnaires, which are designed to formally identify specific age-related executive abilities and abnormalities by means of standardized neuropsychological tests (e.g., BRIEF ™).[22] Problems with visual and verbal memory are the most commonly reported complaints by patients. Tests of visual learning and memory have been designed to assess a variety of potential stimuli including simple designs, complex designs, ambiguous figures, objects, faces, scenes, spatial location, and topographical location. Assessment paradigms traditionally utilize single or multiple learning trials, with immediate and delayed recall trials to measure retention. Paradigms that rely on reproducing visual stimuli during stimulus presentation (e.g., copying designs) also require reproducing the stimuli during recall trials. Such paradigms often utilize an additional delayed, multiple-choice recognition trial to differentiate a learning dysfunction (e.g., a problem with encoding and consolidating information into long-term memory) versus a retrieval dysfunction.

The assessment of general intelligence (*g*) as a measure of cognitive efficiency has long been central to neuropsychology. Despite recent criticism regarding the theoretical validity of a single indicator of general cognitive ability,[23,24,25] its pragmatic value has been well documented, for example, as a robust premorbid predictor of rehabilitative success following brain trauma and neurological disease.[26] Most measures of general intelligence, however, rely substantially (e.g., K-ABC; WISC-IV; WAIS-III; WJ-III) or exclusively (e.g., C-TONI; Leiter-R; TONI-3; UNIT)[16] on visually mediated subtests. Thus, to the degree an individual's visual processing may be compromised, measured intelligence will underestimate general cognitive potential.

Lastly, the neuropsychological assessment of academic abilities (e.g., WIAT-II, WJ-III, WRAT-III)[16] is critical for evaluating the downstream affects of visual processing deficits on reading, writing, math, and other acquired academic skills. For similar reasons, the assessment of emotional, behavioral and adaptive factors (e.g., BASC-2™) [17] are critical, as visual impairments can negatively impact social perceptions, emotional regulation, psychological defenses, functional skills, and overall social stability.

Neurophysiological Rehabilitation of Visual Processing Deficits

The value of employing behavioral methods to modify and modulate the abnormal electroneurophysiology associated with specific conditions was first demonstrated by Barry Sterman, PhD, in landmark experiments: one with cats that were trained to control their brainwaves,[27] and a subsequent study of a patient with epilepsy who learned to suppress her seizure activity using EEG biofeedback.[28] Since then, EEG biofeedback, conventionally referred to as neurofeedback or neurotherapy, has been clinically and empirically validated as an efficacious therapy for improving or remediating many clinical conditions that present with associated abnormal electroneurophysiology. These include attention deficit hyperactivity disorder (ADHD), autistic spectrum disorders, learning disabilities, dyslexia, dyscalculia, dysgraphia, cognitive disorders, traumatic brain injury (TBI), sleep dysregulation, anxiety, depression, obsessive-compulsive disorder (OCD), post-traumatic stress disorder (PTSD), bipolar disorder, conduct disorder, anger and rage, substance abuse, chronic pain, fibromyalgia, migraine, headache, and epilepsy. Additionally, neurofeedback is a non-invasive, painless, and safe treatment; it has been demonstrated to have lasting and permanent benefit without side effects.

In the following section, neurofeedback, the operant conditioning of abnormal electroneurophysiology, as a rehabilitation modality for neuropsychological impairment will be presented. The significant benefits of including neuropsychological and neurophysiological evaluation and treatment, such as neurofeedback, alongside treatment protocols by neuro-optometrists will be emphasized.

Neurofeedback: A Primer

Feedback, the process by which a system modulates itself in response to the output it produces, is a naturally occurring, adaptive phenomenon in biological and ecological systems at all levels of analysis. Biofeedback, as a clinical technique, measures normally occurring, involuntary physiological activities (e.g., breathing, heart rate, blood pressure, muscle tension, skin electrical conductance, and skin temperature) with electrodes, and displays the information on a monitor in real-time so a patient can learn to change it. For example, biofeedback can be used to provide real-time information about blood pressure so the patient can learn to lower it. Although this type of learning is often described as the result of *coming under conscious control*, it is generally believed that feedback modulation is *under operant control*, with varying degrees of conscious and unconscious awareness, depending on the physiology being shaped. Under operant control, desired behaviors are more likely to occur in the future when rewarded, and less likely to occur when not rewarded. This is a type of learning that occurs naturally under various degrees of conscious awareness.

The core healing mechanisms of neurofeedback therapy involve retraining the identified abnormal EEG frequencies, amplitudes, and dynamics (e.g., coherence, phase lag). This facilitates structural reorganization in the brain via neuroplasticity, which promotes or restores healthy neurophysiological functioning. The emergent stable changes in healthy EEG activity are accompanied, correspondingly, by abatement in symptoms and by improvement in performance of the abnormal brainwave counterparts.

A simple single-channel, monopolar or bipolar neurofeedback therapy session involves placing one or two active sensors, which read electroencephalographic (EEG) activity, on the scalp and then clipping one or two sensors on the ears (e.g., reference and ground). An amplifier and a computer collect and analyze the EEG data providing real-time, instantaneous audio-visual feedback about brainwave activity. This feedback can be displayed to the patient as a game such as a car racing on a track, dolphins swimming in the ocean, or a complex cube spinning. The feedback display is programmed by the therapist to respond to and activate remedial brainwave activity. In other words, while the targeted brainwave activity is being produced, the car races, the dolphins swim, or the cube spins. If the targeted brainwave activity is not being produced, the car, the dolphins, or the cube remain inactive. This way, a patient receives both feedback that reflects his or her real-time brainwave behavior, and reinforcement for changing it in the desired direction.

Quantitative EEG neuroimaging (QEEG) involves signal processing of a digitally recorded EEG so that specific wave forms can be highlighted. QEEG can thus identify the significant excesses or deficiencies (i.e., abnormalities) in brain electrical patterns that are most likely associated with a patient's predominant clinical complaints and that are in the greatest need of remediation. The abnormal brainwave patterns are determined by means of normative database comparisons. The results of the QEEG are presented in the form of topographical maps and analyses, which identify statistically deviant brainwave frequencies, amplitudes, and dynamics (e.g., coherence and phase lag) illustrated at 19 locations that correspond to specific cortical surface areas. Low-resolution brain tomography analysis (LORETA) produces additional two and three dimensional images of deeper signal generators, or sources, of the EEG signal. Thus the QEEG and its derivatives are instrumental in planning neurofeedback training.

Brainwaves differ in frequency (speed), amplitude (height), and morphology (shape). Frequencies are measured in waves per second or hertz (Hz), and, although they can be defined in single 1-Hz bins (e.g., 1 Hz, 2 Hz, 3 Hz, etc.), they are conventionally delimited by their traditional frequency bands of delta, (1-4 Hz), theta (4-8 Hz), alpha (8-12 Hz), and beta (13-21 Hz). The actual band pass may vary depending on the comparative normative database or the system used. Other conventional band passes include sensorimotor rhythm (12-15 Hz), high beta (20-32 Hz), and gamma (38-42 Hz), among others. In general, delta is associated with sleep; theta with hypnagogic states (drowsiness before sleep); alpha with relaxation; and beta with cognitive focus. (Theta has also been associated with creativity and spontaneity. Alpha is synchronous at posterior EEG sites when a person is meditating or praying, or in a calm or peaceful state. Anterior beta is predominant while individuals are reflecting, deliberating, synthesizing, and analyzing.)

Pathology is associated with EEG abnormalities, including the following: (1) deficient or excessive frequency amplitudes; (2) asymmetrical frequency amplitudes between different surface locations (i.e., hemispheric asymmetries); (3) low or high synchronous connectivity within frequency bands between surface locations (i.e., coherence, hyper- or hypo-), and (4) slow or fast conduction time within frequency bands between surface locations (i.e., phase lag, high or low). For example, high amplitude rhythmic delta is evident at sites that correspond to the functional neuroanatomy of specific learning disabilities (e.g., dyslexia, dysgraphia, dyscalculia); central auditory processing disorders; central visual processing disorders; and at the locations of coup and contrecoup brain trauma. Excessive anterior theta is associated with daydreaming, inattention, and distractibility; whereas inter-hemisphere asymmetries in anterior theta are associated with depression and anxiety, as are asymmetries in anterior alpha. Excessive anterior slowing (e.g., alpha and theta) diminishes attentional, behavioral, and emotional regulation; impedes learning, memory, and retrieval; and reduces control of impulses, mood, and activity level (e.g., hyperactivity). Children and adults with ADHD, head injuries, brain injuries, seizure disorders, chronic fatigue syndrome, and chronic pain disorders also tend to display excessively slow theta and alpha brainwaves.

Anterior deficient beta, as well as high theta-to-beta and alpha-to-beta ratios, are correlated with inattention and distractibility. Paradoxically, excessive anterior or central beta is also associated with inattention and distractibility, as well as impulsivity, when beta 1 (SMR, 12-15 Hz) is deficient over the sensorimotor strip. However, these deficient versus excessive beta phenotypes differ in their clinical presentation, the former as unfocused and the later as over-focused. Indeed, as many as 16 different QEEG phenotypes have been proposed for ADHD. Correspondingly, several common comorbidities of ADHD are also associated with excessive beta activity, including learning disabilities, oppositional defiant disorder, conduct disorder, Tourette's syndrome, anxiety, obsessive compulsive disorder, depression, bipolar disorder, and sleep disorders; possibly contributing to the differential ADHD EEG patterns. Four decades of QEEG research have identified the complexities of abnormal brainwave activity and its associations with many cognitive, social, emotional, and behavioral disorders.

Neurotherapy protocols are developed relative to the QEEG findings that represent the most clinically relevant neurophysiological abnormalities, those that are most likely associated with the patient's predominant clinical complaints. As simple protocol examples, a patient with a primary complaint of attentional difficulty and QEEG findings of excessive anterior theta plus deficient anterior beta would be treated by up-training beta and down-training theta in the indicated area at the front of the brain. A patient with anxiety and excessive central high frequency beta would be treated by down-training the excessive high frequency activity at that location; whereas, a patient with a visual processing disorder and moodiness, with evidence of EEG slowing over the right temporoparietal area, would be treated by up-training and activating higher frequencies at that location.

Case Studies

Case 1

This case involves a 10-year-old girl in the 5th grade whose parents expressed concern about her general disorganization at home and her difficulty performing chores and homework. They were also particularly concerned about their daughter biting her nails. The parents reported her longstanding distractibility and difficulty paying attention in the classroom. Initial observations were of a girl who was pleasant and cooperative although timid, highly distractible, and notably restless and fidgety. Behavioral assessment indicated inattention, distractibility, impulsivity, and hyperactivity as well as problems organizing, initiating, and persisting in goal-oriented activities. Neuropsychological testing revealed severely impaired attention and response control in both the auditory and visual modalities, each, respectively, below the 1st percentile level.

Quantitative EEG revealed excessive slow wave activity (alpha) and deficient high frequency activity (beta, high beta) in the right anterior cortices, as evident on topographic maps, and on two-dimensional and three-dimensional LORETA images. Excessive slow wave activity (theta) and deficient fast wave activity (beta) were evident on the same images in the right prefrontal gyrus and right parietal regions.

The following neurofeedback protocols, using the International 10-20 System of Electrode Placement, were developed to treat the patient's identified EEG abnormalities: decrease alpha and increase beta and high beta at the right frontal site (Fz-Fp2); and, decrease theta and increase beta at the right sensorimotor site (C4-T4). The patient received neurofeedback therapy, 2 sessions per week, for 10 weeks, with 15-minutes of training at each site per session.

After 20 sessions of therapy, the patient's parents reported that she responsibly completed her homework, and her academic grades had dramatically improved. The patient reported greater ability to concentrate with less distractibility and said that she frequently completed deskwork and school tests ahead of her classmates. Her hyperactive symptoms (including nail biting) reportedly abated both at home and at school; these symptoms were not evident during her latter neurotherapy sessions. Objective neuropsychological testing revealed a significant improvement in auditory and visual attention, from the *deficient range* prior to treatment, to the *average range* following treatment. All indicators of visual attention—inattention as measured by omission errors (vigilance), momentary loss of attention (focus), and reaction time (speed)—improved to equal to and greater than the 50th percentile level. Response control for visual stimuli improved from the deficient range prior to treatment, to the *high end of the low average range*. Components of response control in the visual modality improved to the average range for ability to stop and think before automatically reacting (prudence), ability to stay on task and sustain a reliable effort (consistency), and to the *low average range* for maintaining speed and sustaining attention and effort over time (stamina). Likewise, response control in the auditory modality improved overall from the deficient range prior to treatment, to the *high end of the borderline range* with average prudence and consistency and borderline stamina.

Case 2

This case involves a 16-year-old girl who suffered two concurrent head injuries, the result of a rowing accident. As a crew member of a rowing team she was hit twice with an oar blade: once to the left back of the head, and once to the left front of the head, when a competing boat drifted too close and crashed her boat during a high school race. This most likely resulted in coup and contrecoup blunt instrument type injury to all four quadrants of the cortical and subcortical anatomy involved. On the day of the accident, she was transported by motorboat and, subsequently, by ground transportation to the local area hospital's emergency department for evaluation. She complained of significant post-traumatic amnesia in the form of disorientation and dizziness for more than 48 hours, substantiating potential brain injury.

The patient was described as a high functioning, straight-A student prior to the accident without any premorbid history of cognitive, social, emotional, behavioral, or medical difficulties. She enjoyed a flourishing social life and was considered an accomplished student and a skilled athlete. In the year and half following the accident, the patient suffered consistent post-traumatic headaches and dizziness. She slept only 1 to 2 hours per night. Her cognitive abilities for learning, memory, attention, concentration, and reading were described as severely impaired. Previously described as a voracious reader, the patient's reading ability post the accident was described as extremely slow, labored, and limited. Functionally, she had been unable to attend school or to socialize with her friends since the time of the accident.

The patient was evaluated at the beginning of the summer, the end of what otherwise would have been her sophomore year. At that time, she presented as an attractive, casually dressed, well groomed, young lady, suggesting relatively preserved self-care adaptive skills. However, she complained of a chronic headache and displayed nonverbal signs of such (e.g., grimacing, squinting) throughout her initial interview. A brief neuropsychological examination at that time evidenced an unstable station, weaving gait, and a posture that appeared tilted forward with her shoulders rounded in the same direction. She had a positive Romberg test. On observation, her gaze was not conjugate, and a succeeding vision screening suggested a *midline shift syndrome*. She was subsequently referred to a neuro-optometrist for further evaluation and, in fact, was found to have visual midline shift syndrome with a significant vertical imbalance between her eyes affecting binocularity, posture, and balance. Prism glasses were prescribed to compensate for her binocular dysfunction and visual midline shift syndrome.

Testing before the patient received her yoked prism glasses revealed attention and response control for visual and auditory stimuli were severely impaired in the deficient range below the .1 percentile level, as were all valid component measures including vigilance, focus, speed, prudence and consistency. Post testing, wearing the yoked prism glasses, the patient improved her attentional performances for vigilance and focus in the visual modality to the high average range and low average range, and demonstrated improved posture and balance. Moreover, collateral improvement was noted from below the .1 percentile level, without prism glasses, to the average range with prism glasses for focus in the auditory modality. Testing also revealed improved response control performances in the visual modality from below the .1 percentile level, prior to glasses, to the borderline range for prudence, the low average range for consistency, and the superior range for stamina. Response control for auditory stimuli also improved to the low average range for prudence and consistency and to the high average range for stamina.

The patient's Quantitative EEG revealed global and diffuse under-activation of brainwave activity across all band passes with greatest attenuation of activity noted in alpha as displayed on the three-dimensional LORETA orthoview. The patient underwent advanced live Z-Score neurofeedback training 5 days per week. Live Z-Score neurofeedback allows multiple sites and frequencies to be trained simultaneously. Sessions were bifurcated into two 15-minute rounds, one to normalize alpha at posterior sites (Pz, P3, P4, O1, O2) and the other to normalize beta at frontal sites (Fp1, Fp2, Fz, F3, F4, F7, F8, Cz, C3, C4).

Following 50 sessions of neurofeedback therapy all areas of functioning improved substantially. The patient was able to return to the classroom at the beginning of the fall semester for three-quarter-length school days. She began interacting with her friends regularly and eventually fully reintegrated back into her social life. Follow-up neuropsychological testing revealed improvement in attention for both visual and auditory information to the high average range. Similarly, response control for both visual and auditory information improved to the average range. Follow-up neuro-optometric examination indicated a significant improvement in accommodation, bifocal fusional ranges, and visual midline. New glasses were prescribed with the appropriate adjustments given the patient's improvements. Sleep improved from one and a half hours per night to six to eight hours per night. Academic performance improved to the "A" and "B" range. The patient reported that learning, memory, and reading had improved substantially, although not to pre-morbid levels; she continued to receive neurofeedback training aimed at further remediation. Likewise, her headache and balance improved modestly, and she continued to receive physical therapy and vision therapy for their treatment.

Conclusions

All of our sensory awareness and our ability to think and to carry out actions is the result of information processing in the brain. Foundationally differentiated on the processing level and highly amalgamated on the experiential level, our system for processing visual information is inextricably intertwined in our social, emotional, cognitive, and behavioral experiences of everyday life.

As put forth in this chapter, our experiences are sub-served by neuroanatomy responsible for simple perception of basic visual elements and for attributes at the front end via the eyes, subcortical vision pathways, and primary visual cortex, and subsequently organized upstream by parietal and temporal cortices (i.e., dorsal occipitoparietal and ventral occipitotemporal streams), creating a world of culturally meaningful objects and persons acting within a three-dimensional visual framework. At the back end, via cortical and subcortical frontal structures (i.e., dorsal parietofrontal and ventral temporofrontal networks), what we see occurs within a social, emotional, and personal landscape.

Correspondingly, the quality of our lives very much depends on how well we are seeing. When the visual system, as well as the extant information processing system, is healthy and operating efficiently, we enjoy relatively happy and productive lives. When they are not, adaptive functionality is usually compromised in some fashion, depending on what, when, how, for how long, and to what degree something has negatively affected different brain structures. In children, the earlier the injury the more pervasive the consequences for the related yet-to-develop, higher-order abilities; in adults, the more diffuse the injury the greater the loss of function.

Relatively circumscribed anatomy can also have formative influences on daily experiences as described, for example, by the negative effect of increased activation in the anterior cingulate on visual processing for flicker fusion threshold; fixation of focal spatial attention; and visual perception, attention, and memory of complex scenes. The anterior cingulate arbitrates demands for attentional resources between top-down, executive-driven self-actualization; and bottom-up, arousal-driven self-preservation. When bottom-up processes predominate, the information processing system constricts an otherwise opulent perceptual field into a relatively fixated attentional zone in the service of accomplishing a relatively narrow purpose (e.g., pain-avoidance).

Analogously, anatomy disturbed by trauma may greatly impair visual processing. For example, a traumatically induced disconnection between ambient visual processes and sensorimotor systems (i.e., kinesthetic, proprioceptive and vestibular) in the midbrain may cause a disability for organizing spatial information, along with spatial disorientation, over focalization, overstimulation and anxiety.[29]

The goal of rehabilitation is to restore or to develop an individual's respective previous or potential maximum independence in activities of daily living. A neuropsychological examination can help elucidate the causes and effects of visual processing impairments in the hierarchically nested processes, abilities, and skills involved in cognitive, social, emotional, and behavioral functioning. Likewise, augmenting vision therapy and neuro-optometric interventions with state-of-the-art clinical technologies such as QEEG and neurofeedback can provide a more comprehensive approach to rehabilitation. In this way, we can formulate the broadest and most effective interventions necessary for promoting or restoring healthy, contented, and productive lives.

Chapter 16

FACILITATING LOW VISION UTILIZATION

William V. Padula

This chapter discusses vision as it relates to function and performance for the child with vision impairment. Perception develops in a logical manner. Understanding how visual impairment interferes with this development is of primary importance to the development of a higher level of efficiency in vision.

Low-Vision Utilization

According to the American Foundation for the Blind, "approximately 90% of individuals with visual impairment have functional or low vision; just 10% are functionally blind. However, students with low vision are often an overlooked majority in the population of children who are visually impaired."[1]

Low-vision utilization, as stated here, pertains to function and performance within the environment but relates to the definition of vision discussed in a previous chapter. The snare that we often encounter when discussing function is to consider only muscle mechanisms or sensory systems, and to relate difficulties in performance solely to isolated problems without considering the interrelationship of sensory, motor, and perceptual processes which stem from a sensorimotor base. For example, the child who is classified as a "toe-walker" is one who walks without touching his heels to the ground. His walking pattern is characterized by short steps during which only the balls of the feet and toes touch the ground and his weight is shifted forward. One common diagnosis based on functional abilities is that the tendons in the back of the legs are too short, causing an inability to extend the legs when walking to obtain a heel-to-toe gait.

It has been noted that when specially designed prisms (base-down, yoked) are introduced before the eyes of many of these children, the gait is changed from toe-walking to heel-to-toe gaits, and that the weight becomes distributed more equally over both feet.[2] The common diagnosis of shortened tendons was based on function and isolated to the supposed inability to extend the heel. That approach does not take into account the profound relationship between sensory and motor processes, particularly the role of vision, in performance.

To consider the alternative approach, one must begin by examining behavior as a reflection of the visual process, whether for the sighted or non-sighted individual. When this is done, function and performance become an interaction of physiology, psychological disposition, and the environment, all of which are part of vision and the mainstay of development.

When working with children it is important to realize that the interaction between sensory and motor processes is structured by development. We cannot effectively improve the child's low vision utilization without understanding the developmental level of abilities along with sensorimotor interaction. For this reason, the author has chosen to outline some important considerations of both development and sensorimotor interaction at various ages when attempting to affect low vision utilization. The purpose of any therapy is to reduce the interferences affecting development and to allow the child to advance at his own rate. It is not an attempt to make the child advance his development, thereby reducing a manifested developmental lag.

Note: The most effective tools that the optometrist or ophthalmologist has to affect function and performance are the lens and the prism. Unfortunately, the lens and prism have been regarded by many only in their compensatory capacities to correct myopia, hyperopia or astigmatism. The lens and prism have the potential to actually change the relationship of the kinesthetic, proprioceptive, vestibular and other senses to the visual process. When plus lenses or yoked prisms (prisms with the base or thick end in the same orientation before both eyes) are used properly with a person of any age, the use of the ambient and focal processes will change, thereby affecting other motor and sensory modalities. Therefore, the clinician who is attempting to provide rehabilitation for a visually impaired or motorically disabled person should not miss the opportunity to work with plus lenses and yoked prisms concurrently with various activities.

In this chapter various activities designed to affect the developmental nature of the child's vision will be discussed. Appropriate therapeutic lenses and prisms should be used during these activities to obtain the full and dynamic effect of this treatment. The activity alone cannot be expected to elicit changes without the proper use of lenses and prisms concurrently. Lenses are usually only used for their effect on the focal aspect of vision. However, lenses and prisms also influence the ambient function as it relates to motor organization. The young infant or child has a very plastic visual system. Appropriate lenses or prisms can be used effectively to accent relationships between the ambient visual process and the motor system. As the child begins to experience differences in visual and motor relationships often his performance in other sensory modalities will be affected.

The First Year

The sight-impaired infant develops rudimentary forms of perception which will form the base for more complex perceptual processes. Since the child's processing abilities are simple during the first year of life, so should be the design of any methods of therapy or stimulation. Overstimulation at any age is as detrimental as understimulation. Overstimulation places demands on the child above his level of abilities. When this happens the child must either push himself beyond his developmental level of abilities or he will show compensating behavior such as avoidance, fatigue or irritability. The long-term result of overstimulation may be physiologic compensation.

Since perception of figure-ground relationships is essential for focalization and because a child younger than 8 weeks is primarily developing monocular fixations, an overhead, non-glaring light may be very effective in providing a figure. The light, being the figure, will elicit a fixation that establishes a figure-ground perception. Of course, the light should not be of an intensity that will cause discomfort when looked at directly. Switching the light on and off slowly may also provide variations for perceptual enhancement. Two overhead light sources will permit changes in fixation. They may be constant or slowly alternated. Plus lenses and yoked prisms may be used to provide change to oculomotor and sensory orientation.

Room illumination for the sight-impaired infant should be varied to provide different levels of light stimulation. Lamps should be moved occasionally enabling the child to experience light from different directions. Variations in the formation of shadows will offer added figure-ground dimensions in the room. While mobiles are effective in stimulating fixation, they may be overstimulating to many children, causing prolonged fixation on the figure without a release to the ground. It is recommended that mobiles not be used until after 8 weeks of age when the child is developing binocular fixation, and then the mobile should be used only for short periods of time.

Since the newborn infant may still be in the position of asymmetric tonic neck reflex, focal behavior can be observed on the infant's outstretched hand. This behavior may be enhanced by providing indirect background illumination so that the hand is the highlighted figure. The opposite method of shining a flashlight directly on the hand in a semi-darkened environment will also provide stimulation for fixation.

Because the newborn is essentially ambient in visual function, tracking movements may be elicited by moving a light or brightly colored object ahead of the child's fixation. Fluorescent objects under ultraviolet light in a semi-darkened environment may be useful for the sight-impaired child. The ultraviolet light should be positioned to shine on the object being moved, and not directly at the child's eyes. Audible objects (rattles, bells) will also provide good stimulation. All objects should be at close (near-range) distances for the newborn.

The vestibular system is very important for reinforcing eye alignment and direction. Eye movements, in response to position change by the mother, have been monitored in the unborn infant. From a matching of information received through vision, vestibular, kinesthetic, and proprioceptive stimulation, the infant learns balance and coordinates motor and eye movement skills. Once the infant has achieved binocularity, the information received through vision is no longer segmented and begins to be readily matched with information received through other modalities. However, difficulty in achieving the state of binocularity often occurs because of an inability to utilize various modalities to reinforce visual processing. In turn, processing of information often occurs between isolated senses rather than through multimodality matching.

Moving the child from side to side or rocking the child while the child lies on a large ball will allow vestibular reactions to be matched with vision as the child fixates on a toy. The vestibular stimulation produced will reinforce ocular movements, leading to rudimentary binocular function. The less ability the child has to control focal visual functioning, the more likely it will be that one can observe shifting eye movements during this activity. It has been noted that strabismic children (particularly exotropes) have demonstrated ocular alignment during these procedures, which have been found useful for children through preschool age. Also, cradling the infant and rocking side to side or varying directions while the infant fixates on the clinician's face will provide visual-vestibular matching of information. Coordinating therapy with an approach of neuro-developmental treatment by occupational and/or physical therapists will be helpful and will provide follow-through.

When the child is able to accommodate, focalization may be further improved by lifting him above the head of the clinician and moving him away from and then towards the clinician's face. The infant will enjoy this activity if the clinician talks to him. Turning the child from side to side while this activity is performed will stimulate tracking movements along with convergence and accommodation if he is fixating on the clinician's face.

As focal visual behavior improves, tracking activities should be slowed to allow the child the opportunity to track with fixation. The same strategies described previously will be effective in eliciting tracking responses.

The 32-week-old infant, as you may recall, is able to begin to localize objects at greater distances. Activities can be performed by starting at a near range with visual and audible objects, and backing away while monitoring the infant's fixation and attention. Introducing plus lenses at this time can assist the child in fixating and releasing on near and far objects.

As the infant progresses, the fixation on the object can be stimulated at a distance by making a sound next to a luminous object (i.e., a flashlight) and having the infant localize the object auditorily, with visual fixation being the endpoint of the activity.

> *Note: With all of these activities, the visual abilities of the child will be affected by his particular sight impairment. Working distances that depend on acuity levels and field restrictions must be considered. As this chapter offers suggestions for the individual working with sight-impaired children, it is assumed that refractive considerations have been addressed through a proper clinical examination. The activities may need to be altered for individual children. If the child has reduced acuity or a field restriction, working distances should be shortened or larger objects used based on the child's acuity. In the case of peripheral field restrictions, smaller objects may be more beneficial than larger ones. If there is a field restriction impairment on a particular side, the therapist may need to design his activities to approach from the sighted side.*

Activities should be designed to enable the child to reinforce vision with motor movement as soon as the child begins to coordinate limb function.[3] Touching, tapping, hitting and pushing movements enable the child to continually match information through vision and its relationship to motor concerning distance, size, shape, form, etc.

When the child is able to crawl, movement should be encouraged. The child may begin to rock back and forth, seeking kinesthetic stimulation. It is not necessary to discourage this. This symptom means the child is not establishing relationships through other modalities to stimulate movement. The therapist must provide reinforcements to develop movement, and once the relationships are established, the rocking behavior will diminish or stop completely. Sounds from several feet away, such as the mother's voice, coupled with visually stimulating objects will develop directionality concepts. By moving one arm of the child forward, an asymmetrical position of balance will be created that may cause the child to shift forward in an attempt to gain back balance. A large ball in front of the child may provide the tactile reinforcement. As the child crawls, bumping into the ball will reinforce the concept of direction through touching. If the ball is bright in color (a fluorescent ball under ultraviolet light is effective), it will stimulate visual regard and provide further structure, enabling the child to develop an understanding of the spatial environment.

The Second and Third Year

When the child begins to walk, reinforcement may be needed depending on the impairment. The same techniques used during crawling will be effective. The large ball again will reinforce movement as the child shuffles his feet forward. While crawling and walking, the child is associating peripheral and central visual-motor processes. The central fixation establishes direction and localization. The peripheral awareness yields organization of field along with the concept of awareness of space. When these are combined with motor movement, which includes kinesthetic, proprioceptive and vestibular cues, the infant reinforces balance and coordination. At all ages, therapy should present the child with situations whereby information may be matched through various motor actions and sensory inputs.

As the child advances, the concept of tridimensional activities should be developed to enable him to manipulate objects by pushing them through holes. It is important to encourage tactual manipulation with visual reinforcement at whatever working distance the child needs to involve vision. Backlighting to illuminate the hole and/or fluorescent objects enhances the contrast for the sight-impaired child.

Rolling activities will enable the sight-impaired child to maintain much support from the tactual stimulation of being on the floor while exploring body movement initiated from trunk and torso extension. It is important to utilize vision to lead all responses. To accomplish this, it is first necessary to analyze the movements needed to complete a roll. On his back, in order to roll to the right the child must tuck his chin and turn his head to the right while crossing the left arm over to the right. This will shift the balance to the right. As the child rolls onto his right side, he will need to extend his chin so that the roll onto the stomach will be completed. Once the child is on his stomach, the chin must be tucked to initiate a roll to the right. A follow-through brings the child onto his back again.

An object that stimulates visual regard may be moved in a way to cause the child to move his head into the desired positions. For example, with the child on his back, if an object is moved to the right and down, causing the child to look down and to the right, the desired chin tuck and head turn to the right will be achieved. As the light is moved out and up, causing the child to have to extend his head to follow it, the extension of the head will be completed, stimulating the movements necessary to continue the roll.

Activities should be designed to encourage the child to explore his space world. During this period of development, spatial relationships are being established by matching information about distance between vision and movement. The visually-impaired child who has a sight loss will need added reinforcement through other modalities such as audition. An auditory cue coupled with a visual cue provides an understanding of distance when the child matches this information with motor movement.

Visual loss may greatly affect a child's balance, particularly if the loss involves peripheral fields. Peripheral vision provides information concerning location of the self in the environment. A sense of balance is established through the matching of information from vision, vestibular stimulation and kinesthetic information. Since vision is dominant, a loss of this process may impede the child's ability to utilize information from other modalities.

To help the child organize sensorimotor information, activities should be designed to incorporate motor and sensory function. For example, hold the child in your lap while you rock from side to side. As the child moves with you, the vestibular stimulation will be reinforced by the kinesthetic system. By placing a fixed light source in front of the child, the change in location of the light as the child rocks will provide visual reinforcement. Many other techniques and activities may be developed by the creative therapist who understands the need to reinforce information received through more than one modality. Again, lenses and yoked prisms should always be considered.

Walking will be enhanced by providing tactual cues for the child. Rails, chairs and tables to hold on to all provide reinforcement. Of course, lighting is extremely important. Too much light is as ineffective as not enough light. Overhead light floods an environment, and shadows are cast beneath the object. Shadows are very important in determining depth relationships. For example, shadows cast by early morning or late afternoon sun provide us with information concerning distance of objects because shadows are cast horizontally. Likewise, room lighting that casts shadows to the side of an object will give the child information about depth and his relationship to objects.

Note: For activities involving visual fixation, the use of a flicker bulb will greatly stimulate visual fixation. A flicker bulb is a special light bulb with an oscillating filament within. When electrified, the filament will vibrate at a very rapid rate. Flicker bulbs come in many colors, however, the red bulb has been found most effective in stimulating visual regard. For his protection, place a sheet of Plexiglas between the hot bulb and the child.

By 2½ years the developmentally mature sighted child will begin to use himself as a reference point in his environment by relating sound and sight to distances. The sighted child will delight himself by throwing objects around the room and listening to the impact. The developmentally mature, visually-impaired child may have difficulty establishing himself as a reference point. Variations in behavior, such as the child holding an object close to his eye to look at it and then holding it in his hand while banging it on the table, is an indication that the child is reinforcing spatial concepts with tactual and kinesthetic stimulation, but lacks the necessary understanding of space to expand his reference point. This type of behavior indicates that the child requires greater structure to enable him to explore space. For example, if the child were to throw an object into the distance, the sound of the impact may not be related to the action if the child is unable to experience the continuity of space. Having the child first explore the surroundings with motor movement will establish boundaries. The time lapse between the thrown object and sound of impact will now have a motor reference base. Vision can be reinforced further by using highly stimulating visible objects (i.e., fluorescent balls) coupled with a brief flash of light at the moment of impact coming from the direction of the sound. The child will then use many modalities to develop a concept of space, cause and effect. The simple return of the object by the therapist will help the child establish concept permanence or perceptual constancy. Manipulating it tactually and visually will help the child realize that the object is the same.

Language Development

For the visually-impaired child, descriptive concept formation will be difficult because he is unable to visually discern the detailed relationships necessary to establish experience. Because of this, language development may be affected. Language is a symbol code given to some form, object or action. The ability to symbolize occurs when a person perceives some aspect and/or relationship of figure to ground and then represents it by an abstraction. The code of language enables us to relate abstractions to the world that we perceive and vice versa. Being unable to visually discern relationships, an individual will find distorted meanings in abstractions unless he is able to relate the abstraction through another means of sensorimotor exploration and manipulation.

To aid the visually-impaired child with language development, it is important to use only concrete descriptive language to help relate and reinforce the child's activities. This does not mean continually barraging the child with speech, but choosing appropriate language to succinctly describe the activity of the child. A simple word that describes what the child is attending to will enable the child to key into the relationship and begin to utilize abstract symbolisms. The development of language will, in turn, increase the child's ability to further discern relationships visually because it gives the child an abstract dimensionality of experience by which to perceive new and more meaningful visual relationships. It has been noted that low plus lenses can greatly improve the child's ability to organize visual space and movement and to reduce visual stress. The author has observed that the use of low plus lenses in reducing visual stress and balancing the ambient/focal visual process can affect receptive and expressive language abilities in some children.

As the child matures developmentally, spoken language should begin to help him develop new abilities of perceptual transformation (to know how something would look or to understand a thought from another point of view), perceptual constancy (to know how some thing or some thought can be the same while allowing for an aspect of change), and figure-ground (to hold on to some aspect of detail—either concrete or abstract— and release to the background). Language can facilitate the perceptual development of the child by giving the child a multifaceted, abstract way to describe and manipulate his experiences.

The concept development of a ball for a visually-impaired child may begin by the child first visualizing a circular disk. A new dimension may be experienced when the child manipulates it by touch and feels the round nature of the ball. By reinforcing the word "ball" with the description "round," the therapist has given abstract meaning in concrete terms to the child's visual and tactual-motor experience. New perceptual dimensionality may be added when the child is given two balls, one large and the other small. As the child perceives the similarities and differences of the balls, perceptual constancy is developed, i.e., when the child holds on to one aspect (the roundness) but allows for change (the size). At appropriate moments, the words "large ball" and "small ball" will help to develop abstract concepts of size and shape to relate to the concrete perceived qualities. What the ball looks and feels like as it is rotated in his hands helps develop the child's concurrent transformational perceptions.

The older child will eventually use language to describe and reinforce his perception of the environment and to provide a new structural dimension to vision in perceiving new relationships. By 3½ to 4 years of age the visually impaired child should begin to use abstract symbols to develop new dimensions of other symbols. For example, the child may not have the ball available but should be able to describe it as being "round and big" and, when asked through language how else a ball might look, would say "round and small" or "red" or "it rolls."

It is not the purpose of this chapter to describe the relationship between language and visual development for all stages. Rather, it is intended to point out that language, through representative coding, is related to the child's development of visual-perceptual skills and experiences, and that the therapist can and should consider the use of appropriate language in program development as a tool to enhance vision and perception.

The Fourth and Fifth Years

Depending on the amount and type of sight loss and visual abilities, many visually impaired 4 and 5-year-old children will show marked difficulties with perceptual motor activities. Since vision for these children is unstable and lacking experience, difficulties will be observed with movement and coordination. To improve the difficulties the visually-impaired child has with educating his residual vision to lead motor movement and conceptualize space, therapy must be structured to work at the child's level of ability by presenting activities that permit him to explore without fear.

Movement that explores body position in space is an essential component for spatial concept formation.[3] Leading the child into various positions, beginning with the child on his stomach or back, enables him to experience kinesthetic and proprioceptive reinforcement of body position. Initially, he may avoid visual fixation on his own body movement. When the child experiences the feeling of raising a foot or an arm with the help of a therapist, the child should be encouraged to fixate on the elevated arm or leg. A game may be played where the therapist raises or extends an arm or a leg of the blindfolded child and the child must somehow describe or point with the other arm to where the appendage is. As the child succeeds in understanding body movement through feeling, visual fixation can be added by having the child find the elevated or raised appendage visually, and then reach out with the other arm or hand to touch it while fixating on it.

The next step would be to raise the child to a crawling position. Fixation on the fluorescent-colored backs of his hands will be stimulated by overhead ultraviolet light. Using a different color on each hand will allow color differentiation and controlled fixation to auditory commands. Forward and backward directionality concepts can also be examined.

The child can explore balance by raising an arm or leg. Balance occurs when the child develops the ability to counter-balance movement. The motor equivalent movement enables the child to develop stability and coordination. Without the reactive movement, balance is lost.

Progressing to kneeling and finally to standing allows the child to explore new situations from a safe plane of reference. Movement while standing should proceed from first feeling, to being coupled with vision. The reason for this progression is that many children (sighted and sight-impaired) in their attempt to utilize vision will often suppress or suspend information received from motor movement.

At this age it is important to develop projectionality and concepts of direction. In other words, visual space and visual projections do not or should not change when the child closes his eyes. Visual projection should merely be transferred to kinesthetic reinforcement. For example, a child who looks at a ball 10 feet in front of him lines himself up with the ball and proceeds to walk to it. If the child were to be blindfolded after becoming visually oriented, the child would have to rely on feeling motor movement (by means of the kinesthetic and proprioceptive systems) to be able to direct himself correctly.

Seventh, Eighth and Ninth Years

Depending on the visual impairment and how development has been affected, a wide range of behaviors may be observed in the child. The child whose impairment has not interfered with his progress will be ready to learn perceptual skills and should be worked with in a variety of ways. The child whose impairment has interfered with his progress may be delayed several years. To attempt to introduce higher order perceptual skills to this child will push him beyond his level of perceptual abilities. Frustration will be experienced by both child and therapist, for progress will be very slow.

It is necessary, therefore, to observe the child's behaviors in order to know the child through his actions. If the child is still displaying the behaviors and needs of a 4-year-old, then habilitation programming should be organized accordingly. This chapter is not meant to be a "cookbook" for designing habilitation programs for the low-vision child, but to provide the reader with information about the developmental needs of the visually-impaired child. If those needs are met appropriately, habilitation will proceed in a natural manner with a minimum of frustration and trauma to both the child and the therapist.

The 7th, 8th and 9th years are important in developing higher level visual-perceptual abilities in the low vision child. This doesn't mean that visual-motor activities should be discontinued. Rather, the approach should include a variety of activities.

Visual tracking activities should be continued. Flashlight tracking games will stimulate interest, and since projection concepts should be developing at this stage (by 6 years developmentally), the child should be able to perform them. For example, the author has developed a game called "Star Wars." Six large fluorescent numbers (bases one through six) are hung on a wall in two columns. An ultraviolet light suspended from the ceiling will illuminate the numbers if the room lights are dimmed. The child holds one flashlight with a colored filter (red) and the therapist another with a different colored filter (green). The different colors will enable the child to identify his own light. Using some imagination, the child's light may represent a popular hero from a science fiction fantasy and the therapist's light, of course, a villain. The child should shine his light on base number one and proceed to base two, three, four and so on. The therapist's light should move with the child's light. The object of the game is for the child to move his light to each of the bases in sequence without being tagged by the therapist's light when the child is off the base. After two successive tags, the positions are reversed.

This activity develops tracking skills through fixation on the light, but more importantly, it develops a relationship between peripheral and central vision. The base and the therapist's light will both be in the periphery when the child fixates on his own light. One reason for success in moving the light from one base to another without being tagged will occur when the child can utilize the peripheral vision to anticipate change. The low vision child often has difficulty with this. Peripheral and/or central field losses do not mean that the child will be unable to perform this type of activity. However, the visual process must be worked with in order to develop the necessary skills.

As with children without sight impairments, a sight-impaired child will concentrate so intently on one aspect of vision that he may not process important information from another aspect of vision. For example, the child engrossed in watching a bicyclist go by may trip over the rock that lies in his path. Relating peripheral vision to central vision is important to developing timing, coordination and balance. Perceptually, the peripheral field is the ground to fixation and should relate constancy through which the individual can compare size, distance and motion to other sensorimotor functions to develop an understanding of space-volume. When there is a mismatch of information, understanding the relationship between space and time is distorted. This is usually an unconscious distortion. For example, the person who swings the bat at a pitched ball too early or too late may actually perceive the ball to be at a different location than where it is.

Rail walking activities (walking on a board placed on the floor) while fixating on an object ahead are good for developing visual and kinesthetic awareness. A metronome beat for each step can be incorporated.

Strip fixations will also help develop visual efficiency between peripheral and central vision. Two strips of letters are mounted on the wall approximately seventy five centimeters apart. The child should stand four to five feet from the letters and proceed to read a letter from each column, starting first with the top left letter, then to the top right letter, and so on. The quick eye movements that are made when looking from one letter to another are a motor match of information received from peripheral and central vision concerning direction and distance. Losing one's place will indicate inappropriate sensorimotor matching and/or suspension of information. Also, a metronome beat can add rhythm as progress is achieved. Lenses and prisms provide a means to directly affect vision, timing, and spatial concepts during these activities.

Developing visual imagery and memory is important at this stage of development. Through visualization, problem solving and thought processing continue to develop. Recognizing part and whole relationships are an important part of visualization and memory. Activities should be used to develop these skills. For example, blocks may be organized in a design. The child is to explore the design through visual and tactual-kinesthetic means and then reconstruct it with other blocks from memory. Perceptual transformation and constancy skills can be worked with by asking the child to construct the design as if he were sitting on the other side of the table. The child will have to visualize the design and transpose it in his mind. A child who is having difficulty with laterality (knowing his left from his right) will have difficulty with transformations because perceptual constancy has not been established. The child cannot perceive a difference between an orientation of blocks one way or the other. Color coding the table and the child's hands may help. For example, a piece of red tape on the right hand and green tape on the left hand will help to visually reinforce the laterality concept.

To develop laterality skills, other activities may be performed using red and green tape on the child's hands and feet (red on the right). Activities such as "Simon Says" can require matching the right and left hand to auditory commands. Directionality concepts (projecting left and right into the field) can be developed through visual cues from the leader of "Simon Says." To determine a correct movement, the red or green tape on the child and the therapist should be matched.

Another visual memory activity that is effective in building laterality, directionality, and imagery skills is to play tic-tac-toe from memory (without writing down the moves). This will be a challenge for both the child and the therapist.

Activities such as these will help the child develop skills of visual processing that will improve his efficiency and organization of thought and problem solving. The therapist who understands some of the basics behind the visual and perceptual processes can develop activities pertinent to the needs of the low vision child.

The reader may question what feeling, kinesthetic movement, spatial relationships, and other perceptual developments have to do with getting the child to see and use optical aids. The following section is devoted to explaining these relationships.

The Use of Optical Aids

Visually-impaired children usually do not respond successfully to optical aids until at least 3 years of age (developmental age). It takes that long for a child to develop the perceptual skills necessary to understand visual space through the impairment that he has. If a telescope or magnifier which further distorts space is placed before the child's eyes, matching of information from other sensory modalities is greatly hindered. By 3 years of age those children who have exceptional perceptual skills should be able to adapt to some simple forms of near magnification. There is no magic age. It depends on the child's visual-perceptual flexibilities and, most importantly, on his ability to match information. However, introducing children to optical devices at an early age can encourage independence and participation in a greater variety of activities.[4]

As mentioned previously, it is very important to detect the visual impairment as early as possible. A visual examination by a qualified optometrist or ophthalmologist is recommended within the first four weeks after the child is born. If an impairment is diagnosed, medical and low vision treatment and a habilitation program may be developed to meet the child's present and future needs. In the case of planning for low vision services, the optometrist, parents and other involved professionals should discuss the child's potential future needs for optical aids.[3] They need to decide what can be done to develop the necessary perceptual skills to use the optical aid(s) prior to the prescription of the aid(s). An interdisciplinary approach including therapy will make the introduction of optical aid(s) less demanding and stressful on the child.

The type of therapy designed to prepare the child to use optical aids may vary considerably, depending on the child's developmental age, physical abilities, perceptual abilities, intelligence and environmental surroundings. A basic understanding of the optics of the aid, how space is distorted through the aid and, most importantly, what perceptual skills are needed to reinforce successful use of the aid will enable the therapist to design a program to meet the child's needs. The following procedures are basic functional processes involved in utilizing optical aids successfully. These techniques have been developed through an understanding of the perceptual skills involving organization of field and the interactions among the various sensorimotor functions. The therapist, through creative thinking and an understanding of the basic functional processes involved, should be able to adapt these techniques to the developmental needs of the child and his environment.

Training for Utilization of Distance Optical Aids

Telescopic aids vary greatly in magnification and field of view. They also differ in size and type (e.g., hand-held, head-borne, spectacle-mounted). Since all telescopes (except for a reverse telescope) distort space by magnifying the object, reducing the field of view, and projecting the image of the object closer, many children and adults will become greatly disoriented initially. The disorientation occurs because the sensory information received through the eye from the optical aid has not been matched or has been inappropriately matched with information received through other sensorimotor feedback systems. Experience has not been supportive enough to enable the person to adapt to a new spatial construct. For example, the reduction of the field of view and magnification cause the person to view a relatively small island in the environment. The peripheral vision that is now sacrificed was important to the person for establishing a total organization of field or a part-to-whole concept. The peripheral vision helped to reinforce balance as well as develop an understanding of time and distance relationships.

Initially, the child may hold the telescope before his eye to look through it, but he does not know at what or where he is looking. If the child is standing, he will often begin to wobble because of loss of balance. Sometimes this initial disorienting experience can be a negative one despite all the hard work and good intentions of the optometrist and parents to give the child an optical aid. The failure in use of the optical aid and the negative experience may be avoided by some preliminary work with the child. The developmental activities described earlier are important to stimulate and develop sensorimotor processing. They should be performed regardless of whether or not optical aids are to be used.

If a telescope is to be prescribed for a child, the parent, educator, or other therapist might engage in some game-like activities to develop some of the specific skills needed.[5] Spatial direction and projection are developmentally established through motor reinforcement. Therefore, the maintenance of motor and kinesthetic feedback is extremely important for success with optical aids. Kinesthetic awareness coupled with tactual and auditory stimulation will enable the child to maintain organization of the spatial environment. The first procedure (Stage One) to stimulate this process is for the child to close his eyes and reach out and grasp a pencil that the optometrist is holding. The child is then told that the optometrist is going to move the pencil. The object of the activity is to see if he can keep his head pointed directly at the pencil. As the pencil is moved, the child will be aware of the position of the pencil by kinesthetic reinforcement through his extended arm. Success in head orientation to the position of the pencil is the goal of this procedure.

Stage Two repeats the procedure, but this time instructs the child to hold his head still and follow the pencil only with his closed eyes. At some point after the pencil has been stopped, the optometrist should say "open your eyes," and success is rated on how close the child's eyes are to the pencil. Once the child can maintain the appropriate direction in relation to the moving pencil through kinesthetic reinforcement from the extended arm, the next procedure should be tried.

Stage Three uses auditory and kinesthetic reinforcement of visual direction. A bell is used instead of a pencil. The child holds the bell and Stages One and Two should be performed again for transitional purposes. After the child has adapted to the sound of the bell, remove the child's hand and ask him to point to the bell, first with head movement and then eye movement. (Remember, the eyes should be closed during the procedures and should only be opened as reinforcement to the child.) Successful orientation to the direction and position of the bell indicates that the child is utilizing audition to reinforce the kinesthetic position sense.

In Stage Four the bell is moved farther and farther from the child to determine if directional concepts can still be maintained. Variations in these procedures should be performed by having the child stand and balance on one foot, rather than being seated. As success is achieved, the child may be turned around and around in the center of the room with his eyes closed. He is instructed to stop turning, face and point in the direction of the bell.

The older child (8 to 9 years developmentally) may enjoy playing the game "North, South, East and West." The child stands in the center of the room and memorizes the direction of each wall marked North, South, East and West. When he closes his eyes, the optometrist asks the child to point to the wall that is called out. If the child correctly points to all of the walls, turn him 180 degrees (face him opposite the original direction) and repeat the procedure. A 90-degree change in direction, turning the child around and around, and then stopping, will require the child to rely on kinesthetic movement to maintain spatial orientation.

Several days, weeks, or even months of repeating these procedures, and other similar procedures, may be necessary before an optical aid should even be tried. When success is achieved with these activities, similar therapy with the telescope itself can begin.

Begin using the telescope in the same manner described in Stage One, only have the child hold the telescope to one of his closed eyes while reaching out and holding the pencil with the other hand. Do the procedure. Since the pencil will be too close for the child to view it through the telescope, the idea is to simply set up a procedure that causes the child to continue utilizing the kinesthetic and vestibular systems to reinforce directional concepts. Most importantly, it is success-oriented because the demands are within the level of the perceptual abilities of the child.

Proceed to auditory stimulation at a near range, still not requiring the child to find the bell visually but requiring the child to use localization of auditory sounds to reinforce kinesthetic directional awareness. With success, move the bell to a distance farther away, as outlined in Stage Four. Success is not measured on finding the bell visually through the telescope, but only on directional orientation.

When directional orientation is achieved, the child should be asked what he sees. The child may have difficulty describing what he sees because of the lack of experience in understanding things through magnification.

The therapist may attempt to help bring the child's fixation through the telescope to the desired position by flashing a light or making a movement to enable the child to see some change in contrast and in figure-ground relationship. Changing fixation from one point to another at distance should be the next step. Auditory stimulation at the fixation point, together with pointing first in the direction of the sound, should precede attempting to locate the object visually.

In summary, kinesthetic and auditory reinforcement is very important in establishing and maintaining spatial direction and perception. The child who does not succeed in using telescopic aid prescriptions fails because he is unable to maintain an organization of space through reinforcement from sensorimotor processing. By practicing these procedures daily, and by encouraging and reinforcing the child's responses, the optometrist will be developing the basic functional processes necessary for utilizing the optical aid which will maximize the child's vision.

Training for Utilization of Near Optical Aids

The great variation between the types of near optical aids (i.e., stand magnifiers, hand-held magnifiers, spectacle-mounted binoculars and monoculars, and electronic magnification devices) makes a single, general approach for therapy difficult. This section will be concerned only with the basic functional processes needed to use the aid.

Since the near optical aid distorts space through magnification and reduces the field of view, it brings the projection of an image closer, and disorientation may occur with the child or adult for the same reasons as occur with telescopic aids. The type of disorientation, however, will be in loss of place in near space. Since near optical aids are used mainly for reading, indications of difficulty using the aid may appear as behavioral symptoms. For example, the child may experience loss of place, have difficulty understanding what he is reading, or have difficulty remembering what he has read.

If a near optical aid is to be prescribed, several procedures may be effective in developing the appropriate perceptual skills needed to use the aid prior to its prescription. For all near optical aid use, tactile-kinesthetic reinforcement is important to maintain spatial organization of the field. When this is lost, disorientation occurs and the person will have difficulty knowing where he is looking. The procedure to begin with is touching, understanding direction through kinesthesia, and then looking through the aid.

Utilizing this approach, the therapist may begin by having the child reach with his hand into a sandbox or onto a table and find an object (block, marble, etc.) by feeling for it. (Having the child close his eyes initially may make the procedure more effective.) Once the child has found the object tactually, have the child do whatever he has to in order to see it. The child may have to bring the object very close. A variation of this activity would be to play the game "What Is It?" Several different but familiar objects should be placed in the child's field. When the child finds one, he must determine what it is only by feeling it. After guessing what it is, the child may then look at it to determine if he is right. At this time the therapist should reinforce the child's decision, and if the guess was incorrect, the therapist should help the child determine what it is, preferably by describing salient features of the object in order to have the child finally determine the correct answer.

These are preliminary activities designed to stimulate tactile and kinesthetic awareness. Both of these processes will be used to reinforce visual organization of the field. This can be accomplished by having the child hold a cardboard tube or a large piece of cardboard with a hole in the center up to one eye (the other eye should be occluded). The tube should touch the face. With the other hand the child should hold a peg, light or small object. The child should be told to be aware of feeling the object and then to find the object while looking through the tube. The purpose of the tactual and kinesthetic stimulation is to reinforce the child's visual organization of the field, thereby enabling the child to "feel" the correct direction before sighting through the tube. Auditory stimulation can also be added to give another dimension to the directional stimulation. Once the child has sighted the object through the tube, have him move the tube toward the object, while still sighting through the tube, until the tube slides over the object. During this step the child should continue to hold the object with the other hand for added reinforcement. This procedure will develop sighting ability while reinforcing vision with tactile and kinesthetic cues.

The following procedures for varying types of near optical aids utilize tactual and kinesthetic reinforcement of vision. These procedures may be adapted to the specific instructions of the aid or the child's special needs. It is important that appropriate lighting be used.

Hand-Held Magnifiers

The variation in power of the magnifier will require specific working distances. Once this has been calculated, the therapist or the examining clinician should organize the activity so that the appropriate working distance for the magnifier can be maintained during the activity.

In the procedure previously described, the hand-held magnifier may be substituted for the tube. The child should touch the object with one hand and hold the magnifier up to touch the face around the unoccluded eye. Since the power of the lens will initially not be at the appropriate working distance, the object will be blurred and out of focus. This is desirable because the child must now key into his tactual and kinesthetic cues to learn where the object is. The child should then, in a similar manner to using the tube, move the magnifier toward the object until the object is clear and the appropriate working distance has been verified. Variations of this activity would be to hold the magnifier on the object being held with the other hand and move the magnifier up toward the eye until the object is in focus. The therapist will have to work with the child to determine where the child's head should be positioned for best viewing.

The proper distance to hold the magnifier from the object is learned through kinesthetic reinforcement to vision. The sense of feeling and knowing the location of the arm and hand that is holding the magnifier develops the understanding of where the magnifier is to be positioned. If the child has continuous difficulty learning where to position the magnifier, the therapist may want to work in some other auditory-tactual-kinesthetic awareness activities involving distance determination. For example, with the child's eyes closed, the therapist should hold a dowel or peg at different distances in front of the child. A bell rung near the dowel will give some directional awareness. The child should reach out and find the dowel with one hand and with the other hand place rings or circular objects over the dowel. Varying the distance of the dowel will stimulate the kinesthetic awareness of different distances.

As the child becomes proficient in focusing the aid, and the therapist begins to advance the child with the magnifier to other activities, the child will proceed more rapidly if the therapist keeps the importance of tactile-kinesthetic reinforcement to visual organization in mind. By having the child simply touch or point to what he is attempting to magnify, the child will be more aware of where in his visual field he is directing the magnifier.

Stand Magnifiers

Since stand magnifiers have their working distances already set by their structure, the therapist need only be concerned with getting the child to place it in the correct location on the page. This may be accomplished by first having the child feel the page and find the upper-left corner both visually and tactually. The magnifier should be brought to the upper-left corner on the page and then moved down until the first print is observed. Depending upon the type of stand magnifier, it can slide across the line of print, allowing the child to read the words through the magnifier. It is important that the child mark the beginning of the line with his finger. Again, this gives the child tactile and kinesthetic knowledge of what line he is on. When the child gets to the end of the line, he only has to move the magnifier back to the finger and drop down one line on the page to be appropriately positioned at the beginning of the next line of print.

Head-borne Magnifiers

These may include clip-on magnifiers, bifocals, reading lenses in glasses, or any microscopic aid that has a limited working distance. These will be more appropriate for older children (8 and above) because of the coordination needed. A younger child with superior perceptual skills may adapt with some training. These aids require that whatever is viewed be placed close to the aid. The therapist should be familiar with the specific instructions for use of the particular aid and then adapt tactile and kinesthetic cues to enable the child to understand distance relationships needed to focus the aid.

Focusing the aid on the child's hand is a good way to begin. As the child's hand comes into focus, an object or a paper with print on it can be placed in his hand. This process may be done along with some of the preliminary distance judging activities described earlier.

Reading sentences may offer more difficulty since the distance will change and the print will be out of focus if the child turns his head. An effective activity in developing this technique involves making a device with an ordinary coat hanger. Bend the wire so that it fits over and around the crown of the child's head. On either side of the forehead attach two pencils that project forward the exact distance of the focal length of the lens (i.e., if a +10 D lens is used, then the 10 cm focal length of the lens would require the pencils to also be 10 cm long). When the child holds the paper in front of his face to read, have him move the paper back and forth. The pencils will always keep the paper at the correct working distance.

Telemicroscopes

These are spectacle-mounted microscopic devices designed to have fixed working distances beyond the characteristic working distance of the dioptric value. The child will have to sight through the aid while keeping the printed material at a specified working distance. These sophisticated devices are usually prescribed for purposes such as reading or working with chemicals that should not be brought close to the face.

Since head positioning is very important for using these aids successfully, some of the activities described earlier may be effective for preliminary training. Another activity that has been found effective is to mount a light on the child's head. (Headlamps with a light attached to an elastic strap are sold at most hardware or sporting goods stores at a minimal cost.) The child should first touch the page to gain tactile and kinesthetic reinforcement, and then move his head so that the light shines on the page. When the telemicroscope is positioned before the child's eye(s), the procedure should be the same: touch first and then align the light. When the light shines on the finger touching the page, the child has only to move himself closer to or farther from the page to position the aid at the correct focal length.

If a typoscope (a black marker with a slit in it that is placed over the reading material) is used to help the child find his place, it should not be used in place of pointing to and touching the page. Pointing and touching give the child multi-sensorimotor experiences that reinforce vision. If the typoscope is used, have the child point at the same time.

Electronic Magnification Devices

The field of electronic magnification devices has been growing rapidly and now includes low vision aids (LVAs) that are fixed, as well as hand-held and head mounted devices (HMDs). Most LVAs are mounted on a table or desk and include a computer screen or CRT screen monitor. These are very helpful for allowing persons with low vision to see a printed page, photos, and labels, write a check, etc. Available software enables those with limited vision to increase the size of computer images, and to change print to voice or to braille. While most electronic amplifying devices are used for near or intermediate viewing distances, some are now being used for more distant vision. HMDs have the advantage of allowing the viewer to have his hands free, and some are flexible over a wide range of viewing distances so that they can be used for a variety of viewing purposes.

Most devices have some controls for viewing size, while some have them for varying luminescence and contrast enhancement. Electronic devices may be ordered through an optometrist or ophthalmologist, and in some areas there are businesses that specialize in selling a variety of magnification devices and other aids for those who are blind or have low vision. Be aware that when using electronic magnification devices with children, training similar to that which has been discussed in this chapter will be needed to help the child learn to use the perceptual skills that are necessary to reinforce successful use of the aid.

Understanding the balance of the focal and ambient processes as they relate to development allows a practitioner to take a more direct approach for habilitation of the visually impaired child. Influencing vision through facilitation of the relationship between the focal and ambient processes will increase the chances of success with low vision aids while also affecting function and performance in general.

Chapter 17

MANAGING THE CHILD WITH LOW VISION IN THE CLASSROOM

Judith A. Padula

Introduction

Rehabilitation for the visually-impaired person has been greatly enhanced since the development of the low vision examination more than 50 years ago. Prior to that development, simple magnifiers were used in a trial and error approach with little or no scientific methodology. The use of magnifiers was not considered part of rehabilitation, and it was primarily left up to the visually-impaired person to find an appropriate magnifier. In many cases, it was not until adulthood that individuals even used magnifiers.

Long ago, the term "blind" for the visually-impaired child was more than just a classification. It de-emphasized the importance of vision. Educational and rehabilitation programs emphasized development of tactile and auditory skills to compensate for the supposed lack of vision. The school-age child with vision impairment was isolated from children who didn't have physical impairments. "Sight-saving" classrooms and schools for the blind were established. Braille was taught and auditory training given because it was thought that further use of vision would cause its eventual loss. Children were actually discouraged from using their vision.[1]

This brief historical review should not be thought of as criticism of the methods that were used. The purpose of these introductory paragraphs is to set a stage so that the reader can understand why our current philosophies and understandings have developed and be able to recognize the importance of the low vision services for the visually impaired child.

When it was recognized that optical aids could actually be beneficial in habilitating the use of residual vision, methodology was developed to equate the magnification needs of the patient with acuity measurements and visual field. The low vision examination during these early years utilized a concept of vision that did not always relate to function. The static measurements of acuity and field are related more to the optical considerations than they are to the functional abilities and/or potentials of the person.

Initially, though, as many individuals became visually rehabilitated, the philosophy for saving sight began to change, and the visual abilities of the patient were emphasized. Programs to improve the visual efficiency of the child were developed. Clinical and experimental research proved that not only could visual functioning be improved, but that vision would not deteriorate further.[2]

Although the concept of a low vision examination gained recognition as an attempt to improve visual functioning of the school-age child, success was limited. Criteria were developed for appropriate referrals that related to age and acuity measurements. It was not until it was understood that there was more to visual functioning than an acuity or field measurement that the concept of low vision and the provision of services began to change. Clinicians found that, given similar pathological conditions, acuities and visual fields, some individuals functioned as if there were almost no impairments, while others were almost totally visually debilitated.

An understanding of the dynamic qualities of vision from observation and clinical and experimental research led the clinician away from the optical model of low vision to a concept that is more rehabilitative and need oriented. This does not mean simply asking the patient about what his needs are, but rather attempting to understand visual function by observing behavior. Behavior represents the way the individual utilizes the visual process to lead motor function.

Optical aids alone do not improve visual function. Acuity may improve but is not an indication of improved function. The optical aid is a tool. If the process of vision can utilize this tool effectively, function can be improved.

The low vision examination has evolved to include new methodology that is adaptive to the needs of the visually-impaired child. In addition, new modes of electrodiagnostic testing permit enhanced detection and refinements in analysis by the clinician. Assessment of visual function in the habitual environment is also recognized as an integral part of the low vision analysis. Information about visual functioning in the home, classroom, and/or environment provides the clinician a greater understanding of the acuity and field measurements in the office setting. In order to accomplish this, educators and rehabilitation professionals can perform functional assessments in the field and relay this information to the clinician.

The information gathered can greatly assist the clinician in determining the most appropriate prescriptive optical aids for the child. Further, training programs for learning to use the aids and improving visual function can be moved from the office setting to the habitual environment of the child. This way, a follow-through is established that enables the clinician to develop an effective means of low vision habilitation for the child. The follow-through by the educator and/or rehabilitation professional also enables the child to be referred back for further clinical assessment and prescriptive devices should some aspect of behavioral function change.

The present concept of low vision habilitation includes a multi-disciplinary philosophy which recognizes that the needs of the visually-impaired child cannot be met by one professional alone.[2] However, it is best if the clinician remains the hub of this service.

The functional abilities of the child should be assessed using varied methods and settings in order to determine the child's critical needs. By utilizing a multidisciplinary approach, a cross perspective of those needs can be established which gives the clinician greater insight into the most effective means of prescribing and designing appropriate training programs for the child. This concept has caused low vision rehabilitation to evolve from solely an examination and prescription of optical aids to a model of service that includes educators and rehabilitation professionals. In the low vision service model, functional assessment, clinical assessment, prescription, adaptive training, referral and follow-up are the keys to success. While the low vision clinical examination remains the integral part of this service model, *the clinician must understand that success will be determined by improved performance, not increased acuity*. Further, the involvement of the educator and rehabilitation professional will increase the potential for success of visual habilitation.

The de-emphasis on acuity relating to improved function has already been made but must be clarified further. Acuity and field measurements still represent important quantitative measurements taken by the clinician of the visually-impaired child. Certainly, refractive corrections and predicted magnification systems are essential components of the clinical assessment. However, a dynamic, qualitative understanding of the visual process of the child must be given greater attention. The acuity measurement is really a function of the visual process. The ability to visually control and manipulate an aspect of the field yields the acuity measurement.

> *Vision is the dynamic and balanced blend of spatial organization which, together with focal detail, yields identification and fixation. Without the spatial format of the visual process the isolation on detail prevails. (W.V. Padula)*

Vision can affect the child's overall development. Therefore, the clinician must attempt to analyze how the child utilizes his vision in a manner that relates to habitual environmental settings, e.g., the classroom. The visual skills used in the classroom, such as near-far fixations, saccadic fixations, spatial relationships, eye-hand coordination, balance and motor coordination, must be analyzed by the clinician. These visual functions should be evaluated as part of the low vision examination so that the clinician can determine where the visual interferences occur and impact these interferences by developing appropriate habilitative programming.

For example, a 10 year old, visually-impaired boy with 20/80 acuity, central serous retinopathy, and no peripheral field loss was referred for a low vision examination by an educator. The reason for referral was the need to improve the child's ability to see the chalkboard for the purpose of copying assignments and taking notes. The functional assessment performed by the educator noted that the child often became disoriented in the classroom. The prescription of a telescope was first considered. In this case a testing situation was developed using large printed letters cut into two vertical strips and mounted on a wall approximately three feet apart.

The child was positioned approximately four feet from the charts and asked to read a letter from each strip, thereby showing saccadic fixations. Similar testing was designed for near-far fixation ability using a large block of letters mounted on a wall 10 feet from the child and a block of printed letters on a card that the child held. The child was asked to read one letter from each chart alternately.

The tests revealed that the child frequently lost his place and quickly became frustrated with the tasks. While acuity measurements with a 4.0x hand-held telescope were improved from 20/80 to 20/20+, the child became very disoriented. Even without the telescope, the child demonstrated difficulty using his vision to orient himself in his environment and difficulty using peripheral visual cues to orient central visual functions. The functional assessment by the educator hinted at this, and the clinical assessment further revealed this interference which extended beyond acuity loss.

To prescribe a telescope that would magnify and reduce the visual field would further limit the ability of the child to utilize peripheral visual cues. Therefore, it was decided that the educational program should compensate for these difficulties initially. Adaptive habilitative programs would then be developed to minimize the visual interferences and improve the child's visual functioning to a level at which a telescope could be prescribed.

It was recommended that copying activities be limited to copying from a paper on the child's desk rather than from the chalkboard. Seating in the classroom was changed so that the child was positioned in the front row. In addition, a training program began that included localizing the sound of a bell by pointing toward the bell with eyes closed, then opening the eyes to correct and reinforce. The pointing served to give kinesthetic reinforcement to establish visual and auditory direction. The purpose of the activity was to develop the integrative process of vision.

As progress was made, activities were developed that included near-far fixations and saccadic fixations at varying distances. With these activities, the child used a flashlight to point to the object or letter he was looking at, again to develop kinesthetic reinforcement. When progress was noted, a cardboard tube was introduced that limited peripheral vision. At first, a large tube offering a minimal field limitation was used, and then the field was reduced, using smaller diameter tubes as progress was made.

These activities were performed by the teacher of the visually-impaired child several times a week, and monthly checkups on progress were made by the clinician. Within four months, a wide-angle telescope was introduced, and training was started in the office and continued by the educator. Within six months the child's skills were improved to the extent that the original 4.0x hand-held telescope was prescribed for use in the classroom.

Early Low Vision Intervention

The clinician must consider developmental aspects when performing a low vision examination since delays in development may interfere with success. Through appropriate low vision habilitation programming the practitioner may actually be able to influence the child's development.

The development of the child is a function of three variables: physical abilities, psychological disposition and environmental influences. Vision is not isolated in one variable but actually is part of all three. It certainly has a physical nature and it includes perceptual aspects, but it is also influenced by the environment.

If a child with a visual impairment has adequate or above-average intellectual and perceptual abilities, and is placed in a stimulating environment, he may be able to compensate for the physical/visual deficit to maintain development.

Conversely, if the child cannot compensate for his physical deficit, a delay in development may occur. Even though a child may be chronologically 7 years old, his developmental age may only be 4 or 5 years. In this case, the practitioner should expect the behavior and functional abilities of a younger child. The clinical implications are that the practitioner may need to consider establishing both short and long-range objectives from the low vision examination. Simple magnifiers may be effective initially to improve general functioning at near ranges. Special training programs may be necessary, however, to improve the visual skills in order to utilize more sophisticated devices such as spectacle-mounted microscope prescriptions and/or hand-held telescopes.

When the practitioner encounters a child who may be developmentally delayed, several symptoms may be identified during the discussion of the history with the educator and/or parent. The child may be a behavioral problem in school, being unable to stay seated for a long period or exhibiting frequent loss of attention and concentration. Sometimes the parent and/or educator may misperceive these symptoms and state that the child is lazy or doesn't work up to potential.

The practitioner should not assume that the lack of ability to see clearly is the reason the child is not functioning up to expectations. In this case the parent and/or educator may think that the prescribed optical aid will solve the problem, when in fact the child's lack of developmental-perceptual abilities may interfere with the use of the aid. Failure to use the aid properly and/or no change in the child's behavior in the classroom may cause the educator and parent to view the low vision examination as a failure.

The practitioner must attempt to differentiate the developmental difficulties from those difficulties caused by acuity interruption. To do this, the history should include a discussion of developmental milestones such as the age the child crawled, walked, and spoke in phrases and sentences. Perceptual-motor testing of balance and motor integration should give the practitioner a general idea of whether the child is behind in expected abilities related to chronological norms. In addition, some developmental tests such as the Gesell Copy Forms Test, the Gesell Incomplete Man Test, or the Beery-Buktenica Test of Visual Motor Integration[3] may be given. Although these tests may need to be adapted somewhat by darkening lines, etc., to meet the visual abilities of the child, the general developmental age level scored on these tests may be helpful in understanding the child's behaviors and abilities.

When a child has developmental interferences, the practitioner should spend time explaining the implications to both the parents and the educator. Extra school work assignments or homework will not serve the child's best interests. What is needed is habilitative programming designed to improve the child's skills and thereby affect his functioning and development.

A complete review of all aspects of designing an appropriate habilitative program cannot be developed within the confines of this chapter. The practitioner should, however, understand that the child's development is greatly influenced by the visual process. Therefore, the key to affecting development lies in improving the visual skills in areas of fixation, pursuit tracking, saccadic fixations, and perceptual-motor abilities. Since the developmental process involves the use of vision to lead motor functions and match information between vision and other senses, habilitative programs must include training the child to utilize the visual process to match information between sensory and motor systems.

The results of this type of habilitative programming may not be immediate, but may take months of consistent training. It is most effective for the practitioner to be directly involved in leading the training and changing programming when necessary. The parent and the educator can and should be involved in carrying out procedures on a daily basis. Prescription of optical aids may need to be limited to the child's abilities until visual skill levels have been improved. At that time more sophisticated devices may be given.

The First Low Vision Examination

A question often asked by educators and parents is how old the child should be for referral for a low vision examination. When taking the developmental nature of the visual process into consideration, the answer to this question varies. The practitioner experienced in low vision evaluation should be consulted as soon as possible after the visual impairment is diagnosed because he may be able to prescribe spectacles, contact lenses, bifocals, and even optical aids that will affect the overall development. Also, long-range planning can be started concerning the child's future needs. For example, if it is anticipated that a 3-year-old child will require spotting telescopes for classroom use in the future, the preschool educator of the visually handicapped may be trained in spotting techniques, and additional habilitative programming may be developed. It is also imperative that medical and/or surgical intervention be considered as soon as possible if it will improve the visual state of the child.

In discussing the needs of the visually-impaired child with groups of educators and/or parents, the optometrist must stress the importance of early referral for low vision services.[2] Often a child is not referred until he is 8 years of age or older.

Unfortunately, many years may thus pass before an effective visual program, including refractive corrections and low vision devices, is instituted.

One young man was referred at the age of 16 for his first low vision examination. He had spastic cerebral palsy and was confined to a wheelchair. When he was 3 years old, he was classified as legally blind because acuity testing with best correction did not yield results better than 20/200. Since that time, no visual examinations had been performed. Upon examining this young man, 4 diopters of myopia was objectively determined. The subjective refraction improved his acuity from 20/200 to 20/50, demonstrating that he was not legally blind. Educators and parents should recognize that a low vision examination can greatly improve a child's visual abilities. Often only a careful refraction alone can result in a significant improvement.

This approach may enable the low vision practitioner to prescribe aids for very young children. If aids are prescribed for the preschool child, acceptance is greater. Essentially, the child will grow up with the aids as part of his life. Also, peer pressure in preschool is less than at elementary school levels. By the time the child reaches elementary school, he will have learned to cope with peer pressure situations that will undoubtedly arise.

How the young child can adapt to situations is demonstrated by one who had been using aids since he was 3 years old. The importance of the child's optical aids was illustrated by his behavior. On his first day in the first grade, he took out a 2.5x hand-held spotting telescope to see what his teacher looked like. He told several children who approached him just how things would be when he said (much to their surprise), "I'm gonna deck the first one who makes fun of my telescope." While not all children would deal with the situation as "tactfully" as he did, most children who have used optical aids since preschool will continue to use them throughout their school years and beyond. An older child just receiving aids, however, may not be able to deal effectively with peer influences.

The teacher of the visually impaired can be very helpful in dealing with problems that arise in school over the use of optical aids.[2] Initially the teacher may go directly into the classroom and give a presentation to the other children about what vision impairment is and what optical aids are for. Permitting the children to try them may help to develop their understanding of the aids.

Prescription glasses and aids for the preschool child should not be based solely on improvement in acuity. Often, if the practitioner detects a moderate or even a low amount of myopia, hyperopia or astigmatism, no prescription will be given if a significant improvement in acuity is not demonstrated. If the practitioner were to evaluate perceptual-motor skills and touch-point ability (ability to reach and localize an object accurately), the effects of the lenses might be more readily observed.

Measuring Success

The utilization of optical aids in the practitioner's office should not be considered a success in habilitating the patient. There are too many factors in the classroom and/or home environment that can interfere. The service can only be considered successful after the child has demonstrated improved function and performance in his habitual settings. This can be determined only after a follow-up examination and/or communication with the educator and parent.

The relative nature of success is demonstrated by one 10-year-old girl who had undifferentiated maculas in both eyes, a moderate amount of hyperopia (OU), and nystagmus. She was referred for a low vision examination to determine whether optical aids would be effective in improving her ability to read and see the chalkboard. The result of the examination determined that her acuity at near improved from 20/120 to 20/30 with a 4x stand magnifier. A hand-held magnifier was also prescribed to enable her to have visual flexibility at intermediate ranges (particularly helpful in her science course). Bifocal lenses were prescribed due to her distance and near vision improvement. A hand-held telescope improved her distance vision from 10/80 to 10/30, and she demonstrated proficient use of all three aids after being trained for 30 minutes in the office.

The novelty of the aids soon wore off, and her teacher reported that the girl would not use them or the glasses because several children made fun of her. The girl's teacher attempted to remedy the situation by talking with the other children about vision impairment. Although the ridicule stopped, the girl still refused to use the aids.

Through follow-up visits with the low vision practitioner and communication between the educator, optometrist, parent, and social worker, progress was initiated by having the girl use the aids only at home. Several of her friends began to ask her why she wasn't using her glasses, and for short periods she began to wear them in school. After one year of continued low vision service, the girl began to use the aids in school. Her grades improved and this appeared to reinforce her use of the aids. For this child the initial demonstration that she could use the aids resulted in a false sense of success. The true measurement of success was achieved only after a year of follow-through low vision service by additional professionals.

Success for another child was measured in a different way. A 3-year-old boy was referred for a low vision evaluation. He had spastic cerebral palsy, was previously diagnosed as cortically blind, and speech was not evident. His previous doctor had told the mother that her child could see somewhat, but that there was nothing that could help him.

Upon performing the evaluation, it was determined that the child was able to fixate on a puppet for two to three seconds at approximately a one-foot range. Tracking movements were not elicited, but horizontal saccadic fixations were observed between two lights approximately five inches apart. Reaching for an object was found to be inconsistent and inaccurate. Acuity testing was unreliable. Distance retinoscopy revealed 2 diopters of hyperopia in both eyes and near (Bell) retinoscopy found "with" motion reflexes (no accommodative response) at near ranges. When the hyperopia correction was introduced, intermittent "against" motion reflexes were monitored when he fixated at a 10-inch range. With these lenses, fixation increased to eight to nine seconds and brief tracking movements were made.

Lenses were prescribed for the purpose of investigating their effects on the child's performance. They were to be worn for one or two-hour periods. Several activities were developed for the child to be carried out by the mother. These activities included tracking an object that was placed in his hand while his mother moved his hand passively at first and then attempted to stimulate his active movement. Also, activities were developed to encourage reach and touch. A functional means of testing acuity was developed by the optometrist and carried out daily by the parent.

After three months the parent returned with the child and reported that behavioral changes had been noted in the child's posture and in his awareness. His mother stated that after the first week she noticed that he did not slump in his chair when wearing the lenses for the recommended periods of time. The follow-up evaluation revealed that his fixation period with the glasses had improved to up to 30 seconds, and that he was able to track horizontally and in a circle. Near (Bell) retinoscopy found the "against" motion reflex was sustained during fixation at 10 inches. His reach and object localization improved considerably at an eight-inch range, and he also seemed to fixate on objects around the room. Also, behavioral observations of visual fixation and attention at home enabled the optometrist to equate these factors to acuity of approximately 20/100 (OU).

For this young boy, success was not based solely on the quantitative measurements of retinoscopy, but was measured on a qualitative assessment of the child's performance over a period of time. It is difficult for many practitioners to provide qualitative assessments of vision since educational programs for optometric training emphasize quantitative testing. For many visually-impaired children, however, quantitative measurements offer little advantage. In this case, the behavioral changes from the prescriptive lenses represented progress that the parent had not previously seen. This progress, although it may have been slight in comparison to another child, represented major advancements in his use of vision.

The practitioner should approach the evaluation of low functioning and multiply handicapped children such as this young boy in an investigative, observational manner that attempts to analyze how the child uses his vision. A complete analysis of the use of vision, whether there are peripheral or central scotomas, what the visual acuity is, etc., often cannot be completed during the first visit and actually may take months or even years of repeated assessment for the low functioning child. It is often beneficial to design functional testing activities for acuity and visual field to be performed daily at home by the parent so that so that behavioral responses can be averaged and compared with the child's next visit to the practitioner's office.

The Parent

The effectiveness of early intervention is heavily dependent on the involvement of the family.[2] The home environment is also a valuable component in forming a comprehensive view of the needs of the visually-impaired child. The parents' role in this aspect of the low vision evaluation is important. How a parent views his child's impairment, and what he understands about it, reflects his attitude and gives insight as to how the family is coping with it at home.

The parent must have a good understanding of the purpose of the low vision evaluation. Many parents will experience this concept for the first time. The clinician may meet with some skepticism, or an unrealistic expectation, for example, that the child will "regain" sight. It should not be taken for granted that the parent has a good understanding of the pathology of his child's visual impairment. However, in some cases the parents may have a comprehensive understanding of their child's problem and a positive attitude about it, yet for years they have been told nothing more can be done. Thus they have been asked to understand and accept the child's "blindness," de-emphasizing residual vision and any hope for rehabilitation.

Parents cannot be expected to have an objective view of their child's visual impairment. Some are able to perceive a relationship between the impairment and the child's abilities and limitations. Others, perhaps being overprotective, tend to misperceive the relationship of the pathology to function, and thus project limitations upon the child based on their inaccurate knowledge of the impairment. Still others may underemphasize the impairment, pretending it does not exist, thus presenting a possible barrier to accepting the fact that rehabilitation is needed. In discussing parental views, one can recognize the effort that must be made to form a positive, cohesive relationship between clinician and parent, a task which takes time.

The practitioner must be aware that there are sometimes circumstances in parent/child relationships that will interfere with the low vision examination process. The parent may view his visually-impaired child as lacking in abilities or being very fragile, resulting in overprotectiveness. The child who has overly cautious parents may have had very limited opportunities to explore and experience his environment. This in turn may affect the child's development and self-image. The child may feel inadequate as a result of not being given the chance to succeed, or even fail, at a particular task. These emotions may negatively affect the outcome of the low vision examination. And despite the practitioner's efforts, the optical aid(s) alone may not be the solution to the problem.

The practitioner must be sensitive to situations where the parent may expect too much of the low vision examination. Failure to change behavior may be interpreted by the parent as failure of the examination.

The practitioner may be alerted to an overprotective parent during history taking. The parent and child should be asked about the child's self-help abilities, such as his personal hygiene skills, grooming and dressing skills, and assisting around the house (i.e., cleaning, cooking, and setting the table). The overprotective parent will usually respond that the child is unable to perform these tasks independently, when in fact the child has been given very little opportunity to develop these skills. The interview might also reveal a situation where the parent consistently answers for the child. This indicates that the parent is allowing the child little exposure to varied situations. The practitioner, in discussing parent/child relationships with an educator and/or social worker, may learn about these problems prior to the examination. The expertise of the educator and social worker and/or psychologist should then be incorporated as part of the low vision service to deal with these problems effectively.

Another area of the parent/child relationship that might interfere with the low vision rehabilitation process is denial by the parent that the impairment exists. Consider the following example: a child had cataracts removed at age three following which he received prescriptive lenses as well as other optical aids from a low vision specialist. Hearing aids were prescribed by an audiologist to treat the child's hearing loss. Significant improvement in the child's ability to use his vision and hearing was noted. However, his mother could not accept the appearance of both the aphakic prescription and hearing aids. She consistently removed the glasses and hearing aids significantly increasing the handicapping degree of the child's sensory losses. A combined effort by the educator and social worker, in conjunction with a consultation with the low vision specialist, convinced the parent of the importance of the aids. This situation again emphasizes the need for a multi-disciplinary approach in meeting the needs of many children. Without the team effort and a holistic view of the child, such a misunderstanding on the part of the parent could have gravely affected this child's function and performance.

In dealing with both the overprotective parent and the parent who fails to accept the child's impairment, the optometrist must remain consistent in his counseling about the impairment and low vision recommendations. The explanations should be brief and to the point. Medical and optical terminology should be defined in language that the parents can understand. Too often, the information provided will be in excess of what the parent can comprehend at the time of the examination, resulting in confusion. Also, a parent may leave the examination understanding the optometrist's explanation but experiencing feelings of personal guilt. This guilt may be projected as disappointment about the results of the examination.

The low vision specialist should be aware of these possibilities and be ready to deal with them. A telephone call to the parent a week or so after the examination may uncover some of these problems. A follow-up explanation may be effective in eliminating any misunderstanding, or in the case of defensive projections, counseling for the parent and/or the child might be recommended.

Considering the Classroom and Home Environment

Before prescribing optical aids and devices for the school-age child, the practitioner needs to know how the child functions in the classroom and at home. The educator may be willing to offer this information in a brief report. There are standard functional low vision assessment instruments available. However, a more informal approach may suffice by simply discussing with the educator the type of information that is needed. For example, the optometrist will benefit from information about where the child is seated in the classroom, where the windows are located, whether glare from the windows presents any particular problems, and what the lighting is like in the classroom. Optical aids may be totally ineffective if glare or inadequate lighting interferes with the child's ability to use them.

Information concerning how the child uses his vision in the habitual environment may enable the optometrist to be more precise in the examination. For example, does the child turn his head to one side when viewing at near or at distance, squint when looking at a distance, cover one eye when reading, point to the material being read, or lose his place frequently while reading. Head turns or covering one eye may be an indication of difficulty with binocular alignment, while squinting may indicate an uncorrected refractive error. Loss of place while reading may indicate functional difficulties of fixations, pursuits and/or saccades.

Information about the child's coordination, balance and spatial organization will enable the optometrist to understand how the child uses peripheral vision to match information with motor movement and orientation. Knowing that the child consistently bumps into objects on one side or trips over objects will give the optometrist reason to consider a possible field loss prior to the examination. Regarding personal hygiene and appearance, the child who fails to comb his hair may not be able to see himself in the mirror. This need would then be considered in the low vision examination.

The most important consideration is why this child is being referred for a low vision examination. The educator should discuss what specific aspects of performance need to be improved. Obtaining the answer to this question and other information mentioned above, may save a considerable amount of time during the examination.

Reporting to the Educator

The concept of a low vision service is only as good as the communication between the professionals involved. The best low vision examination can be diminished in quality if the educator and/or parents do not understand the implications of the examination or how the child is to use the aids.

One educator thought that the cap that snapped onto the front of her student's handheld telescope was a dust cover. Two years after the examination, she learned that it was a reading cap. When the child used the telescope with the cap, both teacher and pupil were surprised to find that reading could be performed at an intermediate range. While both were elated to think that the device could be used to view intermediate ranges, it was unfortunate that two years had elapsed without the child benefitting from the prescribed cap.

The low vision specialist must provide basic information concerning the diagnosis and etiology in language that is easily understood. Acuity measurements for both distance and near ranges should be stated along with the testing distance. It may be beneficial to include both uncorrected and best corrected measurements. Visual field measurements for distance, if obtained, and for near should be stated along with an explanation of how they may affect the child's performance. Refractive findings should be included with a brief discussion, if appropriate, about the type of prescription given and whether contact lenses were prescribed or considered.

A discussion of the child's binocular state and how the visual condition may or may not contribute to fatigue levels, loss of attention and reading difficulty may be helpful to the educator.

When aids are prescribed, the improved acuity measurements and an explanation of how they are to be used should be provided along with the visual aid(s).[4] The optometrist should mention any difficulties the child had in using the aid(s) and should suggest, if appropriate, how the educator may effectively assist in training the child. Print size should be discussed. A range of print sizes, rather than just one, should be suggested. The educator may find that the child will work more effectively with certain types of print, depending on the child's fatigue level, lighting provided, quality of print, or subject covered. Magnifying devices are often as cost efficient, less cumbersome and offer access to print that would otherwise have to be enlarged.[5] A final statement should include a recommendation for a follow-up visit.

By communicating with the educator, the low vision specialist can help to insure that the recommendations from the examination will be followed. Also, if a problem develops, such as a misunderstanding about the use of the aids, the report can answer many questions.

Educational Programs for the Visually-Impaired Child

The setting for the education of the visually impaired may vary.[2] This largely depends on the program set up by the state or town and can be influenced by the population of visually-impaired children for whom a city or town must provide services. One means by which a visually-handicapped child receives special education is by attending a school for the blind. Such a school has a staff of specially trained teachers and orientation and mobility instruction for the visually impaired. Schools for the blind are usually residential, with the children going home on weekends. In some instances, children are transported to such schools on a daily basis.

The resource room is another place where the special needs of the visually-impaired child are met. The resource room is usually housed within a regular public school, and a teacher for the visually-impaired is employed to provide special services. The visually-impaired children are transported from throughout the town or district on a daily basis. The objective of the resource room is to place children into everyday classroom settings with non-visually-impaired children. The amount of time the visually-impaired child is in the regular classroom is dependent upon the amount of individualized support service the child needs from the resource teacher. In the resource room the child is instructed in specialized curricula areas and in the use of various adaptive devices.

A third means by which the visually-impaired child can receive special educational services is through the itinerant teacher program. Where such a program exists, the visually-impaired child attends his neighborhood school and the itinerant teacher is an integral part of the regular school day. The teacher for the visually impaired usually travels from school to school to serve the visually-impaired child in his classroom. The regular classroom teacher can expect to receive assistance from and consultations with the itinerant teacher who will also schedule direct tutorial services for the visually-impaired child.

Summary

The low vision specialist must recognize that the examination of a child should include an analysis of function and performance. Further, the needs of the child must be evaluated with an understanding of development and with a qualitative analysis of vision. The traditional quantitative means of vision assessment may be of limited effectiveness if used as the sole means for prescriptive determination.

Early intervention is the key to effectively dealing with the unique difficulties of each child and the negative effects of social pressures. Also, early intervention is the best means for affecting the overall development of the child. The recognition by the optometrist of the dynamic relationship of vision to function and development will enable the practitioner to apply traditional prescriptive techniques to low vision care to meet the developmental needs of the child. The success of the low vision examination should not be measured by the improvement in the child's acuity through use of the aids, but rather by the improvement in the child's performance in his habitual environments.

The challenge of providing low vision services for a child is one in which the low vision specialist must recognize that his effectiveness can be maximized by utilizing the skills of other professionals. Thus, the concept of a multi-disciplinary service can be developed only when all professionals communicate and work toward the common goal of meeting the needs of the child.

Chapter 18

SUMMARY

William V. Padula

The central theme of this book has been that vision is dynamic and influences all aspects of development, cognitive-perceptual function, movement, posture and balance. This idea has been discussed by others and is by no means considered to be this author's hallmark. The concept that vision comprises two separate visual processes, focal and ambient, is the model that has served as the foundation for neuro-optometric rehabilitation. However, it is the ambient process, especially, that deserves attention. In the human race, higher cognitive processes have developed from and reinforce the focal process. However, without the balance of the ambient process, the focal process will often distort or misrepresent space. It is the ambient process that creates stability in our lives and enables us to anticipate change related to movement, posture and balance as well as to experience time relationships, past, present and anticipation of future. The focal process is a linear and sequential process. The ambient process does not necessarily represent time and space in a linear manner. However, the bimodal system can facilitate and balance changes in temporal as well as spatial relationships because of the plasticity between these processes.

Through consideration of the visual bimodal spatial and temporal model, development of the child may also be more completely understood. In addition, disorders of posture, balance, movement, and vision impairment gain new direction when incorporating the concept of the ambient visual process. The Post Trauma Vision Syndrome and Visual Midline Shift Syndrome cannot be understood without knowledge of the ambient visual process, and without this knowledge, professionals may often misinterpret or discount the symptoms in people with neurological impairments.

It is the intention of the senior author for this book to serve as a means to stimulate new discussions and research concerning visual, physical, and cognitive-educational rehabilitation. It is also meant to challenge us not to become complacent with those theories and/or practices that have been developed as a result of previous models. He would like leave the reader with the following thought:

> *"The ambient process provides the foundation for the establishment of the linear and temporal relationships of the physical world, while embracing the emptiness that enables and encourages the focal awareness to seek its own reality. Just as opposing mirrors reflect their own vacuity, our vision is a mirror reflecting both the preconscious and conscious awareness of perceived energy upon its own emptiness." WVP*

AN ADDENDUM ON PRISMS

The optometrist has the ability to affect vision and visual motor behaviors through the use of lenses and prisms. This book has attempted to provide the reader with enough background in the development of motor and sensory systems, emphasizing vision, so that consideration for possible prism use can be identified. While only optometrists or ophthalmologists can prescribe lenses and prisms, a basic knowledge of how they work, when they are used, and what they can achieve is important for all who work with patients who may benefit from them. Thus appropriate referrals can be made and inappropriate therapies avoided. While information on prisms has been described when indicated throughout the text, a review and summary regarding prisms is provided below.

Optometrists speak of prisms as transparent optical lenses that cause light rays to be refracted in some manner. While prisms can be ground into lenses for therapeutic or continuous wear, prisms used during evaluations or therapy are shaped like a wedge with a wide and flat *base* end, converging towards a narrow top or *apex* end. The degree to which light or an image is shifted is measured in prism diopters. Since the image is always shifted away from the base end, the direction in which the image is shifted is described in terms of the base. Thus, for example, base up lenses shift the image downwards, and base left lenses shift the image to the right. (For a discussion of how a prism affects the focal and ambient processes see Chapter 7.)

When two prisms are used in the same orientation (e.g., right eye base-in and left eye base-out) they are referred to as *yoked prisms*, and they affect three dimensional space. The base-end of the prisms will compress space in the lateral direction and expand space in the anterior/posterior direction, while the apex end will expand space in the lateral direction and compress space in the anterior/posterior direction.

The therapeutic use of yoked prisms has also been discussed in Chapters 5 and 7. In chapter 7 their use was described in terms of the direction of prism orientation used to counter visual midline shift. Thus you will recall, for example, that if a person has a left hemiplegia his visual midline and weight bearing will most often be shifted to the right. In this case the orientation for use of yoked prism lenses is bases left to realign the person's concept of the egocenter or visual midline in relation to the physical body. (See Chapter 7.) However, we see many patients who do not have a specific diagnosis such as VMSS yet who may have eye alignment problems, atypical motor patterns, or postural changes, where consideration should be given to the use of prisms to try to improve function.

When considering prisms it is especially important for the optometrist or therapist to be a good observer. While all clinicians should observe gait, posture, body alignment and balance as the patient walks to the examining room, further observation of the patient walking back and forth across a room or down a hall and returning is strongly encouraged. It may be necessary to repeat this several times in order to start to understand the visual-motor and/or visual-postural relationships, gait, etc. (See Chapter 3.) If possible, having a PT and/or OT on the rehabilitation team can be very beneficial.

During patient observation it is also helpful to try to think of the patient's orientation in various body sectors: What is the position of the head and shoulders; is the head flexed, extended, or tilted to one side; is one shoulder lower than the other? What is the position of the pelvis; is it higher on one side than the other? What is the position of the feet; are they turned in or out, do they appear evenly weighted or not? How does movement affect the observed sitting postures, head/neck alignment, and balance? Does the patient lean or veer to the right or left; does posture change when walking vs. sitting? Try to think of the potential use of prisms to modify the observed differences in posture, alignment, movement, gait, etc.

Is also helpful to think of how prisms affect the perception of space in another manner. Yoked prisms with bases right or bases left produce a similar compression and expansion of space for each eye. For lateral yoked prisms the base of the prism compresses the x axis (near-far axis) and expands the z axis (horizontal axis), and the apex expands the x axis and contracts the z axis. (See Chapter 7.) For example, often a person with a hemiparesis will elevate the shoulder and depress the pelvis on the non-affected side causing a lean and/or drift toward the non-affected side. The clinician should observe posture as a behavior related to the shift of the visual midline. Placing the yoked prisms with the base ends opposite the elevated shoulder will realign the visual midline and increase weight bearing on the affected side.

Summary:

Prisms can be a powerful way to effect change in the ambient system and its integration with other sensorimotor systems. While commonly observed reactions to prisms have been described in various chapters of this book, the practitioner should always be alert to the fact that due to variations in visual processing following a neurological event, reactions and behavioral changes related to the use of prisms can vary. In a manner similar to patients' varying responses to medication, some individuals with seemingly similar problems may react quite differently to prisms. This is especially true in cases of traumatic brain injury. It is also important to respect the patient's ability to accept change. While a significant change in posture may be observed with stronger prisms, not all patients will be able to accept the change. Therefore, a thorough understanding of prism use and careful assessment and observation of the patient are critical in order to achieve successful outcomes.

WVP

REFERENCES

Preface

1. Skeffington AM, Lesser SK, Barstow R. *Nearpoint Optometry*. Santa Ana, CA: Optometric Extension Program; 1947-48, 1948-49, 1949-50.
2. Gesell AL, Ilg FL, Bullis GE. *Vision: Its Development in Infant and Child.* (1949) Santa Ana, CA: Optometric Extension Program, 1998.

Chapter 1

1. Gesell AL, Ilg FL, Bullis GE. *Vision: Its Development in Infant and Child.* (1949) Santa Ana, CA: Optometric Extension Program, 1998.
2. Larsen WJ, Sherman LS, Potter SS, Scott WJ. *Human Embryology, 3rd ed.* Philadelphia, PA: Churchill Livingstone, Inc., 2001.
3. Dudek RW, Fix JD. *Embryology, 3rd ed.* Baltimore, MD: Lippincott, Williams and Wilkins, 2005.
4. Skinner BF. *The Behavior of Organisms: An Experimental Analysis.* New York, NY: Appleton-Century-Crofts, 1938.
5. Hull CL. *Principles of Behavior: An Introduction to Behavior Theory.* New York, NY: Appleton-Century, 1943.
6. Liebowitz HW, Post RB. Two modes of processing concept and some implications. In: Beck JJ, ed. *Organization and Representation in Perception*. London, England: Erlbaum, 1982.
7. Trevarthen CB. Two mechanisms of vision in primates. *Psychol Res* 1968;31:299-337.
8. Bishop A. Use of the hand in lower primates. In: Buettner-Janusch J, ed. *Evolutionary and Genetic Biology of Primates.* New York, NY: Academic Press;1964:357-385.
9. Hubel DH. *Eye, Brain and Vision*. Scientific American Library Series: New York, NY, 1988.
10. Wolff E. *Anatomy of the Eye and Orbit, 6th ed.* Philadelphia, PA: WB Saunders, 1968.
11. Nelson C, Senesac C. Management of clinical problems of children with cerebral palsy. In: Umphred DA, ed. *Neurological Rehabilitation, 5th ed.* St Louis, MO: Mosby, 2007:357-85.
12. Nashold B, Seaber J. Defects of ocular motility after stereotactic midbrain lesions in man. *Arch Ophthalmol* 1972;88:245-48.
13. Lettvin JY, Maturana HR, McCulloch WS, Pitts WH. What the Frog's Eye Tells the Frog's Brain. *Proceedings of the IRF*. 1959;47:1940-1951.
14. Gesell AL. *Infant Development: The Embryology of Early Human Behavior.* Westport, CT: Greenwood Press, 1972.
15. Padula WV. *Neuro-Optometric Rehabilitation*. Santa Ana, CA: Optometric Extension Program Foundation, 2000.
16. Padula WV, Wu L, Vicci VR Jr, et al. Evaluating and Treating Visual Dysfunction. In: Zasler N, Katz DI, Zafonte RD, eds. *Brain Injury Medicine*. New York, NY: Demos Medical Publishing, 2006.
17. Schneider GE. Contrasting visuo-motor functions of tectum and cortex in the golden hamster. *Psychol Forsch* 1967;31:52-62.
18. Streff, J. Visual rehabilitation of hemianopic head trauma patients emphasizing ambient pathways. *Neuro Rehab*1996;6:173-181.
19. Posner MI, Raichle ME. *Images of Mind.* New York: Scientific American Library, 1994.
20. Eubank TF, Ooi TL. Improving visually guided action and perception through use of prisms. *Optometry* 2001;72:217-27.
21. Cartwright R, Seth R. Neuronal overstimulation: The pathogenesis of brain insult. *Brain Injury Source* 2000;4:32-35,42.
22. Held R, Hein A. Movement-produced stimulation in the development of visually guided behavior. *J Comp Physiol Psychol* 1963;56:872-76.

23. Held R. Plasticity in sensory-motor systems. *Sci Am* 1965;5:84-95.
24. Liebowitz HW. The relation between the rate threshold for the perception of movement and luminance for various durations and exposure. *J Exp Psychol* 1955;49:209-14.
25. Michon JA. A model of some temporal relations in human behavior. *Psychol Forsch* 1968;31(4):287-98.
26. Ludlum W. Paralytic strabismus. In: Borish IM, ed. *Clinical Refraction, 3rd ed.* Chicago, IL: The Professional Press,1970:1253–83.
27. Shankman AL. *Vision Enhancement Training*. Santa Ana, CA: Optometric Extension Program,1988.

Chapter 2

1. Combs AW, ed. *Perceiving, Behaving, Becoming: A New Focus for Education.* Washington, DC: Assoc. for Supervisors, Curriculum & Development, 1962, reprinted 1971.
2. Flach F. *Rickie.* New York, NY: Fawcett Columbine, 1990.
3. Kavner RS, Dusky L. *Total Vision.* New York, NY: A & W Publishers, 1978.
4. Gilman G. *Behavioral Optometry.* Quincy, CA: Paradox Publishing, 1988.
5. Schwartz JM, Begley S. *The Mind and the Brain: Neuroplasticity and the Power of Mental Force.* New York, NY: Harper Collins Publishers, Inc, 2003.
6. Forrest E. *Stress and Vision.* Santa Ana, CA: Optometric Extension Program Foundation, 1988.
7. Padula WV. *A Behavioral Vision Approach for Persons with Physical Disabilities.* Santa Ana, CA: Optometric Extension Program Foundation, 1988.

Chapter 3

1. Moore JC. *The Neuroanatomy of the Visual System [DVD]*. Las Cruces, NM: Clinician's View; 2001.
2. Shumway-Cook A, Woollacott MH. *Motor Control Theory and Practical Applications*. Baltimore, MD: Williams & Wilkins, 1995.
3. Moore JC. Personal correspondence. 2006.
4. Sparling JW, ed. *Concepts in Fetal Movement Research*. NY: Haworth Press, 1993.
5. Young M. A review on postural realignment and its muscular and neural components. *Exp Brain Res* 2004;159:33-46.
6. Magrun WM. *Evaluating Movement and Posture Disorganization*, 2nd Ed. Las Cruces, NM: Clinician's View, 1996.
7. Adler L. *Improving Function in Children Using NDT, SI, and Motor Learning Frameworks [DVD]*. Las Cruces, NM: Clinician's View, 2005.
8. Adler L. *Beyond Weight Bearing [DVD]*. Las Cruces, NM: Clinician's View, 2009.
9. Young M. A review on postural realignment and its muscular and neural components. *Exp Brain Res* 2004;159:33-46.
10. Kephart NC. *The Slow Learner in the Classroom*. Columbus, OH: Charles E. Merrill Books, 1960.
11. Padula WV. Personal correspondence. 2006.
12. Moore JC, Nelson CA. *Structural and Function Aspects of Intervention for Children with Neuromotor and Sensory Motor Disorders [DVD].* Las Cruces, NM: Clinician's View, 1998.
13. Schmidt RA, Lee TD. *Motor Control and Learning: A Behavioral Emphasis*. 4th ed. Champaign, IL: Human Kinetics, 2004.
14. Gdowski GT, McCrea RA. Neck proprioception inputs to primate vestibular nucleus neurons. *Exp Brain Res* 2000;135:511-26.
15. Falla D, Rainoldi A, Merletti R, Jull G. Spatio-temporal evaluation of neck muscle activation during postural perturbations in healthy subjects. *J Neurophysiol* 2004;92:2368-79.
16. Kogler A, Lindfors J, Odkvist LM, Ledin T. Postural stability using different neck positions in normal subjects and patients with neck trauma. *J Assoc Res Otolaryngol* 2004;5:25-31.
17. Brandt T, Krafczyk S, Malsbenden I. Postural imbalance with head extension: improvement by training as a model for ataxia therapy. *J Neurophysiol* 1995;74:2216-19.
18. Schieppati M, Nardone A, Schmid M. Neck muscle fatigue affects postural control in man. *Neurosci* 2003;121:277-85.
19. Blouin J, Vercher JL, Gauthier GM, Paillard J, et al. Perception of passive whole-body rotations in the absence of neck and body proprioception. *J Neurophysiol* 1995;74:2216-19.

20. Cohen LA. Role of the eye and neck proprioceptive mechanisms in body orientation and motor coordination. *J Neurophysiol* 1961;24:1-11.
21. Moore JC. *The Neuroanatomy of Learning Disabilities [DVD]*. Las Cruces, NM: Clinician's View, 2002.
22. Moore JC. *Perinatal Pathology [DVD]*. Las Cruces, NM: Clinician's View, 2003.
23. Crutchfield CA, Barnes MR. *Motor Control and Motor Learning in Rehabilitation*. Atlanta, GA: Stokesville Publishing, 1993.
24. Young MA. Review on postural realignment and its muscular and neural components. *Exp Brain Res* 2004;59:33-46.
25. Horak FB, Hlavacka F. Somatosensory loss increases vestibulospinal sensitivity. *J Neurophysiol* 2001;86:575-85.
26. Mittelstaedt H. Somatic graviception. *J Vest Res* 1996;6:355-66.
27. Mittelstaedt H. Origin and processing of postural information. *Neurosci Biobehav Rev* 1998;22:473–78.
28. Mittelstaedt H. Evidence of somatic graviception from new and classical investigations. *Percept Psychophy* 1999;61:615-24.
29. Kelso JAS. *Dynamic Patterns: The Self-Organization of the Brain and Behavior*. Cambridge, MA: MIT Press, 1995.
30. Diamond M, Hopson J. *Magic Trees of the Mind.* New York, NY: Penguin Books, 1998.
31. Anand V, Buckley J, Scally A, Elliott DB. The effect of refractive blur on postural stability. *Neurosci Res* 2003;45:409-17.
32. Keshner EA, Kenyon RV, Dhaher Y, Streepey JW. Employing a virtual environment in postural research and rehabilitation to reveal the impact of visual information. *J Neurophysiol* 2002;88:2232-41.
33. Rossingnol S. Visuomotor regulation of locomotion. *Can J Physiol Pharmacol* 1996;74:418-25.
34. Nougier V, Bard C, Fleury M, Teasdale N. Contributions of central and peripheral vision to the regulation of stance: Developmental aspects. *Neurosci Let* 1999:260:109-12.
35. Buchanan J J, Horak FB. Emergence of postural patterns as a function of vision and translation frequency. *Exp Brain Res* 1987;69:77-92.
36. Cullen KE, Roy JE. Signal processing in the vestibular system during active versus passive head movements. *J Neurophysiol* 2004;91:1919-33.
37. Magrun WM. *Neural Systems Integration: Improving Performance in Children with Learning Disabilities.* Las Cruces, NM: Clinician's View, 2006.
38. Jaekl PM, Jenkin MR, Harris LR. Perceptual stability during active head movements orthogonal and parallel to gravity. *J Vestibular Res* 2003;13:265-71.
39. Bles W, Kapteyn TS, Brandt T, Arnold F. The mechanism of physiological height vertigo. II, Posturography. *Acta Otolaryngol* 1980;89:534-40.
40. Roy JE, Cullen K. Dissociating Self-generated from passively applied head motion: neural mechanisms in the vestibular nuclei. *J Vestibular Res* 2003;13:245-53.
41. Allum JH, Honegger F. Interactions between vestibular and proprioceptive inputs triggering and modulating human balance-correcting responses differ across muscles. *J Vestibular Res* 2004;14:307-19.
42. Peterka RJ. Sensorimotor integration in human postural control. *J Neurophysiol* 2002;88:1097-118.

Chapter 4

1. Odom JV, Bach M, Barber C, Brigell M, et al. Visual evoked potential standard. *Documenta Ophthalmologica* 2004;108:115-23.
2. Padula WV, Argyris S, Ray J. Visual evoked potentials: evaluating treatment for post trauma vision syndrome in patients with traumatic brain injuries. *J Brain Injury* 1994;8:125-33.

Chapter 5

1. Gianutsos R, Glosser D, Elbaum J, Vroman G. Visual interception in brain-injured adults: multifaceted measures. *Arch Phys Med Rehab* 1983;64:456-61.
2. Hart C. Disturbances of fusion following head injury. Proc R Soc Med 1969;62:704-6.
3. Rook JL, Rosenquist SD, Helffenstein DA, Sol N. *Whiplash Injuries: Diagnosis and Management.* Boston, MA: Butterworth/Heinemann, 2003.

4. Gianutsos R, Ramsey G. Enabling rehabilitation optometrists to help survivors of acquired brain injury. *J Vis Rehab* 1988;2:37-58.
5. Soden R, Cohen A. An optometric approach to the treatment of noncomitant deviation. *J Am Optom Assoc* 1983;54:451-54.
6. Benabib RM, Nelson CA. Efficiency in visual skills and postural control: Dynamic interaction. *Occup Ther Prac* 1991;3:57-68.
7. Carroll R. Acute loss of fusional convergence following head trauma. *Arch Ophthalmol* 1984;88:57-59.
8. Stanworth A. Defects of ocular movement and fusion after head injury. *Br J Ophthalmol* 1974;58:266-71.
9. Weed H. Divergence paralysis due to head injury. *Trans Am Acad Ophthalmol* 1934;39:189-197.
10. Neger RE. The evaluation of diplopia in head trauma. *J Head Trauma Rehab* 1989;4:27-34.
11. Padula WV, Argyris S, Ray J. Visual evoked potentials: evaluating treatment for post trauma vision syndrome in patients with traumatic brain injuries. *J Brain Injury* 1994;8:125-33.
12. Odom JV, Bach M, Barber C, Brigell M, et al. Visual evoked potential standard. *Documenta Ophthalmologica* 2004;108:115-23.
13. Sarno S, Erasmus LP, Lippert G, Frey M, Lipp B, Schlaegel W. Electrophysiological correlates of visual impairments after traumatic brain injury. *Vis Res* 2000;40:3029-38.
14. Streff J. The use of binasal occluded treatment for patients with head Trauma. *Neuro-Optometric Rehab Assoc Newsletter* 1992;2.

Chapter 6

1. Bobath K. The neuropathology of cerebral palsy and its importance in treatment and diagnosis. *Cerebral Palsy Bull* 1959;1:13-33.
2. Bobath K, Bobath B. The facilitation of normal postural reactions and movements in the treatment of cerebral palsy. *Physiother* 1964;50:264-67.

Chapter 7

1. Streff JW. *Vision Symposium*. Gesell Institute of Child Development. June 1976.

Chapter 8

1. Apell R, Lowry RW. Behavior characteristics of nursery school children. *Optom Wkly* 1959; Dec. 1.
2. Ragnar G. *Charles Scott Sherrington: An Appraisal*. Garden City, NY: Doubleday; 1967.
3. Gesell AL, Ilg FL, Bullis GE. *Vision: Its Development in Infant and Child.* (1949) Santa Ana, CA: Optometric Extension Program Foundation, 1998.
4. Trevarthen C, Sperry RW. Perceptual unity of the ambient visual field in human commissurotomy patients. *Brain* 1973;96:547–70.

Chapter 9

1. Gesell AL, Amatruda CS. *Developmental Diagnosis: Normal and Abnormal Child Development, Clinical Methods, and Pediatric Applications*. New York: PB Hoeber, 1947.
2. Gesell AL, Ilg FL, Bullis GE. *Vision: Its Development in Infant and Child.* (1949) Santa Ana, CA: Optometric Extension Program Foundation, 1998.
3. Fraiberg S, Siegel B, Gibson R. The role of sound in the search behavior of a blind infant. *Psychoanalytic Study of the Child.*1966;21:327-57.
4. Barraga NC. *Increased Visual Behavior in Low Vision Children*. New York, NY: American Foundation for the Blind, 1964.
5. Barraga NC. Learning efficiency in low vision. *J Am Optom Assoc* 1969;40:807-10.
6. Smith AJ, Cote KS. *Look at Me*. Philadelphia, PA: Pennsylvania College of Optometry Press; 1984.
7. Freeman PB, Jose RT. *Art and Practice of Low Vision*. Boston, MA: Butterworth-Heinemann; 1991.
8. Zasler N, Katz DI, Zafonte RD, Eds. *Brain Injury Medicine*. New York, NY: Demos Medical Publishing; 2006.
9. Cowan C, Shepler R. Techniques for teaching young children to use low vision devices. *J Vis Impair Blind* 1990;84:419-21.

10. Corn AL, Koenig AJ. *Foundations of Low Vision.* New York, NY: American Foundation for the Blind, 1996.
11. Barraga N, Erin J. *Visual Impairments and Learning, 4th ed.* Austin, TX: Pro-Ed Inc; 2001.

Chapter 10

1. Borish IM. *Clinical Refraction.* 3rd ed. Chicago, IL: The Professional Press, Inc.:1970.

Chapter 11

1. Bach-y-Rita P. *Recovery of Function: Theoretical Considerations for Brain Injury.* Bern, Switzerland: Hans Heiber Publishers; 1980.

Chapter 12

1. Leekham SR, Nieto C, Libby SJ, Wing L, et al. Describing the sensory abnormalities of children and adults with autism. *J Autism Dev Disord* 2007;37:894-910.
2. Davis RAO, Bockbrader MA, Murphy RR, Hetrick WP, et al. Subjective perceptual distortions and visual dysfunction in children with autism. *J Autism Dev Disord* 2006;36:199-210.
3. Kana RK, Keller TA, Cherkassky VL, Minshew NJ, et al. Sentence comprehension in autism: thinking in pictures with decreased functional connectivity. *Brain.* 2006;129:2484-93.
4. Grandin T. *Thinking in Pictures.* New York, NY: Vintage Books – Division of Random House; 1996.
5. Mottron L, Mineau S, Martel G, Bernier CS, et al. Lateral glances toward moving stimuli among young children with autism: Early regulation of locally oriented perception? *Dev Psychopathol.* 2007;19:23-36.
6. Ozonoff S, Macari S, Young GS, Goldring S, Thompson M, Rogers SJ. Atypical object exploration at 12 months of age is associated with autism in a prospective sample. *Autism* 2008;12:457-72.
7. Denis D, Burillon C, Livet MO, Burguiere O. Ophthalmologic signs in children with autism. *J Fr Ophtalmol* 1997;20:103-10.
8. Scharre JE, Creedon MP. Assessment of visual function in autistic children. *Optom Vis Sci* 1992;69:433-39.
9. Streff JW. Optometric care for a child manifesting qualities of autism. *J Am Optom Assoc* 1975;46:592-97.
10. Milne E, Griffiths H, Buckley D, Scope A. Vision in children and adolescents with autistic spectrum disorder: evidence for reduced convergence. *J Autism Dev Disord* 2009;39:965-75 doi:10.1007/s10803-009-0705-8.
11. Dakin S, Frith U. Vagaries of Visual Perception in Autism. *Neuron* 2005;48:497-507. doi: 10.16/j.neuron.2005.10,018.
12. Trachtman JN. Background and history of autism in relation to vision care. *Optometry* 2008;79:560-61.
13. Mottron L, Mineau S, Dawson M, Soulieres I, et al. Enhanced perceptual functioning in autism: an update and eight principles of autistic perception. *J Autism Dev Disord* 2006;36:27-443.
14. Bertone A, Mottron L, Jelenic P, Faubert J. Enhanced and diminished visuo-spatial information processing in autism depends on stimulus complexity. *Brain* 2005;128:2430-41.
15. Brenner LA, Turner KC, Muller, RA Eye movement and visual search: are there elementary abnormalities in autism. *J Autism Dev Disord* 2007;37:1289-309.
16. Ashwin E, Ashwin C, Rhydderch D, Howells J, et al. Eagle-eyed visual acuity: an experimental investigation of enhanced perception in autism. *Biol Psychiatry* 2008;65:17-21. doi: 10.1016/j.biopsych.2008.06.012.
17. Kemner C, vanEwijk L, Van Engeland H, Hooge I. Brief report: Eye movements during visual search tasks indicate enhanced stimulus discriminability in subjects with PDD. *J Autism Dev Disord* 2008;38:553-57.
18. Vandenbroucke MWG, Scholte HS, vanEngeland H, Lamme VAF, et al. A neural substrate for atypical low-level visual processing in autism spectrum disorder. *Brain* 2008; 131:1013-24.
19. Udden LQ, Davies MS, Scott AA, Zaidel E, et al. Neural basis of self and other representation in autism: an fMRI study of self-face recognition. *PLoS ONE* 2008;3:1-9. doi:10.1371/journal.pone.0003526.
20. Jemel B, Mottron L, Dawson M. Impaired face processing in autism: fact or artifact. *J Autism Dev Disord* 2006;36:91-106.
21. Behrmann M, Thomas C, Humphreys K. Seeing it differently: visual processing in autism. *Trends Cogn Sci* 2006;10:258-64.
22. Klin A, Jones W, Schultz R, Volkmar FR,et al. Defining and quantifying the social phenotype in autism. *Am J Psychiatry* 2002;159:895-908.

23. Dalton M, Nacewicz BM, Johnstone T, Schaefer HS et al. Gaze fixation and the neural circuitry of face processing in autism. *Nature Neurosci* 2005;8:519-26.
24. Deruelle C, Rondan C, Gepner B, Tardif C. Spatial frequency and face processing in children with autism and Asperger syndrome. J Autism Dev Disord 2004;34:199-210.
25. Sugiura M, Watanabe J, Maeda Y, Matsue Y, et al. Cortical Mechanisms of visual self-recognition. *NeuroImage* 2005;24:143-49.
26. Just MA, Cherkassky VL, Keller TA, Minshew NJ. Cortical activation and synchronization during sentence comprehension in high-functioning autism: evidence of underconnectivity. *Brain* 2004;127:1811-921.
27. Hughes JR. Autism: the first firm finding = underconnectivity. *Epilepsy Behav* 2007;11:20-24. doi:10.1016/j.yebeh.2007.03.010.
28. Huebner RA. *Autism: A Sensorimotor Approach to Management.* Gaithersburg, MD: Aspen Publishers; 2001.
29. Padula WV, Argyris S, Ray J. Visual evoked potentials: evaluating treatment for post-traumatic vision syndrome. *J Brain Injury* 1984;8:125-33.
30. Trevarthen CB. Two mechanisms of vision in primates. *Psychogische Forschung* 1968;31:229-337.
31. Kaplan M. Visual management: A physiological approach to rehabilitating autism spectrum disorders. *Autism Research Institute* 2006;2:1-2.
32. Hirstein W, Iversen P, Ramachandran VS. Autonomic responses of autistic children to people and objects. *Proc R Soc Lond* 2001;268:1883-88.
33. Kaplan M, Edelson SM, Seip JL. Behavioral changes in autistic individuals as a result of wearing ambient transitional prism lenses. *Child Psychiatry Hum Dev* 1998;29:65-75.
34. Gallop S. A variation on the use of binasal occlusion. *J Behav Optom* 1998;9:31-35.
35. Allison CL, Gabriel H, Schlange D, Fredrickson S. An optometric approach to patients with sensory integration dysfunction. *Optometry* 2007:78;644-51.
36. Rapin I, Tuchman RF. What is new in autism? *Curr Opin Neurol* 2008;21:143-49.
37. Minshew JN, Williams DL. The new neurobiology of autism: cortex, connectivity and neuronal organization. *Arch Neurol* 2007:64;945-50.
38. Iarocci G, McDonald J. Sensory integration and the perceptual experience of persons with autism. *J Autism Dev Disord* 2006:6:77-90.

Chapter 13

1. Gesell AL, Ilg FL, Bullis GE. *Vision: Its Development in Infant and Child.* (1949) Santa Ana, CA: Optometric Extension Program, 1998.
2. Kanner L. Autistic disturbances of affective contact. *Nerv Child* 1943;2:217-50.
3. Delacato CH. *The Ultimate Stranger.* The Autistic Child. Novato, CA: Arena Press; 1974.
4. Chiao CC, Osorio D, Vorobyev M, Cronin TW. Characterization of natural illuminants in forest and the use of digital video data to reconstruct illuminant spectra. *J Opt Soc Am A Opt Image Sci Vis* 2000;17:1712-21.
5. Parisi A, Buonomo AL. *Children Who Do Not Look You in the Eye: The Secrets of Autistic Behavior.* Naples, Italy: Scientifiche Italiane, 1999.

Chapter 14

1. Clark W, Ohlemiller K. *Anatomy and Physiology of Hearing for Audiologists.* Clifton Park, NY: Thomson Delmar Learning; 2006.
2. Moller A. *Hearing: Its Physiology and Pathophysiology.* San Diego, CA: Academic Press; 2000:15-24.
3. Pfeiffer RR. Classification of response patterns of spike discharges for units in the cochlear nucleus: Tone burst stimulation. *Exp Brain Res* 1966;1:220-35.
4. Helfert RH, Sneed CR, Altschuler RA. The ascending auditory pathways. In: Altschuler RA, Bobbin RP, Clopton BM, Hoffman DW, eds. *Neurobiology of Hearing: The Central Auditory System.* New York, NY: Raven Press, 1991:1-26.
5. Musiek FE, Baran JA. *The Auditory System: Anatomy, Physiology, and Clinical Correlates.* Boston, MA: Pearson; 2007.
6. Ehret G. The auditory midbrain, a "shunting-yard" of acoustic information processing. In: Ehret G, Romand R, eds. *The Central Auditory System.* New York, NY: Oxford University Press; 1997:259-316.
7. Waddington M. *Atlas of Human Intracranial Anatomy.* Rutland, VT: Academy Books, 1984.

8. Musiek FE, Baran JA. Neuroanatomy, neurophysiology and central auditory assessment. I. The brainstem. *Ear Hear* 1986;7:207-19.
9. Streitfeld BD. The fiber connections of the temporal lobe with emphasis on Rhesus monkey. *Int J Neurosci* 1980;11:51-71.
10. Russchen FT. Amygdalopetal projections in the cat. II. Subcortical afferent connections. A study with retrograde tracing techniques. *J Comp Neurol* 1982;207:157-76.
11. Rademacher J, Morosan P, Schormann T, Schleicher A, et al. Probabilistic mapping and volume measurement of human primary auditory cortex. *NeuroImage* 2001;13:669-83.
12. Geschwind N, Levitsky W. Human brain: Left-right asymmetries in temporal speech regions. *Sci* 1968;161:186-87.
13. DeArmond S, Fusco M, Dewey M. *Structure and Function of the Human Brain.* 3rd ed. New York, NY: Oxford University Press, 1989.
14. Mesulam MM, Mufson EJ. The insular of Reil in man and monkey architectonics, connectivity, and function. In: Jones EG, Peters A, eds. *Cerebral Cortex, vol 4.* New York, NY: Plenum Press;1985:179-226.
15. Augustine JR. The insular lobe in primates including humans. *Neurol Res* 1985;7:2-10.
16. Augustine JR. Circuitry and functional aspects of the insular lobe in primates including humans. *Brain Res Rev* 1996; 22:229-44.
17. Martin F, Clark J. *Introduction to Audiology.* Boston, MA: Allyn & Bacon, 2000.
18. Weaver M, Staller S. The acoustic nerve tumor. In: Northern JL, ed. *Hearing Disorders*, 2nd ed. Boston, MA: Little Brown and Company, 1984:171-79.
19. American Speech-Language-Hearing Association. Central auditory processing: Current status of research and implications for clinical practice. *Am J Audiol* 1996;5:41-54.
20. Chermak G, Musiek F. Central Auditory Processing Disorders: New Perspectives. San Diego,CA: Singular; 1997.
21. Odom J, Bach M, Barber C, Brigell M, et al. Visual evoked potentials standard. *Doc Opthalmol* 2004;108:115-23.
22. Brigell M, Bach M, Barber C, Kawasaki K, et al. Guidelines for calibration of stimulus and recording parameters used in clinical electrophysiology of vision. *Doc Opthalmol* 1998;95:1-14.
23. Musiek F, Bornstein S, Hall J, Schwaber M. Auditory brainstem response: Neurodiagnostic and intraoperative applications. In: J Katz, ed. *Handbook of Clinical Audiology,* 4th ed. Baltimore, MD: Williams and Wilkins; 1994:351-74.
24. Hall J. *New Handbook of Auditory Evoked Responses.* Boston, MA: Allyn and Bacon, 2007:27-29, 488-517, 544-47.
25. Quine D, Regan D, Murray T. Degraded discrimination between speech-like sounds by patients with Multiple Sclerosis and Friedreich's ataxia. *Brain* 1984;107:1113-22.
26. Padula WV, Argyris S, Ray J. Visual evoked potentials (VEP) evaluating treatment for post trauma vision syndrome (PTVS) in patients with traumatic brain injuries (TBI). *Brain Injury* 1994;8:125-33.
27. Regan D. *Human Brain Electrophysiology.* London, UK: Elsevier; 1989:8-30, 167-202, 507-61.
28. Kandel E. Nerve cells and behavior. In: Kandel E, Schwartz J, Jessell T, eds. *Principles of Neuroscience.* 4th ed. New York: McGraw-Hill, 2000:19-35.
29. Kilgard M, Pandya P, Vazquez J, Gehi A, et al. Sensory input directs spatial and temporal plasticity in primary auditory cortex. *J Neurophysiol* 2001;86:326-38.
30. Bavelier D, Neville H. Cross-modal plasticity: Where and how? *Nat Rev Neurosci* 2002;3: 443-52.
31. Bavelier D, Dye M, Hauser P. Do deaf individuals see better? *Trends Cogn Sci* 2006;10:512-18.
32. Sur M, Garraghty P, Roe A. Experimentally induced visual projections into auditory thalamus and cortex. *Sci* 1988;242:1437-41.
33. Campbell G, Frost D. Synaptic organization of anomalous retinal projections to the somatosensory and auditory thalamus: Target-controlled morphogenesis of axon terminals and synaptic glomeruli. *J Comp Neurol* 2988;272:383-408.
34. Ptito M, Giguere J, Boire D, Frost F, et al. When the auditory cortex turns visual. *Prog Brain Res* 2001:134;447-58.
35. Piche M, Chabot N, Bronchti G, Miceli D, et al. Auditory responses in the visual cortex of neonatally enucleated rats. *Neurosci* 2007;145:1144-56.
36. Rauschecker J. Substitution of visual by auditory inputs in the cat's anterior ectosylvian cortex. *Prog Brain Res* 1996;112:313-23.

37. Burton, H. Visual cortex activity in early and late blind people. *J Neurosci* 2003;23:4005-11.
38. Finney E, Fine I, Dobkins K. Visual stimuli activate auditory cortex in deaf. *Nat Neurosci* 2001;4:1171-73.
39. Pettito L, Zatorre R, Guana K, Nikelski E, et al Speech-like cerebral activity in profoundly deaf people processing signed languages: Implications for the neural basis of human language. *Proc Natl Acad Sci USA* 2000;97:13961-66.
40. Weeks R, Horwitz B, Aziz-Sultan A, Tian B, et al. A positron emission tomographic study of auditory localization in the congenitally blind. *J Neurosci.* 2000;20:2664-72.
41. Burton H, Snyder A, Diamond J, Raichle M. Adaptive changes in early and late blind: An fMRI study of verb generation to heard nouns. *J Neurophysiol* 2002;88:3359-71.
42. Roder B, Stock O, Bien S, Neville H, et al. Speech processing activates visual cortex in congenitally blind humans. *Eur J Neurosci* 2002;16:930-36.
43. Elbert T, Sterr A, Rockstroh B, Pantev C, et al. Expansion of the tonotopic area in the auditory cortex of the blind. *J Neurosci* 2002;22:9941-44.
44. Neville H, Lawson D. Attention to central and peripheral visual space in a movement detection task: An event related potential and behavioral study. II. Congenitally deaf adults. *Brain Res* 1987;405:268-83.
45. Lessard N, Pare M, Lepore F, Lassonde M. Early-blind human subjects localize sound sources better than sighted subjects. *Nature* 1998;395:278-80.
46. Rice C. Early blindness, early experience, and perceptual enhancement. *Am Found Blind Res Bull* 1970;22:1-22.
47. Stevens A, Weaver K. Functional characteristics of auditory cortex in the blind. *Behav Brain Res* 2009;196:134-38.
48. Knudsen EI Early auditory experience aligns the auditory map of space in the optic tectum of the barn owl. *Sci* 1983;222:939-42.
49. Watson AB. *Windows of Visibility*. NASA, 2009.
50. Bulkin DA, Groh JM. Seeing sounds: Visual and auditory interactions in the brain. *Curr Opin Neurobiol* 2006;16:415-19.
51. Bronkhorst AW, Plomp R. The effect of head-induced interaural time and level differences on speech intelligibility in noise. *J Acoust Soc Am* 1988;83:1508-16.
52. Neher T, Behrens T, Beck DL. Spatial hearing and understanding speech in complex environments. *Hearing Rev* 2006;15:22-25.
53. Knudsen EI, Knudsen PF. Vision calibrates sound localization in developing barn owls. *J Neurosci* 1989;9:3306-13.
54. Knudsen EI, Brainard MS. Creating a unified representation of visual and auditory space in the brain. *Annu Rev Neurosci* 1995;18:19-43.
55. King AJ. Sensory experience and the formation of a computational map of auditory space in the brain. *BioEssays*1999;21:900-11.
56. King AJ. Visual influences on auditory and spatial learning. *Phil Trans R Soc B* 2009;364:331-39.
57. Balslev D, Miall RC. Eye position representation in human anterior parietal cortex. *J Neurosci* 2008;28):8968-72.
58. Razavi B, O'Neill WE, Paige GD. Auditory spatial perception dynamically 58.realigns with changing eye position. *J Neurosci* 2007;27:10249-58. doi:10.1523/jneurosci.0938-07.2007.
59. Werner-Reiss U, Kelly K, Trause AS, Underhill AM, et al. Eye position affects activity in primary auditory cortex of primates. *Curr Biol* 2003;13:554-62.
60. Vliegen J, Van Grootel TJ, Van Opstal A. Dynamic sound localization during rapid eye– head gaze shifts. *J.Neurosci* 2004;24:9291-302. doi:10.1523/JNEUROSCI.2671-04.2004.
61. Welch RB, Warren DH. Immediate perceptual response to intersensory discrepancy. *Psychol Bull* 1980;88:638-67.
62. Recanzone, GH. Auditory Influences on visual rate perception. *J Neurophysiol* 2003;89:1078-93.
63. Alais D, Burr D. The ventriloquist effect results from near-optimal bimodal integration. *Curr Biol* 2004;14:267-62. doi:10.1016/j.cub.2004.01.029
64. Knudsen EI. Instructed learning in the auditory localization pathway of the barn owl. *Nature* 2002;417:322-28.
65. Zwiers MP, Opstal JV, Paige GD. Plasticity in human sound localization induced by compressed spatial vision. *Nature Neurosci* 2003;6:175-181. doi:10.1038/nn999.

66. Okada K, Hickok G. Two cortical mechanisms support the integration of visual and auditory speech: A hypothesis and preliminary data. *Neurosci Lett* 2009;452:219-23. doi:10.1016/jneulet.2009.01.060.
67. McGurk H, MacDonald J. Hearing lips and seeing voices. *Nature* 1976;264:746-48.
68. Schorr EA, Fox NA, vanWassenhove V, Knudsen EI. Auditory-visual fusion in speech perception in children with cochlear implants. *PNAS*.2005;102:18748-50. doi:/10.1073/pnas.0508862102.
69. Repp BH, Penel A. Auditory dominance in temporal processing: New evidence from synchronization with simultaneous visual and auditory sequences. *J Exp Psychol* 2002;28:1085-99.
70. Shimojo S, Shams L. Sensory modalities are not separate modalities: Plasticity and interactions. Curr Opin Neurobiol 2001;11:505-09.
71. Guttman SE, Gilroy LA, Blake R. Hearing what the eyes see. *Psychol Sci* 2005;16:228-35.
72. Shams L, Kamitani Y, Shimojo S. Visual illusion induced by sound. *Cogn Brain Res* 2002;14:147-52.
73. Watkins S, Shams L, Tanaka S, Hayes JD, et al. Sound alters activity in human V1 in association with illusory visual perception. *NeuroImage* 2006;31:1247-56.
74. Chen Y-C, Yeh S-L. Catch the moment: multisensory enhancement of rapid visual events by sound. *Exp Brain Res* 2009;198:209-19. doi: 10.1007/s00221-009-1831-4.
75. Stein BE, London N, Wilkinson LK, Price DD. Enhancement of perceived visual intensity by auditory stimuli: A psychophysical analysis. *J Cogn Neurosci* 1996;8:497-506.
76. Vroomen J, deGelder B. Sound enhances visual perception: cross-modal effects of auditory organization on vision. *J Exp Psychol* 2000;26:1583-90.
77. Wang, Y, Celebrini S, Trotter Y, Barone P. Visuo-auditory interactions in the primary visual cortex of the behaving monkey: Electrophysiological evidence. *BMC Neurosci* 2008;9:79.
78. Driver J, Noesselt T. Multisensory interplay reveals crossmodal influences on sensory specific brain regions, neural responses, and judgments. *Neuron* 2008;57:123. doi:10.1016/j.neuron.2007.12.013.
79. Ghazanfar AA, Schroeder CE. Is neocortex essentially multisensory? *Trends Cogn Sci* 2006:10:278-85.

Chapter 15

1. Underleider LG, Mishkin M. Two cortical visual systems. In: Ingle MA, Goodale MI, Mansfield RJW, eds. *Analysis of Visual Behavior*. Cambridge, MA: MIT Press;1982.
2. Goodale MA, Milner AD. Separate visual pathways for perception and action. *Trends Neurosci* 1992;15:20-25. doi: 10.1016/0166-2236(92)90344-8.
3. Goodale MA, Wolf M. Vision for action. In: Dedrick D, Trick L, eds. *Computation, Cognition, and Pylyshyn*. Cambridge, MA: MIT Press; 2009:103.
4. Kastner S, Ungerleider LG. Mechanisms of visual attention in the human cortex. *Ann Rev Neurosci* 2000;23:315-41.
5. Pessoa L, Ungerleider LG. Neural correlates of change detection and change blindness in a working memory task. *Cerebral Cortex* 2004;14:511-20.
6. Fichtenholtz HM, Dean HL, Dillon DG, Yamasaki H, et al. Emotion-attention network interactions during a visual oddball task. *Cogn Brain Res* 2004;20:67-80. doi:10.1016/j.cogbrainres.2004.01.006.
7. Morris JS, Friston KJ, Buchel C, Frith CD, et al. A neuromodulatory role for the human amygdala in processing emotional facial expressions. *Brain* 2007;121:47-57. doi: 10.1093/brain/121.1.47.
8. Golden GS. Strokes in children and adolescents. *Stroke* 1978;9:169-71.
9. Alpers GW, Gerdes AB M, Lagarie B, Tabbert K, et al. Attention and amygdala activity: An fMRI study with spider pictures in spider phobia. *J Neural Transm* 2009;116:747-57. doi:10.1007/s00702-008-0106-8.
10. Simmons A, Matthews SC, Feinstein JS, Hitchcock C, et al. Anxiety vulnerability is associated with altered anterior cingulate response to an affective appraisal task. Neuroreport 2008;19:1033-37.
11. McClure EB, Monk CS, Nelson EE, Parrish J M, et al. Abnormal attention modulation of fear circuit function in pediatric generalized anxiety disorder. *Arch Gen Psychiatry* 2007;64:97-106.
12. Gupta S. Effects of white noise on critical flicker fusion scores in high and low anxious individuals. *J Pers Clin Studies* 2001;17:50-57.
13. MacLeod C, Mathews A. Anxiety and the allocation of attention to threat. *J Exp Psychol Hum Exp Psychol* 1988;38:659-70.
14. Tuller M, Pinto J. Effects of anxiety on attention and visual memory. *J Vis* 2005;5:389. doi: 10.1167/5.8.389.
15. Damasio AR. Descartes' Error: Emotion, Reason, and the *Human Brain*. New York: Avon; 1994.

16. Lezak MD, Howieson DB, Loring DW. *Neuropsychological Assessment, 4th ed.* New York: Oxford University Press, 2004.
17. Reynolds CR, Kamphaus RW. *Behavior Assessment System for Children, 2nd ed.* (BASC-2). Circle Pines, MN: American Guidance Service, 2004.
18. Sparrow SS, Cicchetti DV, Balla DA, *Vineland Adaptive Behavior Scales, 2nd ed.* Circle Pines, MN: American Guidance, 2005.
19. Dean RS, Woodcock RW *The Dean-Woodcock Neuropsychological Battery*. Itasca, IL: Riverside Publishing, 2003.
20. Sandford JA, Turner A. *Manual for the Integrated Visual and Auditory Continuous Performance Test.* Richmond, VA: Braintrain, 1995.
21. Delis DC, Kaplan E, Kramer JH. *The Delis-Kaplan Executive Function System (D-KEFS).* San Antonio, TX: The Psychological Corporation, 2001.
22. Gioia GA, Isquith PK, Guy SC, Kenworthy L. *Behavior Rating Inventory of Executive Function™ (BRIEF™).* Los Angeles, CA: Western Psychological Services; 2000.
23. Kaufman AS. Cerebral specialization and intelligence testing. *J Res Dev Educ* 1979;12:96-107.
24. Detterman DK. Does "g" exist? *Intelligence* 1982;6:99-108.
25. Naglieri JA, Das JP. Planning-arousal-simultaneous-successive (PASS): A model for assessment, *J School Psychol* 1988;26:35-48.
26. Goldin P, Manve T, Hakimi S, Canli T, et al. Neural bases of social anxiety disorder. *Arch Gen Psychiatry* 2009;66:70-180.
27. Sterman MB, Clemente CD. Forebrain inhibitory mechanisms: Sleep patterns induced by basal forebrain stimulation in the behaving cat. *Exp Neurol* 1962;6:103-17.
28. Sterman MB, Friar L. Suppression of seizures in epileptic following sensorimotor EEG feedback training. Electroenceph. *Clin Neurophysiol* 1972;33:89-95.
29. Padula WV. *Neuro-Optometric Rehabilitation.* Santa Ana, CA: Optometric Extension Program Foundation; 2000.

Chapter 16

1. Educational Interventions for Students with Low Vision. American Foundation for the Blind. Website accessed December 3, 2010.
2. Kaplan MK. Vertical Yoked Prisms. Optometric Extension Program Continuing Education Courses, Vol. 51. Santa Ana, CA: Optometric Extension Program Foundation; 1979.
3. Barrage NC. *Increased Visual Behavior in Low Vision Children.* NY: AFB Press; 1964.
4. Barraga NC, Erin JN. *Visual Impairments and Learning* 4th ed. Austin, TX: Pro-Ed Inc; 2001.
5. Cowan C, Shepler R. Activities and games for teaching children to use magnifiers. In: D'Andrea FM, Farrenkopf C, eds. *Looking to Learn: Promoting Literacy for Students with Low Vision.* New York, NY: AFB Press; 2000.

Chapter 17

1. Corn AL, Wall RS, Jose RT, Bell JK, et al. An initial study of reading and comprehension rates for students who received optical devices. J Vis Impair Blindness. 2000:96;322-34.
2. Beery KE, Buktenica NA, Beery NA. *The Beery-Buktenica Developmental Test of Visual-Motor Integration. 5th ed. (Beery VMI-5)* San Antonio, TX: Pearson, 2006.
3. Barraga NC, Erin JN. *Visual Impairments and Learning, 4th ed.* Austin, TX: Pro-Ed Inc, 2001.
4. Corn AL. Optical aids in the classroom. *Education of the Visually Handicapped.* 1980;12:114-21.

INDEX